Radionuclide Peptide Cancer Therapy

Edited by

Marco Chinol
European Institute of Oncology
Milan, Italy

Giovanni Paganelli
European Institute of Oncology
Milan, Italy

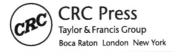

CRC Press
Taylor & Francis Group
Boca Raton London New York

CRC Press is an imprint of the
Taylor & Francis Group, an **informa** business

A TAYLOR & FRANCIS BOOK

CRC Press
Taylor & Francis Group
6000 Broken Sound Parkway NW, Suite 300
Boca Raton, FL 33487-2742

© 2006 by Taylor & Francis Group, LLC
CRC Press is an imprint of Taylor & Francis Group, an Informa business

First issued in paperback 2019

No claim to original U.S. Government works

ISBN 13: 978-0-367-45355-8 (pbk)
ISBN 13: 978-0-8247-2887-8 (hbk)

Library of Congress Cataloging-in-Publication Data

Radionuclide peptide cancer therapy / edited by Marco Chinol, Giovanni Paganelli.
    p. cm.
Includes bibliographical references and index.
ISBN-13: 978-0-8247-2887-8 (alk. paper)
ISBN-10: 0-8247-2887-4 (alk. paper)
    1. Cancer--Radioimmunoimaging. 2. Peptides--Therapeutic use. 3. Radioisotopes--Therapeutic use. I. Chinol, Marco. II. Paganelli, Giovanni.

RC271.R26R33 2006
616.99'407575--dc22   2005046649

Visit the Taylor & Francis Web site at
http://www.taylorandfrancis.com

and the CRC Press Web site at
http://www.crcpress.com

Foreword

Selectively killing tumor cells while sparing normal tissues has been the goal of research in nuclear medicine ever since Paul Ehrlich's theory of the "magic bullet."

For the last two decades monoclonal antibodies have been regarded as the ideal vector for delivering high loads of radioactivity to tumor cells disseminated throughout the body.

Despite the fact that two radiolabeled monoclonal antibodies have finally been launched on the market for the treatment of hematologic tumors, fundamental issues, such as the very low concentration of radiolabeled antibodies in the neoplastic tissues, their potential unspecific accumulation in normal organs, and production of immunologic reactions preventing multiple cycles of therapy still remain to be resolved before we see an antibody-based radio-pharmaceutical against solid tumors.

In contrast to larger molecules, peptides have the advantage of being flexible messenger molecules with easy penetration into all tissues. Therefore, peptide research has been and still is heavily focused on developing metabolically stable peptides which eventually could be radiolabeled for clinical use. The discovery that tumors originating from the neural crest overexpress somatostatin receptors has spurred the development of somatostatin analogs designed to target tumor cells so that the enhanced radiation delivery will occur mostly at the receptor expressing tumor cells.

In this book the Editors have brought together outstanding studies by experts in the field, providing basic background, latest clinical applications, dosimetric aspects, and regulatory requirements.

This comprehensive book on these new radiolabled molecules, which are in the forefront of the fight against cancer, comes at a time when we are celebrating the first ten years of the European Institute of Oncology, whose primary goal is research into innovative treatments to combat cancer.

The combination of antitumor efficacy and high "quality of life" treatment regimens represents a fundamental and achievable goal which, with the advent of radiolabeled peptides, seems well within our reach.

I believe that this book will not only be warmly welcomed by scientists working in this field but will also benefit those investigators working in centers that focus more and more on this new approach to the treatment of cancer.

Umberto Veronesi

Preface

Over its extensive period of development, the field of radioimmunotherapy has enjoyed much progress, including the selection of suitable radionuclides, chelation chemistry, and novel targets on tumor cells. The knowledge accrued has accelerated the advancement of radiolabeled peptides, which have already demonstrated their pivotal role in the fight against cancer. Despite just a few years of development, a large amount of data is available in the literature to support their clinical applications.

This book provides a comprehensive set of chapters that describe the state of art in the field of radiolabeled peptides for cancer therapy. Included are chapters reviewing the technology of peptide production, aspects of radiolabeling, and the results of their clinical applications obtained in outstanding institutions. This book also includes two perspective sections presenting novel strategies to enhance the spectrum of application of peptides.

The progress described in these chapters offers strong and compelling evidence of the success of radiolabeled peptides and foresees the potential development which the field will undergo in the coming years.

We wish to express our heartfelt gratitude to all the authors who contributed to the writing of this book and we thank the European Institute of Oncology for its continuous and unstinting support towards our research efforts.

Marco Chinol
Giovanni Paganelli

Contents

3. **Developments of Radiolabeled Peptides** *41*
   Ronald E. Weiner and Mathew L. Thakur

4. **The Labeling of Peptides with Positron-Emitting Radionuclides: The Importance of PET in Cancer Diagnosis** *87*
   Stefano Papi, Nicoletta Urbano, Esteban R. Obenaus, and Marco Chinol

5. **Radiolabeling DOTA-Peptides with ^{90}Y and ^{177}Lu to a High Specific Activity** *119*
   Wouter A. P. Breeman, Erik de Blois, Willem H. Bakker, and Eric P. Krenning

Contributors

Horacio Amaral Nuclear Medicine Center, Clinica Alemana and A. Lopez Perez Foundation, and Faculty of Medicine, Universidad del Desarrollo, Santiago, Chile

Willem H. Bakker Department of Nuclear Medicine, Erasmus MC Rotterdam, Rotterdam, The Netherlands

Bert Bernard Department of Nuclear Medicine, Erasmus MC Rotterdam, Rotterdam, The Netherlands

Lisa Bodei Division of Nuclear Medicine, European Institute of Oncology, Milan, Italy

Wouter A. P. Breeman Department of Nuclear Medicine, Erasmus MC Rotterdam, Rotterdam, The Netherlands

Astrid Capello Department of Nuclear Medicine, Erasmus MC Rotterdam, Rotterdam, The Netherlands

Marco Chinol Division of Nuclear Medicine, European Institute of Oncology, Milan, Italy

Ana Maria Comaru-Schally Department of Medicine, Endocrine, Polypeptide, and Cancer Institute, Veterans Affairs Medical Center and Section of Experimental Medicine, Tulane University School of Medicine, New Orleans, Louisiana, U.S.A.

Marta Cremonesi   Medical Physics Department, European Institute of Oncology, Milan, Italy

Erik de Blois   Department of Nuclear Medicine, Erasmus MC Rotterdam, Rotterdam, The Netherlands

Marion de Jong   Department of Nuclear Medicine, Erasmus MC Rotterdam, Rotterdam, The Netherlands

Mahila Ferrari   Medical Physics Department, European Institute of Oncology, Milan, Italy

Michael Gabriel   Department of Nuclear Medicine, Innsbruck Medical University, Innsbruck, Austria

David A. Goodwin   Stanford University, Stanford and VA Palo Alto Health Care System, Palo Alto, California, U.S.A.

Dirk Heute   Department of Nuclear Medicine, Innsbruck Medical University, Innsbruck, Austria

Eric P. Krenning   Department of Nuclear Medicine, and Department of Internal Medicine, Erasmus MC Rotterdam, Rotterdam, The Netherlands

Dik J. Kwekkeboom   Department of Nuclear Medicine, Erasmus MC Rotterdam, Rotterdam, The Netherlands

Michelle Masullo   Division of Pathology and Laboratory Medicine, European Institute of Oncology and University of Milan School of Medicine, Milan, Italy

Claude F. Meares   Chemistry Department, University of California Davis, Davis, California, U.S.A.

Giancarlo Morelli   InterUniversity Center on Bioactive Peptides (CIRPeB) at University of Naples "Federico II" and Institute of Biostructures and Bioimaging, C.N.R.—Via Mezzocannone, Napoli, Italy

Jan Müller-Brand   Institute of Nuclear Medicine, University Hospital Basel, Basel, Switzerland

Attila Nagy   Department of Medicine, Endocrine, Polypeptide, and Cancer Institute, Veterans Affairs Medical Center and Section of Experimental Medicine, Tulane University School of Medicine, New Orleans, Louisiana, U.S.A.

Esteban R. Obenaus   Division of Nuclear Medicine, European Institute of Oncology, Milan, Italy

Giovanni Paganelli Division of Nuclear Medicine, European Institute of Oncology, Milan, Italy

Stefano Papi Division of Nuclear Medicine, European Institute of Oncology, Milan, Italy

Carlo Pedone InterUniversity Center on Bioactive Peptides (CIRPeB) at University of Naples "Federico II" and Institute of Biostructures and Bioimaging, C.N.R.—Via Mezzocannone, Napoli, Italy

Giuseppe Pelosi Division of Pathology and Laboratory Medicine, European Institute of Oncology and University of Milan School of Medicine, Milan, Italy

Jean Claude Reubi Division of Cell Biology and Experimental Cancer Research, Institute of Pathology, University of Berne, Berne, Switzerland

Margarida Rodrigues Department of Nuclear Medicine, Innsbruck Medical University, Innsbruck, Austria

Michele Saviano InterUniversity Center on Bioactive Peptides (CIRPeB) at University of Naples "Federico II" and Institute of Biostructures and Bioimaging, C.N.R.—Via Mezzocannone, Napoli, Italy

Andrew V. Schally Department of Medicine, Endocrine, Polypeptide, and Cancer Institute, Veterans Affairs Medical Center and Section of Experimental Medicine, Tulane University School of Medicine, New Orleans, Louisiana, U.S.A.

Michael G. Stabin Department of Radiology and Radiological Sciences, Vanderbilt University, Nashville, Tennessee, U.S.A.

Diego Tesauro InterUniversity Center on Bioactive Peptides (CIRPeB) at University of Naples "Federico II" and Institute of Biostructures and Bioimaging, C.N.R.—Via Mezzocannone, Napoli, Italy

Mathew L. Thakur Department of Radiology, Thomas Jefferson University Hospital, Philadelphia, Pennsylvania, U.S.A.

Giampiero Tosi Medical Physics Department, European Institute of Oncology, Milan, Italy

Tatjana Traub-Weidinger Department of Nuclear Medicine, Innsbruck Medical University, Innsbruck, Austria

Nicoletta Urbano Division of Nuclear Medicine, European Institute of Oncology, Milan, Italy

Giuseppe Viale   Division of Pathology and Laboratory Medicine, European Institute of Oncology and University of Milan School of Medicine, Milan, Italy

Irene Virgolini   Department of Nuclear Medicine, Innsbruck Medical University, Innsbruck, Austria

Christian Waldherr   Institute of Nuclear Medicine, University Hospital Basel, Basel, and Department of Diagnostic Radiology, University Hospital Bern, Bern, Switzerland, and Department of Molecular and Medical Pharmacology, Ahmanson Biological Imaging Center, David Geffen School of Medicine, University of California, Los Angeles, California, U.S.A.

Ronald E. Weiner   Department of Diagnostic Imaging and Therapeutics, University of Connecticut Health Center, Farmington, Connecticut, U.S.A.

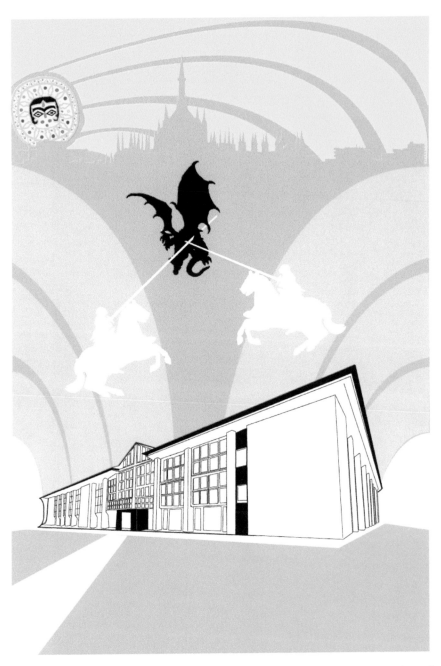

The fight against cancer in Milan: the building in the foreground is the European Institute of Oncology and the Milan skyline is in the background. The two white horsemen are fighting cancer (black dragon) with accurately-wielded spears representing targeted therapy. Above all is the Hope represented by the "woman sun," an ancient image from Eastern mythology.

Drawing by Nicoletta Montanari

1

Peptide Structure and Analysis

Carlo Pedone, Giancarlo Morelli, Diego Tesauro, and Michele Saviano

InterUniversity Center on Bioactive Peptides (CIRPeB) at University of Naples "Federico II" and Institute of Biostructures and Bioimaging, C.N.R.—Via Mezzocannone, Napoli, Italy

INTRODUCTION

Peptides of natural or synthetic origin are compounds involved in a variety of biological functions. They are hormones, opioides, sweeteners, antibiotics, protein substrates, inhibitors, releasing factors, regulators of biological functions, citoprotectors, and so on (1).

From the chemical point of view peptides are formed when two or more amino acid residues are condensed together, leading to a secondary amide bond, and, consequently, to a peptide unit. Peptides are, then, chains of a certain number of covalently linked amino acid residues, each of which is intrinsically asymmetric because of the optically active α-carbon atoms. The amino acid sequence along the chain, the spatial configuration of the asymmetric C^α atoms of each residue, and the local conformation of part of the molecule or the overall conformation of the entire peptide, together with the intra-molecular and inter-molecular interactions of various types, are all important factors in determining the biological activity and the mechanism of its action.

Establishing the molecular and structural formula, the stereo-configuration of the atoms, and the molecular conformation and inter- or intra-molecular interactions is often the key to discovering the relationships between structure and properties of the compounds under investigation, especially for natural substances such as protein and biologically active compounds.

The structural characteristic of the peptide unit formed through the linkage of residues i and i+1 are fully described in terms of geometry of bonds, conformation, and non-planarity of chemical bonds. Molecular conformation is most conveniently and precisely characterized by torsion angle as described in Figure 1. The shape of a particular peptide molecule is the consequence of a certain succession of torsion angles ϕ_i, ψ_i, ω_i, for each amino acid residue, while the torsion angles χ_i, fully describe the side chain conformation (2). The ω_i angles in linear peptides usually present values close to 180° corresponding to a *trans* arrangement of the peptide bond, which is energetically more stable than the *cis* arrangement ($\omega_i = 0°$) by about 2 Kcal/mol (3). Of course the *cis* arrangement is a necessity in small cyclic peptides, while it is a very rare conformation in large cyclic peptides and in linear chains. Consequently the molecular conformation of a peptide can be visualized in the (ϕ, ψ) space by energy of the molecule as function of these torsion angles. The maps obtained show that all best known secondary structures assumed by a peptide chain, such as the β-structure, the α-helix, and the 3_{10}-helix, occur within energy minima.

A complete description of the most common secondary structure is reported below within the description of the conformational restrains that can be introduced in a peptide sequence to force the peptide molecule in assuming the wished conformation.

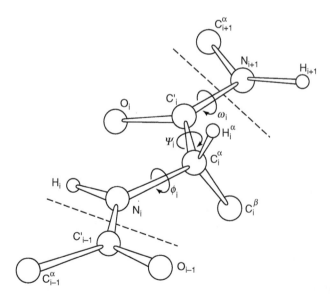

Figure 1 The structural characteristic of the peptide unit formed through the linkage of residues i and i+1 described in terms of torsion angles. The shape of a particular peptide molecule is the consequence of a certain succession of torsion angles ϕ_i, ψ_i, ω_i, for each amino acid residue, while the torsion angles χ_i, fully describe the side chain conformation.

PEPTIDE CONFORMATION AND STRUCTURES

Over the past several years, a set of empirical potentials and parameters has been developed to calculate the relative conformational energies of peptides, polypeptides, and proteins. These parameters were obtained by considering first the intermolecular interactions in x-ray crystal structures of model compound; they were then applied to the analysis of the 20 naturally occurring amino acid residues, because of the importance of the conformational character of individual amino acid residues in studies of larger peptides. These conformation studies were carried out analyzing the low-energy structures of the N-acetyl-N′-methylamides of the 20 naturally occurring amino acids (4). Zimmerman et al. developed an effective method of searching conformational space for low-energy minima (4). At each energy minimum, it was calculated the conformational energy, entropy, and conformational free energy, assigned a conformational letter code, and checked for the presence of hydrogen bonds.

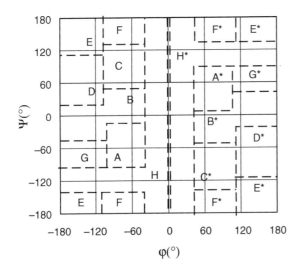

Figure 2 ϕ-ψ map showing the regions defining the conformational letter code. The entire ϕ-ψ map is subdivided into regions denoted by capital letters. On the left-hand half of the map ($\phi \leq 0°$), six of the regions (A, C to G) comprise the distinct ϕ-ψ areas in which energy minima are found for various amino acid residues, while one region (B) is defined around the moderate-energy bridge region. On the right-hand half of the map ($\phi > 0°$), regions are defined by inversion of the left-hand half around the center of the map, i.e., around the point (0°, 0°), and an asterisk is appended to the letters. A denotes the region which contains the right-handed α-helical conformation, B is the bridge region, C contains the C_7 ring (a seven-membered hydrogen-bonded ring, with the side chain in the equatorial position), E contains the extended conformations (e.g., C_5, a five-membered hydrogen bonded ring), and H is the high-energy region. D, F, and G were assigned to the remaining regions to indicate contiguity.

Conformations are classified in terms of the regions of the φ-ψ map in which they occur (Fig. 2) (4). These regions are identified by a letter code, giving rise to a low-energy structure. The entire φ-ψ map is subdivided into regions denoted by capital letters, as shown in Figure 2. On the left-hand half of the map ($\phi \leq 0°$), six of the regions (**A**, **C** to **G**) comprise the distinct φ-ψ areas in which energy minima are found for various amino acid residues, while one region (**B**) is defined around the moderate-energy bridge region. On the right-hand half of the map ($\phi > 0°$), regions are defined by inversion of the left-hand half around the center of the map, i.e., around the point (0°, 0°), and an asterisk is appended to the letters.

In defining the letter code, the boundaries of the regions were selected so that all related minima would fall within the same region. The letters denoting each region were chosen so that they are easy to remember: A denotes the region which contains the right-handed α-helical conformation, B is the bridge region, C contains the C_7 ring (a seven-member hydrogen-bonded ring, with the side chain in the equatorial position), E contains the extended conformations (e.g., C_5, a five-member hydrogen bonded ring), and H is the high-energy region. D, F, and G were assigned to the remaining regions to indicate contiguity. All amino acid computed minima fall in the allowed regions of conformational map. These results were in general agreement with experiments, and encouraged continued refinement of the energy parameters from experimental data on intramolecular interactions. In fact, the analysis of the conformation assumed by the 20 natural amino acids in x-ray protein structures underlines that almost all of the φ-ψ dihedral angles fall in the allowed regions of conformational map.

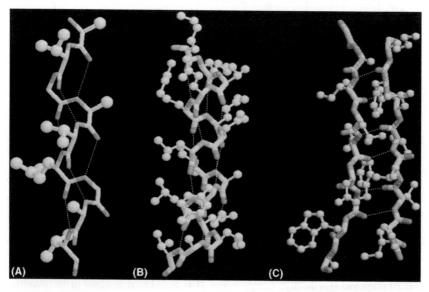

Figure 3   Three-dimensional structures of (**A**) a 3_{10} helix, (**B**) a α-helix, and (**C**) a β-sheet.

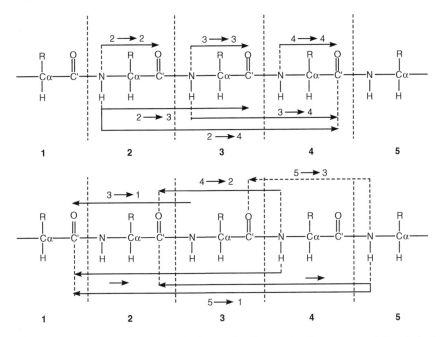

Figure 4 Possible intramolecular hydrogen bonds occuring in a system of four linked peptide residues.

In proteins it is well-known that α-helices and β-sheets (Fig. 3) are the major stabilizing structures in proteins. In peptides, the classification of secondary regular structures is more complex, and is related to the hydrogen bond pattern that stabilizes the structure (5). An H bond between N-H of an amino acid sequence number m, and C=O of a residue of the sequence number n is designated as m→n (Fig. 4). Then, the possible structures in the systems of four linked peptide units are the 2→2 (or 3→3, or 4→4), the 2→3 (or 3→4), the 2→4, the 3→1 (or 4→2 or 5→3), the 4→1 (or 5→2), and the 5→1 intramolecular H-bonded conformations. On the basis of the number of atoms in the ring formed by closing the H-bond, the aforementioned conformations are also called the C_5, C_8, C_{11}, C_7, C_{10}, and C_{13} conformations. The C_5 conformation is extended, and the others are of the folded type. A nomenclature of common use for C_7, C_8, C_{10}, C_{11}, and C_{13} conformations is γ-, δ-, β-, ε-, and α-turn, respectively. The C_8, C_{10}, C_{11}, ad C_{13} forms may include *cis* peptide configurations. The presence of consecutive α-turns or β-turns gives rise to α-helical or 3_{10} helix secondary structures, respectively.

METHODOLOGIES FOR PEPTIDE DESIGN

Rational molecular design, whether it is aimed at generating novel pharmaceuticals or other bioactives, is at heart a knowledge-based activity. At a structural level, the molecular modeler requires answers to some very basic questions regarding any proposed lead molecule:

1. How big is the molecule- what are its molecular dimensions?
2. What shape is this molecule - what is its likely conformation(s), and what are the relative conformations of its functional substructures?
3. How is this molecule likely to interact at its binding site (if the structure is known) or can this molecule mimic the ligand binding properties of existing known activities?

This knowledge, usually combined with other chemical, physical or biological information, can lead to modification of the original proposal, and reiteration of the modeling experiments. However, a thorough knowledge of 3D structure in all its aspects is a crucial factor in the total process (6).

There are two basic methods of obtaining 3D structural knowledge: computational and experimental. The computational techniques include conformational search, energy minimization, and molecular dynamics (MD) simulations, with a variety of semi-empirical and ab initio force fields. All of these methods have practical limitations, e.g., in the cpu-intensity required for conformational search or in the accuracy of some semi-empirical force fields, and only the most advanced and expensive ab initio methods are capable of treating non-covalent interaction or metal ions interactions with biomolecules.

The wide application of crystallographic analysis makes it the method of choice for the experimental determination of 3D structures (for more details see below in this chapter). Thus, crystallography can contribute significantly to the molecular design process, either through analysis of specific key molecules, or through the knowledge that can be acquired from systematic studies of existing structures, as stirred in the crystallographic databases (Cambridge Structural Database for small and medium size molecules, Protein Data Bank for proteins, and oligo-nucleotides).

In the last decade, the technological and theoretical advances in nuclear magnetic resonance (NMR) spectroscopy have increased the accuracy of 3D structures from NMR data, and their use in the drug design process.

Structure-activity relationship (SAR) studies in bioactive peptides have as their main objective the understanding of biological phenomena at the molecular level with the aim to produce and possible develop new materials relevant to pharmacology and medicinal chemistry, which might mimic biological processes by enhancing or somehow modulating their effects. The peptide pharmaceutical targets of these studies have been among others hormones, enzymes, G-protein coupled receptors, neurotransmitters, etc. The number of native and modified peptides used as drug is constantly increasing. However, the use of peptides as drugs is limited by some factors:

1. Their low metabolic stability towards proteolysis in the gastrointestinal tract and in the serum

2. Their poor absorption after oral ingestion, in particular due to their relative high molecular mass or the lack of specific transport systems or both

3. Their rapid excretion through liver and kidneys

4. Their undesired effected caused by interaction of the conformationally flexible peptides with various receptors.

In recent years, intensive efforts have been made to develop peptides or peptidomimetics that display more favorable pharmacological properties then their prototypes. Most of the research carried out is concerned with the preparation of analogs with different chemical structure, and possibly modified conformational preferences in solution. All biomolecular binding processes involve MD, even those apparently corresponding to the rigid lock-and-key model. Therefore, one of the goals of the design of new compounds is the introduction of some constraints to reduce the conformational flexibility, and to stabilize biologically active conformations of native peptides. This rational design can led to molecules endowed with high affinity, and/or selectivity for one class of receptors. Structural changes and different dynamic behavior can be obtained in a peptide in two ways: (1) modifying the sequence using coded amino acids with specific conformational preferences or uncoded amino acids, and amino acids with D configuration, (2) cyclization of the N-terminal with the C-terminal, of the N-terminal with a side-chain, of the C-terminal with a side-chain, and of the side-chain with another side-chain (7).

An example of a new compound with reduced flexibility obtained by cyclization is the cyclo(Met-Asp-Trp-Phe-Dap-Leu)cyclo(2β-5β) (Fig. 5) (8), a selective and potent Tachykinin NK2 receptor antagonist. Now a glycosilated peptide analogue, NEPADUTANT (MENARINI Group) is in phase IIa trials in Belgium and Sweden for the potential treatment of asthma and irritable bowel syndrome.

Structural changes with the aim of inducing specific secondary structure in a peptide can be obtained with non-coded α- or β- amino acids (Figs. 6 and 7). Appropriate constrained non-coded amino acids are of particular interest as "building blocks" for the preparation of analogs, since their inclusion in a peptide sequence could maintain the pharmacological properties of the native peptide, and possibly enhance resistance to biodegradation with improved bioavailability and pharmacokinetics. Several solid state studies have been carried out to define the conformational preferences in solution, and in the solid state of specific classes of non-coded α-amino acids, as for example the symmetrical and unsymmetrical α,α-disubstituted glycines (α,α-dialkylated residues). A growing "arsenal" of non-coded α-amino acids of this class is being built by means of which specific structural changes can now be induced in bioactive molecules, in order to modulate or appropriately mimic biological effects. The explosive interest in the study of the α,α-disubstituted glycine residues (9–11) finds its origin in the analysis of the prototype of this class of non-coded residues α-aminoisobutyric acid (Aib) (Fig. 6),

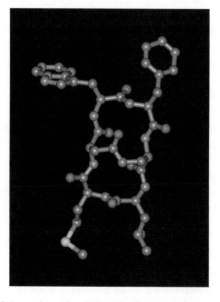

Figure 5 Schematic and solid state structure of a neurokinin A receptor antagonist cyclo(Met¹-Asp²-Trp³-Phe⁴-Dap⁵-Leu⁶)cyclo(2β-5β).

commonly found in a family of natural antibiotics produced by microbial sources, such as alamethicin, tricozianine, antimoebin, etc, called peptaibols, which are able to alter the ionic permeability of biological membranes by the formation of channels. The conformational studies on Aib residue underlined that the replacement of the hydrogen atoms of the C^α carbon of glycine with methyl groups produces severe restriction on the conformational space, as shown in Fig. 8. As a consequence, folded, and helical structures of two well-defined, almost isoenergetic helical types, the 3_{10}-helix ($\phi = -60°$, $\psi = -30°$ or $\phi = 60°$, $\psi = 30°$ for right- or left-handed screw sense, respectively), and the α-helix ($\phi = -55°$, $\psi = -45°$

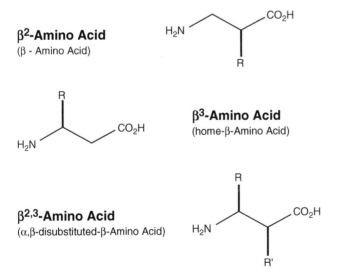

Figure 6 Some $C^{\alpha,\alpha}$-symmetrically disubstituted glycines.

Figure 7 Schematic representation of non-coded β-amino acids.

or $\phi=55°$, $\psi=45°$ for right- or left-handed screw sense, respectively) are significantly more stable than fully extended structures ($\phi=\psi=180°$). Starting from these experimental evidences, researchers have designed new $C^{\alpha,\alpha}$ disubstituted residue with specific conformational behavior.

Examples of new bioactive peptides with non-coded amino acid in the sequence are somatostatin analogs (see below in the text), and synthetic analogs of the aspartame sweeteners (12). Using this arsenal of building blocks we can proceed to the rational design of new molecules with specific structure, conformation, and activity in a sort of "molecular meccano." What are the methods for the peptide de novo design? If the three dimensional structure of the ligand-receptor

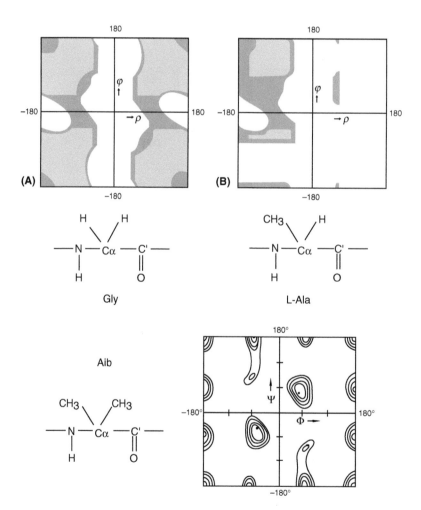

Figure 8 ϕ-ψ maps of glycine (Gly), alanine (Ala), and α-aminoisobutyric acid (Aib).

complex is known at atomic resolution, the ligand structure is modified, using backbone or side-chain modification including cyclization, preserving the ligand-receptor interactions (hydrogen bond, Wan der Waals interactions etc). If the structure of the complex is unknown, conformational studies of the ligand and of the receptor, in solution and/or in solid state, can be used as the starting point in molecular design. In this procedure, before the design stage, docking programs were used to simulate the active ligand-receptor complex. If only the ligand structure is known, the design stage must be preceded by an accurate conformational analysis of the molecule. This phase is performed carrying out MD simulations in solution to have statistical data on the dynamic behavior, and on the possible conformational families assumed by the ligand (13).

METHODOLOGIES FOR PEPTIDE SYNTHESIS

The well-known peptides solution or liquid phase peptide synthesis is the "classical" method to obtain a peptide sequence. The synthetic procedure to obtain in solution a peptide bond between two amino acids is known since the beginning of the last century (14). These "classical" methods for synthesis in solution are labor, time, and skill intensive, largely due to the unpredictable solubility characteristics of intermediates. These procedures are now applied only for large scale synthesis of well known peptides for pharmaceutical applications. Most peptide hormones, usually small molecules up to twelve/fifteen residues, are produced by solution methods by pharmaceutical industries.

In 1984 Bruce Merriefeld, an American chemist of Rockefeller University, won the Nobel Prize for his contribution to the advancement of peptide chemistry. Merrifield introduced the technique known as solid phase peptide synthesis (SPPS) in 1963 (15). The concept of the SPPS can be illustrated by Figure 9 where the first protected amino acid is attached to an insoluble polystyrene solid support via an acid labile linker. He developed a SPPS methodology of peptides, which uses a polymer with reactive sites (solid supports, insoluble resin supports) that chemically combine to the developing peptide chain. That solved the problem of previous peptide chemistry. Using Merrifield's technique, the problems associated with low yields due to separation and purification are avoided. The polymer can be filtered and washed without mechanical losses because the polymer is very insoluble.

Solid-phase peptide synthesis consists of three distinct sets of operations: (1) chain assembly on a resin; (2) simultaneous or sequential cleavage, and deprotection of the resin-bound, fully protected chain; and (3) purification and characterization of the target peptide. Various chemical strategies exist for the chain assembly and cleavage/deprotection operations, but purification and characterization methods are more or less invariant to the methods used to generate the crude peptide product.

Two major chemistries for SPPS are 9-fluorenylmethoxycarbonyl (Fmoc) (base labile protecting group) (16) and *tert*-butoxycarbonyl (*t*-Boc) (acid labile

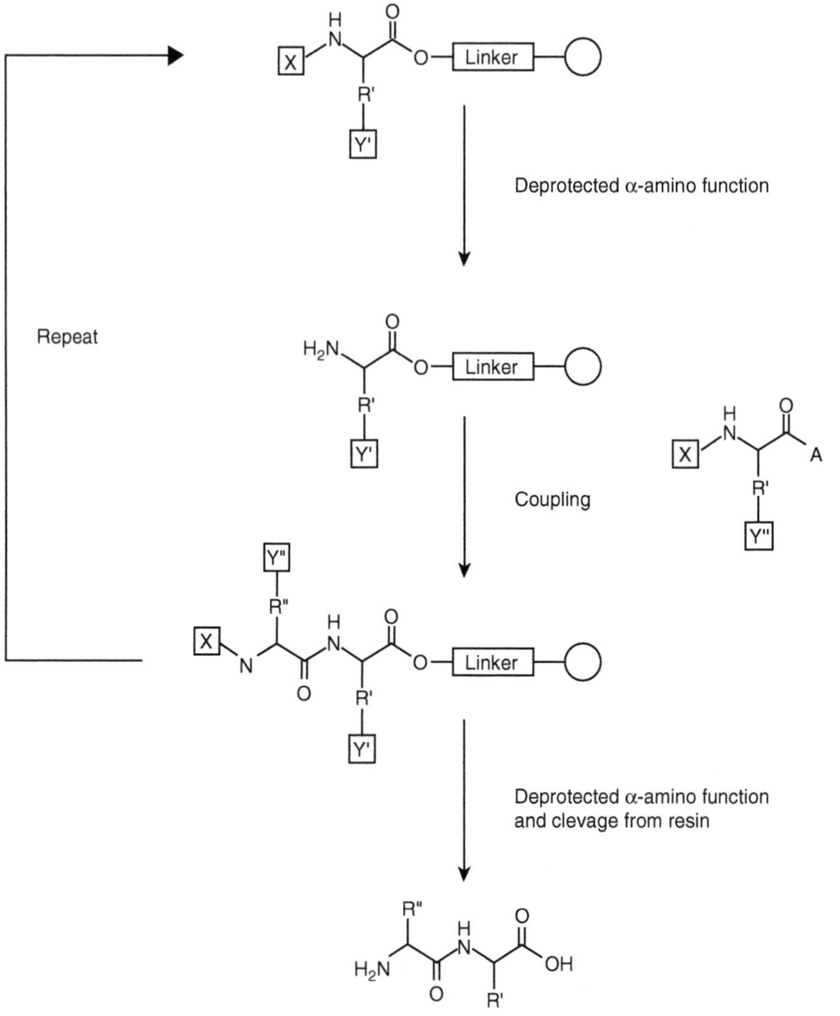

Figure 9 A schematic representation of the chemical steps in solid phase peptide synthesis.

α-amino protecting group) (15). Each method involves fundamentally different amino acid side-chain protection, and consequent cleavage/deprotection methods and resins.

In the *t*-Boc strategy the amino acids are protected by a temporary acid labile protecting group, *t*-butoxycarbonyl (*t*-Boc), on the α-amino position, and by a more acid stable benzyl type protecting group on the functionality of the side chain. The *t*-Boc group is deprotected by trifluoroacetic acid (TFA), followed by the neutralization and washing steps, and then the next protected amino acid couples to the amino peptide resin in the presence of activator. The deprotection and coupling steps are repeated until the desired sequence of the peptide is assembled. The final peptide is cleaved, and deprotected from the resin simultaneously by liquid hydrogen fluoride which requires a special apparatus for its safe handling. Impurities in *t*-Boc-synthesized peptides can be found, and they are mostly attributed to cleavage problems, dehydration, and *t*-butylation.

The SPPS strategy with a temporary base labile α-amino protecting group, Fmoc, was introduced by Carpino in 1972 (16). In Fmoc SPPS, α-amino group of each amino acid is protected by Fmoc, and the side chain functionality is protected by the acid labile t-butyl type protecting groups. Fmoc-based SPPS provided an alternative to the *t*-Boc based SPPS, and offered the advantage of a milder acid cleavage process. Fmoc chemistry is known for peptide synthesis of higher quality, and in greater yield than *t*-Boc chemistry. This strategy is actually the most widely used to obtain standard and modified peptide sequences.

The developments in Fmoc SPPS (17) can be summarized by the following categories: solid supports, linkers, the first residue attachment, protecting groups, Fmoc deprotections, coupling reagents, monitoring, cleavage and removal of protecting groups, peptide evaluation, peptide modifications, and peptide ligation. The advances in the Fmoc SPPS allowed the synthesis of some long peptides. Examples include human parathyroid hormone (84 residues) (18), HIV-1 aspartyl protease (99 residues) (19), and interleukin-3 (140 residues) (20). Some of the crucial points in SPPS with Fmoc strategy are discussed in details below.

Solid Support

The SPPS requires a well-solvated gel to allow the reactions to take place between reagents in the mobile phase, and functional groups on chains throughout the interior of a resin. The original resin was developed as a polystyrene polymer cross-linked with 1% of 1,3-divinylbenzene with a swelling capacity 3 fold in volume in N,N-dimethylformamide (DMF). A polyamide resin was introduced by Atherton and Sheppard (21) under the concept that the solid support and peptide backbone should be of comparable polarities. Recently, resins based on grafting of polyethylene glycol (PEG) to low cross-linked polystyrene were developed such as Tentagel (22) and PEG-PS resins (23), with a swelling capacity 5 fold in volume in DMF. More recently, resins based on cross-linked PEG have also been available such as PEGA (24) and CLERA resins (25) with a swelling capacity 11, and 6.5 fold in volume, respectively. Due to their excellent swelling property, Tentagel and PEGA resins have shown superior performance, especially on peptides with long and difficult sequences.

Linkers

The function of the linker is to provide a reversible linkage between the peptide chain and the solid support, and to protect the C-terminal α-carboxyl group.

The commonly used resins to provide peptides acid are Wang (26), Hydroxymethyl-phenoxy acetyl (24), Rink acid (27), and 2-Chlorotrityl chloride (28). The most commonly used resin for peptide amide is Rink amide resin (29).

The First Residue Attachment

The esterification of the first amino acid to the hydroxyl group on the resin is one of the key steps to producing a high quality peptide. The incomplete loading and racemization will cause truncated and epimeric peptides, respectively, as a result of slow esterification reaction. The commonly used loading methods are the 1-hydroxybenzotriazole (HOBt) active ester, symmetrical anhydride, and dichlorobenzoyl chloride procedures. The first amino acid residue can be loaded to trityl-based resins with no racemization.

Protecting Groups

For routine synthesis, the global protecting strategy is employed to all reactive functionalities of the side chains. For instance, hydroxyl and carboxyl functionalities are protected by *t*-butyl group, lysine and triptophan are protected by *t*-Boc group, asparagines, glutamine, cysteine, and histidine are protected by trityl group, and arginine is protected by the pentafluoro-phenyl ester (Pbf) group. A wide range of protecting groups are also available for different applications such as 2-oxy-4-methyloxybenzyl (Hmb) group used as an amide protecting group to alleviate aggregation during SPPS.

Fluorenylmethoxycarbonyl Deprotection

The removal of the Fmoc group is usually accomplished by treatment with 20–50% piperidine in DMF for 20 minutes. In the case of incomplete Fmoc deprotection, a stronger base such as 1,8-diazabicyclo[5.4.0]undec-7-ene (DBU) with 2% piperidine can be used.

Coupling

Amide bond formation involves activation of the carboxyl group of the amino acid. There are four major coupling techniques: (1) in situ coupling reagents such as carbodiimide-mediated coupling, benzotriazol-1-yl-oxy-tris-pyrrolidino-phosphonium (PyBOP), 2-(1H-Benzotriazole-1yl)-1,1,3,3-tetramethyluronium hexaflurophosphate (HBTU) as well as O-(7-azabenzotriazol-1-yl)-1,1,3,3-tetra-methyluronium (HATU), (2) preformed active esters such as pentafluorophenyl (Opfp), (3) preformed symmetrical anhydrides, and (4) acid halides such as acyl fluoride as well as acyl chloride.

Monitoring

The completion of the deprotection and coupling needs to be monitored to ensure the success of the SPPS. The most widely used monitoring reaction is the Ninhydrin test to examine the presence of free amino group as a result of incomplete coupling. Other methods such as the TNBS and the Chloranil test can be used as complementary methods to the Ninhydrin test.

Cleavage and Removal of the Protecting Groups

Fmoc SPPS is designed for simultaneous cleavage of the anchoring linkage and global deprotection of side-chain-protecting groups with TFA. The most commonly used cleavage cocktail is Reagent K (TFA/thioanisol/water/phenol/ethandithiol (EDT): 82.5:5:5:5:2.5 v/v).

Peptide Evaluation

Nowadays, the peptide quality is examined routinely by the analytical High Performance Liquid Cromatografy (HPLC) to determine the purity in conjunction with mass spectral analysis to determine the identity. Most of the crude peptides can be purified alone by the reversed phase HPLC to achieve the desired purity. The combinations of anion or cation HPLC purification followed by the reversed phase HPLC purification provide a powerful technique to purify a crude peptide with inferior quality. The peptide purity needs to be determined by analytical HPLC with two different buffer systems or even further by capillary Electrophoresis. Mass spectrum by MALDI-TOF (Matrix Assisted Laser Delayed Induced—Time of Flight) methodology is the standard analytical procedure to assess peptide identity, moreover, data from sequence analysis and amino acid analysis can provide further detailed information on peptide homogeneity.

Recent Advances in Peptide Synthesis: Peptide Ligation

The introduction of the ligation strategy (chemoselective coupling of two unprotected peptide fragments) by Kent (29) provides the tremendous potential to achieve protein synthesis which is beyond the scope of SPPS. Many proteins with the size of 100–300 residues have been synthesized successfully by this method. Synthetic peptides have continued to play an ever increasing crucial role in the research fields of biochemistry, pharmacology, neurobiology, enzymology, and molecular biology because of the enormous advances in the SPPS. The ligation approach further enhances the capacity for synthetic peptides. With future developments in the SPPS, and ligation methodology, synthetic peptides will continue to be an indispensable tool for the research communities.

METHODOLOGIES FOR PEPTIDE MODIFICATIONS TOWARD THE OBTAINMENT OF A PEPTIDE-BASED RADIOPHARMACEUTICAL

By using orthogonal protecting group strategy, resins with novel linkers, and customized cleavage protocols, modified peptides can be synthesized routinely. These modified peptides can be catagorized as N-terminal modified, C-terminal modified, and peptides containing side-chain modifications. The most important peptide modifications allow to obtain peptides with a single or multiple disulfide bond, branched and/or cyclic peptides, and peptides derivatized with a non-amino acidic molecule. Among the non-amino acidic molecules that can be bound to a peptide sequence, much interest is devoted to chromogenic and flurescent probes that allow localizing the peptide derivative in biological media and tissues. Other modifications concern the obtainment of biotinylated peptides, glycosilated peptides, fatty acid containing peptides, and phosphorilated or sulfated peptides.

Chemical modification of the N-terminus of a peptide is often necessary to accomplish a variety of objectives. First, it can be useful as a device for simplifying the synthesis of difficult sequences; second, it can assist the purification of synthesized peptide; third, it can provide a useful tag by which to identify the peptide. Finally, peptides bearing a chemically modified N-terminus are not recognized by aminopeptidases, and therefore exhibit a longer half-life in vivo. Examples of N-terminus modifications are: formylation, acetylation, tert-butoxycarbonylation, and pyroglutammic formation. Moreover, most of the non-amino acid molecules, such as biotin, PEG, or fatty acids, are attached to a peptide using the N-terminus position. In fact, solid phase methodologies can be easy applied by reacting a carboxylic moiety of the non-amino acid molecule with the N-terminus of the peptide present on the solid support.

The most common C-terminal modification include peptidyl amides and N-alkyl amides. Several important hormones such as oxytocin, secretin, and LHRH are peptidyl amides. This modification, as well the acetylation of the N-terminus, is often chosen to obtain a peptide sequence more stable in vivo, and more close to the part of protein that the peptide molecule represent; in fact the presence of the amide group and of the acetyl moiety prevent the formation of charges in the terminal ends. Furthermore, to facilitate the survival of synthetic peptidyl amides in vivo, an obvious defense against the action of carboxy-peptidases is the N-alkylation of the carboxylic amide terminus. Anyway, C-terminal peptide modifications need more difficult synthetic approaches, and therefore, unless structure/activity relationship studies don't indicate this position as the unique possibility, peptide modifications by the presence of a non-amino acid molecules are preferred on the peptide N-terminus or on the side-chains.

Peptide modification on amino acid side chains can be obtained using synthetic approaches compatible with the Fmoc strategy of SPPS. Recently, there has been a concerted effort to develop side-chain protecting groups that utilize a different mechanism of cleavage to achieve selectivity: the protecting groups must remain chemically inert throughout the synthesis, and must be removed in a facile manner to liberate the appropriate side chain functional group. As the lysine residue is a bifunctional amine, differential protection for the N^α, and N^ε amino groups represents the most advantageous tool for peptide modification. Using this opportunity, many modified peptides have been obtained; they carry on the lysine side-chain or a peptide sequence to give branched or cyclic peptides, or a non-amino acid molecule such as fluorescent probes, porphyrin moieties, and other chelating agents.

Peptide modification with a chelating agent gives the very important opportunity to prepare stable metallo-peptides. Among the several applications of metallo-peptides, such as the modeling of metallo-proteins, or their catalytical behavior, the obtainment of peptide-based metallo radiopharmaceutical represents a new, exciting opportunity (30).

To obtain peptide-based radio pharmaceuticals the critical steps are: (1) the individuation of the peptide sequence with the appropriate biological activity: in vivo stability, binding affinity, and selectivity to target cells, biodistribution profiles, etc.; (2) the individuation of the point, where, within the peptide structure, modifications may be performed without affecting binding affinity of the molecule; and (3) the individuation of the method to radiolabel the peptide molecule.

As it concerns the labeling of the new peptide-based molecule, direct radiolabeling methods have been found to be less desirable, particularly for small peptides or in the case of peptide analogs. Such labeling schemes require rather complex chemistry and fairly sophisticated analytical methods to assess radiochemical purity and labeling efficiency. In most cases these methodologies are not readily available in nuclear medicine pharmacies. Therefore compounds that are directly radiolabeled, such as ^{123}I labeled radiopharmaceuticals, are centrally produced in commercial radiopharmacies where all necessary quality control is performed, and the radiopharmaceutical is then distributed ready for injection. This type of approach has obvious logistical complications. A more adequate way of solving this issue is to synthesize compounds bearing a chelating group in order to complex commonly used radioactive metals utilized in nuclear medicine applications. In this way one can keep stock of the peptide that can be labeled with the appropriate metal on demand using simple and reproducible methods that are very efficient. The concept of a kit formulation of the unlabeled radiopharmaceutical has been widely applied for virtually all nuclear medicine applications. Most peptide-based agents currently in development and in clinical use utilize this sort of approach for labeling. Figure 10 shows some of the commonly utilized chelating agents that are capable of coordinating radioactive metals. The most widely used chelating agents are polyamino-polycarboxylic ligands with a branched (DTPA like) or a cyclic (DOTA like) structure. These compounds and their modified analogs give very stable complexes with many metals and their radioactive isotopes are utilized for nuclear medicine applications (31,32). In particular they include complex isotopes such as

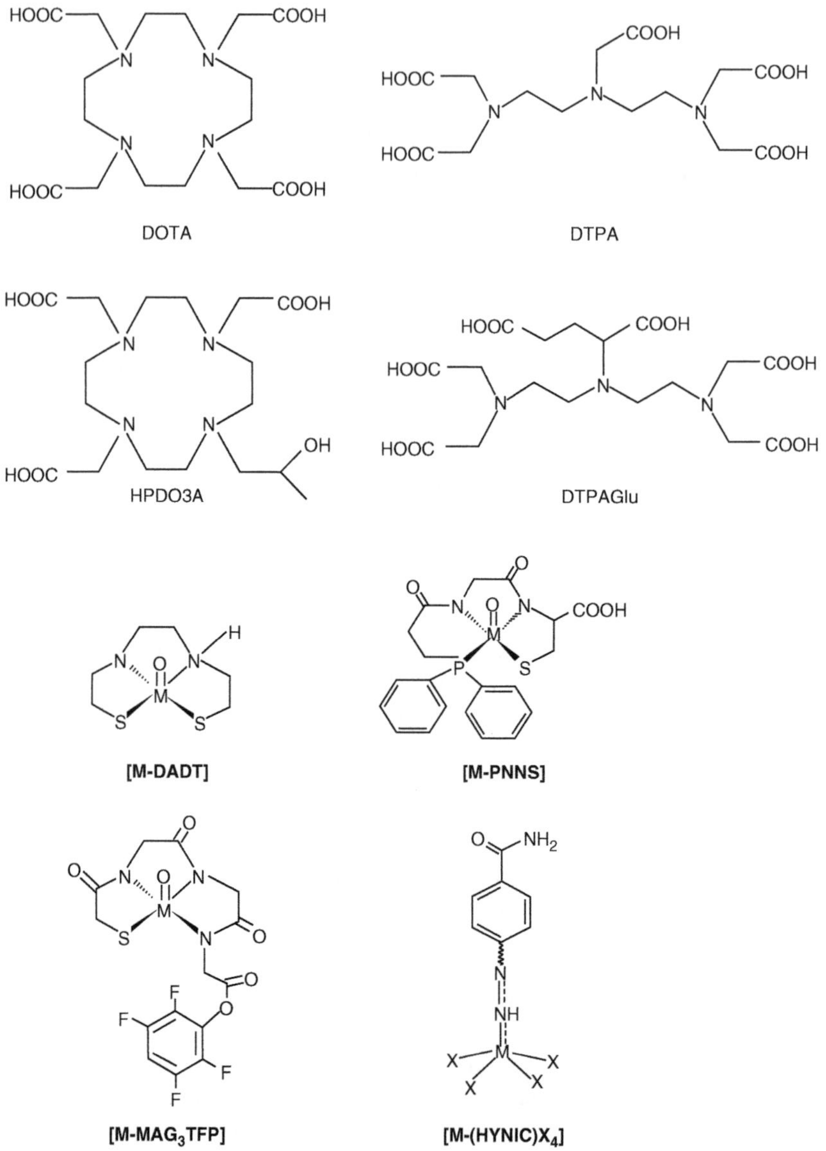

DOTA

DTPA

HPDO3A

DTPAGlu

[M-DADT]

[M-PNNS]

[M-MAG₃TFP]

[M-(HYNIC)X₄]

Figure 10 The most widely used chelating agents are polyaminopolycarboxylic ligands with a cyclic (DOTA like) (*top left*) or branched (DTPA like) structure (*top right*). Two derivatives of these chelating agents are also given: HPDO3A (*left*) and DTPAGlu (*right*). The chelating agents DADT, PNNS, MAG₃TFP and (HYNIC)X able to chelate metals of group VII of the periodic table are also reported. These last compounds are used to form stable complexes with ^{99m}Tc(V), ^{186}Re(V) and ^{188}Re(V).

^{111}In(III), ^{90}Y(III), ^{177}Lu(III), ^{68}Ga(III), and ^{153}Sm(III). These compounds use most of their carboxylic functions and all the amino groups to form a stable coordinative set for the metal. A carboxylic function is used to form a covalent amide linkage with one of the peptide amino groups. Also reported in Figure. 10 are another class of chelating agents that can be utilized to coordinate ^{99m}Tc(V), ^{99m}Tc(I), and ^{186}Re(V) (33–35).

SPECTROSCOPIC STUDIES

Fluorescence Studies

Steady-state fluorescence spectroscopy, based on continuous excitation of the fluorescent sample, has been used for more than two decades to investigate structural and rotational parameters of fluorophore-containing peptides (36–38). More recently improvements in the fluorescence decay measurement by nanosecond fluorometry have made possible the elucidation of conformational and dynamic aspects of polypeptides in greater detail. We are able to obtain three types of information: (1) characterization of the immediate environments of the fluorophore by determining fluorescence emission maxima and quantum yields or by measuring fluorescence lifetimes; (2) determination of the rotational characteristics of the fluorophore by fluorescence anisotropy measurements; and (3) estimation of the intramolecular distances between two fluorophores contained in the peptide by a singlet-singlet resonance energy transfer experiment.

The advantages of this technique over other physicochemical techniques currently used in studies of peptide conformations and interactions are the high temporal resolution (it is allowed to monitor motions in order of nanoseconds), the high sensitivity (measurements can be performed in concentration lower than 10^{-5} M avoiding the aggregations), and the feasibility of fluorescence (measurements in the presence of complex biological systems by use of appropriate fluorescence probes).

Since the fluorescence transition always occurs from the ground vibronic level of the lowest excited singlet state S_1 to any vibronic level of the ground state S_0, a spectral distribution of the fluorescence intensity, characterized by emission maximum, is observed. The fluorescence emission spectrum is obtained by recording the fluorescence intensity as a function of wavelength upon excitation at a given wavelength (usually the wavelength corresponding to the maximum of the longest wavelength absorption band).

Fluorescence measurements require the presence of the amino acid residues among the natural tryptophan, tyrosin, and phenylalanine (39), or a fluorescent probe (sulfonyl chlorides, isothiocyanates, spirofurans) covalently attached to the peptide (40). Tryptophan, tyrosin, and phenylalanine show fluorescence emission maxims at 348 nm, 303 nm, and 281 nm, respectively. The quenching and the shift give information about the structural elements. Numerous studies with tryptophan and tyrosine derivatives or containing peptides have led to identification of structural elements. Many factors, such as the proximity of a histidinum moiety to a tryptophan; can modify the fluorescence quantum yield of the residue in a peptide. A sulphide bridge, sulphydryl groups and protonated form of N-terminal amino groups quench the fluorescence in a distance-dependent way. The emission maximum is affected by exposition to solvent; for example cyclo, (Gly-Trp) shows a blue shift due to the interaction of the indole moiety with the dipeptide ring in a folded conformation, which produces a less hydrophilic environment (40). These studies carried out in different conditions of pH and solvent give information about many biologically active peptides such as adrenocorticotropin (ACTH 1–24) (41), α MSH (42), Glucagon (43), Melittin (44), Enkephalin (45), and Angiotensin II (46). It is significatively worth a comparison of the biologically active somatostatin fragments (47). The inversion of the configuration of the tryptophanyl residue 8 from L to D produces a threefold increase in the tryptophan florescence quantum yields, and a blue shift of 1,5 nm because the hydrophobic interaction with the side chain of Lys^9 are more favorable in $DTrp^8$ diastomer than in $LTrp^8$. The estimation of intramolecular distances by singlet-singlet resonance energy transfer was performed for the first time with a fully active n-terminal 24 peptide fragment of ACTH 1–24. This property allows evaluation of the distance between Tyr, Trp or other chromophore in the peptide, and the contribution to the determination of the conformation in different media. Studies were carried out for Angiotensins, Enkephalins, and other peptides in different conditions of solvent or pH (48).

Fluorescence quantum yield or lifetime determination, anisotropy measurements, and energy transfer experiments can also be used to study the interaction of peptides with complex biological systems, for example, protein, membrane, or receptor. Such studies not only permit the determination of binding parameters, but also may reveal conformational aspects of the interaction between the peptide and the macromolecular system under investigation. A number of these investigations were reviewed by Edelhoch (49). The interaction of glucagons, calcitonin, and ACTH with micelles of lysolecithin, a natural constituent of lipoproteins, and membranes (50), the interaction of melittin with various lipids (51) have been extensively studied. In recent years, because of its high sensitivity, fluorescence spectroscopy is the method choice for the characterization of well-defined solubilized receptors. All relevant binding parameters can be detected, as well as the conformational changes in the peptide ligand and/or receptor protein due to binding. An excellent example in the paper related to the galactose receptor which changed conformation at least 30 ang from the binding site of galactose (52). More recent studies were carried out to study the interaction between peptide ligands and G-protein membrane fragments in the presence of surfactant to mimic the membrane environment. The titration of receptor analogue CXCR4(29–39) with chemokine analogue SDF-1(1–17) (53), performed in presence of 2.5 mM DPC, allowed estimation of the apparent dissociation constant (Kd') in 2.6 ± 0.2 μM. Fluorescence changes were originated exciting at 250 nm, and monitoring at 305 nm. They include the excited-state energy resonance contribution transferred from phenylalanine donors to the tyrosine acceptor SDF-1(1–17). The dissociation constants of the interaction between 1–47 N-terminus fragment of cholecystokinin receptor and the nonsulfated cholecystokinin octapeptide (CCK8) was valued in the same way (54). In this case the quenching of fluorescence intensities of tryptophan residues of both peptides was diagnostic of the binding (Fig. 11).

Circular Dichroism Studies

The Circular dichroism (CD) and the optical rotatory dispersion (ORD) have a unique sensitivity to the molecular conformation and stereochemical relationships that makes them ideally suited to the detection of conformational differences and changes. They provide information about the absolute conformations in many cases, and can be a powerful probe into the conformation of peptides in solution. The CD and ORD are a chiroptical spectroscopy; the chiroptical term refers to differential interactions between matter, and the two forms (right, and left) of circularly polarized light. A chiral compound will absorb the right and left polarized light with different molar ext coefficients (ε). The measurement of the difference of the $\varepsilon(\Delta\varepsilon)$ in the electron transitions allows plotting of graphics depending the wavelength. The are several advantages to CD that have made it the predominant method. The relatively narrowness of CD bands, in contrast to the much broader Cotton effects in ORD, is the most

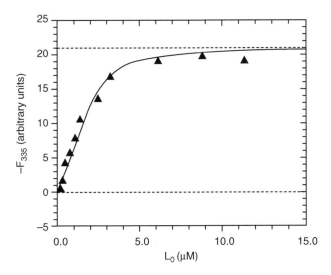

Figure 11 Titration of CCK_A-R(1–47) with CCK8 in phosphate buffer, pH 7.2 containing SDS micelles. The binding curve was obtained monitoring fluorescence intensities at 335 as a function of the total octapeptide concentration. Intensities were obtained by the difference between the fluorescence of a solution containing both receptor and CCK8 and the fluorescence of a solution containing the same amount of octapeptide as that added to the receptor. Data allow to calculate a K_d value of 56 nM.

important, followed by the contributions of signals of aromatic side chains or prostestic groups in far-UV spectra (178–250 nm). The chromophore in peptide far UV spectrum is the electron transition in the amide group. Two electron transitions of the amide group fall in this region of the spectrum: i) the $n\pi^*$ involving the promotion of electron from a nonbonding orbital on the carbonyl oxygen to the antibonding π^* orbital of the amide observed 230 nm, and ii) the $\pi\pi^*$, observed near 190 nm in secondary amides, involving the electron transition from the highest fill orbital to the π^* orbital.

The signals of these transitions are affected by the hydrogen-bonding environments. Many common conformational motifs of peptide chain show characteristic feature. The α-helical conformations display large CD bands with a negative ellipticity at 222, and 208 nm, and a positive ellipticity at 193 nm. As long as the amino acid side chain does not contain a chromophoric substituent on the β-carbon (such as Phe, Tyr, and Trp), the CD spectra are qualitatively independent of the side chain and of the solvent. β-sheets features are a negative band near 216 nm and a large positive band near 195 nm, while disordered extended chains have a weak broad positive CD band near 217 nm and a large negative band near 200 nm. The spectrum of peptide is basically the sum of the spectra of its conformational elements, and thus the CD can be used to estimate secondary structure. In addition, the chromophores of the aromatic amino acid proteins are often in very dissymmetric environments resulting in distinctive CD spectra in the near UV (250–300 nm), which can serve as useful probes of the tertiary structure. When there is a predominant type of secondary structure, the CD will be generally be diagnostic of conformation. The presence of an α-helix CD pattern can be taken as strong evidence for the presence of a significant amount of this motif. Many effects has gone into deducing the CD spectra and the contents of β sheet, β turn, and unordered sequence. Conformational analysis of cyclic peptide are reported in literature using diketo-piperazines as important model systems, for testing and developing theoretical approachs.

Conformational analysis of linear peptides is considerably more difficult than that of cyclic peptides because of the absence of the cyclization constraints. In general, small linear peptides exist in solution as ensemble of conformers, the relative concentrations of which depend on solvent and temperature. Many peptide are studied and many configurations are reported as Enkephalins (55), Bradkinin (56), Angiotensin II (57), and Glucagon (58).

BIOMOLECULAR THREE-DIMENSIONAL STRUCTURES FROM X-RAY AND NUCLEAR MAGNETIC RESONANCE TECHNIQUES

The most important structural determination technique of biomolecules is the x-ray diffraction analysis on single crystals (59). Crystallography was, as already described, the decisive line of development of molecular modeling. This is due to the power of this technique that is able to give at atomic resolution the atom position in the three-dimensional structures of biomolecules. If we want to determine the position of atoms, we need a probe which is able to detect distances of the order of 1 Å (10^{-10} m). The three kinds of radiation used in crystallography are X-rays, electrons, and neutrons. It is possible to tune the wavelength of each of them, such that an optimal wavelength is used for the experiment related to the sample being analyzed.

X-rays are created by bombarding a metal plate with electrons accelerated to some 40 kV. If the metal is copper, then the main wavelength (λ) of the x-rays is CuKα at 1.54 Å, incidentally the same as the length of the C-C single bond, the most important bond for life. When X-rays pass through matter, they interact with the electrons surrounding the atomic nuclei, but not with the nuclei themselves. Yet since most electrons are located very close to the atomic nuclei, x-rays give information mainly about the position of atoms rather that about the more diffuse shapes of valence electrons. Another radiation used for small or medium size compounds containing heavy metals is the wavelength (λ) of MoKα at 0.71 Å. For polypeptides, standard x-ray experiments are sufficient to obtain diffraction data, while for proteins or more complex molecules it is necessary to use special sources of x-ray such as synchrotron beam lines. In solid state analysis there are two crucial steps: the obtainment of crystals of appropriate size for diffraction experiment, and the phase problem to solve the structure.

In many cases, various crystallization experiments at controlled conditions of pH and temperature in various buffer systems are needed to obtain single crystals. Single crystals are required with the infinite ordered structure in the solid state (in the crystal cell) to obtain data suitable for structural analysis. Despite numerous trials, in many cases (specially for peptides) these crystallization procedures aren't able to give single crystals for diffraction studies.

Once crystals of appropriate size are obtained, x-ray diffraction data will be collected, when necessary also at low temperature. The crucial next step is represented by the structure solution. In a diffraction experiment intensities are measures (I_{hkl}) whereas the magnitudes of another quantity (containing the information on the atomic coordinates-the structure factor F_{hkl}) are necessary to image the electron density. The F_{hkl} is mathematic imaginary quantity [$F_{hkl} = |F_{hkl}|\exp(i\phi_{hkl})$]. The Now $|F_{hkl}|$ can be straightforward from I_{hkl} (the diffraction data), but the relative phases ϕ_{hkl} are lost in the experiment, and cause the so-called phase problem. Many methods (direct methods, patterson analysis, molecular replacement) are used for polypeptides to solve the phase problem. Now with the low price of high-speed computers, programs that search the correct phases of all diffraction data with a random procedure have been implemented. These programs have the ability to solve almost all the structures of medium size molecules (until 1000 atoms). The last step is represented by the refinement of the structure to obtain the final high resolution data. The resulting structural data are of great utility in order to verify the previous rational design, and to obtain new synthetic molecules.

Over the last decade, NMR spectroscopy has emerged as an important tool for structural determination of bimolecular in solution. In addition, with advances in magnet technology, the increase of NMR analysis is due to the improvements in the speed and data storage capacity of modern computers. This has allowed the development of powerful two- and multi-dimensional NMR methods (60,61) which offer the possibility to solve the resonance assignment problem (62), an important problem in any detailed NMR study of biomolecules.

NMR structures are based primarily on a set of short proton-proton distances obtained from the nuclear Overhauser effect (NOE) (63). The origin of the NOE is dipolar cross-relaxation between protons. Because of the weak proton magnetic moment, and the r^{-6} distance dependence of the effect, NOEs can only be measured between protons at relatively short distances (<5 Å). Using distance calibration procedures, the NOEs can be transformed into constrains on proton-proton distances. Different computational methods can be used now for structural determination using these distance constraints such as distance-geometry (64) and restrained MD (65). The NOE is a spin-relaxation phenomenon, strictly related with the dynamic behavior of the molecule in solution. Therefore the structure and the dynamics of a biomolecule as seen by NMR are intimately connected. These considerations underline that the three-dimensional structures determined by NMR spectroscopy are average structures computed on an ensemble of biomolecular conformations from NOE data. The inherent flexibility of peptides with respect to proteins is a a hindrance to the accurate determination of three-dimensional structure. From the point of view of an experimentalist, this requires that as much experimental data as possible be utilized in the refinement of the conformation. In this regard, measurement of NOEs is the most important. However, for peptides the number of NOEs is rather limited, when compared to proteins, because of a large ratio of surface area to core. For this reason, other experimental conformational information are actively used in NMR structure determination, such as J-coupling constants and temperature coefficients (66) The coupling constants, obtained from 2D experiments, are related with ϕ backbone dihedral angles, and with side chains' conformation. The temperature coefficients, determined from ^{1}H experiments at different temperatures, give information on the NH involvement in hydrogen bond interactions.

The protocol for peptide structure determination from NMR can be summarized in four steps:

1. Assign ^{1}H resonances
2. Determine proton-proton distance constraints, and dihedral angle constraints from NOEs, and J-couplings, respectively, using 2D experiments (COSY, TOCSY, ROESY, HOHAHA) (67–69)
3. Calculate family of structures using constraints only (experimental constraints plus covalent structure) using computational procedures
4. Refine these structures using geometrical constraints, and potential energy functions with restrained energy minimization, and restrained MD
5. Analysis of the average structures obtained from refined conformational families.

The first two steps, consisting of ^{1}H resonances assignment and determination of distance, and dihedral angle constraints, are common to all NMR procedures. For peptides, the sequential assignment of the proton resonances is performed using two main classes of 2D NMR experiments, COSY (correlated spectroscopy), and TOCSY (total correlation spectroscopy). Proton-proton distance constraints are most conveniently derived from cross-peak intensities in 2D NOE spectra. For the dynamic behavior of macromolecule in solution, the approach that is used is that of translating the NOE information into distance ranges rather than attempting to obtain precise distances. The 2D COSY experiments give also the value of J-coupling constants and related dihedral angles.

The other steps are dependent from the experimental results obtained in the first two steps. In general, all NMR data are used as constraints in distance geometry (DG) programs. Thus far, it is the only method that does not rely on some starting conformation and is therefore free from operator bias. In the DG procedures, two matrices with upper and lower bond are set up for all atom-atom distances of the molecules. These matrices contain standard bond lengths and bond angles of the covalent structure, and the experimentally found distance ranges form NOEs and J-coupling constants. Then the DG algorithm computes the 3D structures corresponding to the used constraints. After the structure generation, usually the best structures are refined using energy minimization and restrained MD procedures.

An example of the active use of three-dimensional structure information using NMR and x-ray data to determine SAR for bioactive molecules is the conformational studies on somatostatin, and its analogs. Somatostatin (H-Ala^1-Gly^2-c[Cys^3-Lys^4-Asn^5-Phe^6-Phe^7-Trp^8-Lys^9-Thr^{10}-Phe^{11}-Thr^{12}-Ser^{13}-Cys^{14}]-OH), a cyclic tetradeca-peptide, inhibits the release of several hormones, including growth hormone, glucagon, insulin, secretin, and gastrin. (70). It also plays a vital role in neurotransmission and neuromodulation (71,72), and has antiproliferative effects, regulating cell proliferation and differentiation. The diverse biological activities of somatostatin are mediated by a family of five different receptors, sst1-sst5 (sst's). Due to its broad spectrum of physiological activities, and its short duration of action due to rapid proteolytic degradation in vivo (73), somatostatin continues to be a target for the development of small subtype specific analogs.

Indeed, over the past three decades, hundreds of somatostatin analogs have been reported, and tested for their affinity and selectivity toward the five receptor subtypes. Furthermore, extensive structural studies, including NMR and X-ray diffraction, (74–79) have been carried out to elucidate the pharmacophore and the consensus sst2/sst5 (and sst3) receptors. The analysis of the three-dimensional structures obtained have demonstrated the specific involvement of the side chains of all residues but Phe^7-DTrp^8-Lys^9-Thr^{10} for biological recognition (Fig. 12), with a β-turn structure in the backbone of the segment Phe-DTrp-Lys-Thr. In addition, the comparison of the conformational behavior of sst-selective analogs has allowed to propose pharmacophore models for the

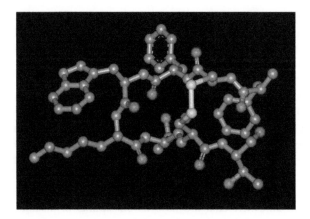

Figure 12 Molecular model of octreotide molecule.

different somatostatin receptors. For example, the proposed consensus structural motif at the binding pocket for the sst4-selective analogs (80) requires a unique set of distances between an indole/2-naphthyl ring, a lysine side chain, and another aromatic ring. This motif is necessary, and sufficient to explain the binding affinities of all of the analogs studied, and it is distinct from the existing model suggested for sst2/sst5 selectivity.

These studies also indicate that the backbone conformation is not important in binding to the receptor but forms a scaffold to orient the sidechains of the essentially important residues, namely indole at position 8, aminoalkyl function at position 9, and an aromatic ring.

REFERENCES

1. Hruby VJ, Matsunaga TO. Applications of synthetic peptides. Synthetic Peptides. 2nd ed. New York: Oxford University Press, 2002:292–376.
2. Benedetti E, Morelli G, Nemethy G, Sheraga HA. Statistical and energetic analysis of side-chain conformations in oligopeptides. Int J Pept Prot Res 1983; 22:1–15.
3. Ramachandran GN, Kolaskar AS, Ramakrishnan C, Sasisakharan V. Mean geometry of the peptide unit from crystal structure data. Biochem Biophys Acta 1974; 359:298–302.
4. Zimmerman SS, Pottle MS, Némethy G, Scheraga HA. Conformational analysis of the 20 naturally occurring amino acid residues using ECEPP. Macromolecules 1977; 10:1–7.
5. Toniolo C. Intramolecularly hydrogen-bonded peptide conformations. CRC Crit Rev Biochem 1980; 9:1–44.
6. Allen FH, Pitchford NA. Conformational analysis from crystallographic data. In: Codding PW ed. Structure-Based Drug Design. The Netherlands: Kluwer Academic Publishers, 1998:5–26.

7. Benedetti E, Iacovino R, Saviano M. The use of uncoded α-amino acids residues in drug design. In: Codding PW ed. Structure-Based Drug Design. The Netherlands: Kluwer Academic Publishers, 1998:103–112.
8. Pavone V, Lombardi A, Nastri F, et al. Design and structure of a novel neurokinin a receptor antagonist cyclo(Met1-Asp2-Trp3-Phe4-Dap5-Leu6)cyclo(2β-5β). J Chem Soc Perk Trans 1995; 2:26–29.
9. Toniolo C, Benedetti E. Old and new structures from studies of synthetic peptides rich in C$^{\alpha,\alpha}$-disbstituted glycines. ISI atlas of science. Biochemistry 1988; 1:225–230.
10. Karle IL. Flexibility in peptide molecules and restraints imposed by hydrogen bonds, the Aib residue and core inserts. Biopolymers (Pept Sci) 1996; 40:157–180.
11. Benedetti E. Molecular engineering in the preparation of bioactive peptides. In: Doniach S ed. Statistical Mechanics. Protein Structure and Protein Substrate Interactions. New York: Plenum Press, 1994:381–400.
12. Isernia C, Bucci E, De Napoli L, et al. Synthesis and conformation of dipeptide taste ligands containing homo-β-aminoacid residues. J Phys Org Chem 1999; 12:577–587.
13. Wade EC, Lüdemann S. Computational strategies for modeling receptor flexibility in studies of receptor-ligand interactions. In: Codding PW ed. Structure-Based Drug Design. The Netherlands: Kluwer Academic Publishers, 1998:41–52.
14. Fisher E. Synthesis of polypeptide derivatives. Ber Deut Chem Ges 1903; 36:2094–2106.
15. Merrifield RB. Solid phase peptide synthesis. I. The synthesis of a tetrapeptide. J Am Chem Soc 1963; 85:2149–2154.
16. Carpino LA, Han GY. 9-Fluorenylmethoxycarbonyl amino-protecting group. J Org Chem 1972; 37:3404–3409.
17. Fields GB, Noble RL. Solid phase peptide synthesis utilizing 9-fluorenylmethoxycarbonyl amino acids. Int J Pept Prot Res 1990; 35:161–214.
18. Olstad OK, Morrison NE, Jemtland R, Jueppner H, Segre GV, Gautvik KM. Differences in binding affinities of human PTH(1-84) do not alter biological potency: a comparison between chemically synthesized hormone, natural, and mutant forms. In: Peptides, Vol. 15. New York: Tarrytown, 1994:1261–1265.
19. Hoeprich PD. Polypeptide/protein synthesis using Fmoc/tert-butyl protection strategy. Innovation perspect solid phase synth collect pap. Int symp. Forster City: Appl Biosystems Inc, 1992:49–55.
20. Dawson PE, Muir TW, Clark-Lewis I, Kent SB. Synthesis of proteins by native chemical ligation. Science 1994; 266:776–779.
21. Atherton E, Sheppard RC. Solid phase peptide synthesis: a practical approach. Oxford, U.K.: IRL Press, 1989:1–203.
22. Bayer E, Rapp W. New polymer supports for solid-liquid-phase peptide synthesis. Chem Pept Prot 1986; 3:3–8.
23. Barany G, Albericio F, Biancalana S, et al. Biopolymer syntheses on novel polyethylene glycolpolystyrene (PEG-PS) graft supports. Pept Chem Biol Proc Am Pept Symp 1992:603–604.
24. Meldal M. PEGA: a flow-stable polyethylene glycol-dimethylacrylamide copolymer for solid-phase synthesis. Tetrahedron Lett 1992; 33:3077–3080.
25. Kempe M, Barany G. CLEAR: a novel family of highly cross-linked polymeric supports for solid-phase peptide synthesis. J Am Chem Soc 1996; 118:7083–7093.

26. Wang S. *p*-Alkoxybenzyl alcohol resin and *p*-alkoxybenzyloxycarbonylhydrazide resin for solid phase synthesis of protected peptide fragments. J Am Chem Soc 1973; 95:1328–1333.

27. Rink H. Solid-phase synthesis of protected peptide fragments using a trialkoxy-diphenyl-methyl ester resin. Tetrahedron Lett 1987; 28:3787–3790.

28. Barlos K, Gatos D, Kapolos S, Papaphotiu G, Schaefer W, Yao W. Esterification of partially protected peptide fragments with resins. Synthesis of Leu15-gastrin I using 2-chlorotrityl chloride resin. Tetrahedron Lett 1989; 30:3947–3950.

29. Schnolzer M, Alewood P, Jones A, Alewood D, Kent SB. In situ neutralization in Boc-chemistry solid phase peptide synthesis. Rapid, high yield assembly of difficult sequences. Int J Pept Prot Res 1992; 40:180–193.

30. Aloj L, Morelli G. Design, synthesis, and preclinical evaluation of radiolabeled peptides for diagnosis and therapy. Curr Pharm Des 2004; 10:1–23.

31. Anderson CJ, Pajeau TS, Edwards EB, Sherman ELC, Rogers BE, Welch MJ. In vitro and in vivo evaluation of copper-64-octreotide conjugates. J Nucl Med 1995; 36:2315–2325.

32. de Jong M, Bakker WH, Krenning EP, et al. Yttrium^{90} and Indium^{111} labeling, receptor binding and biodistribution of [DOTA0- Dphe1, Tyr^3]octreotide, a promising somatostatin analogue for radionuclide therapy. Eur J Nucl Med 1997; 24:368–371.

33. Baidoo KE, Scheffel U, Stathis M, et al. High-affinity no-carrier-added 99mTc-labeled chemotactic peptides for studies of inflammation in vivo. Bioconjug Chem 1998; 9:208–217.

34. Hnatowich DJ, Qu T, Chang F, Ley AC, Rusckowski RC. Labeling peptides with technetium-99m using a bifunctional chelator of a N-hydroxysuccinimide ester of mercaptoacetyltriglycine. J Nucl Med 1998; 39:56–64.

35. Schwartz DA, Abrams MJ, Hauser MM, et al. Preparation of hydrazino-modified proteins and their use for the synthesis of technetium-99m-protein conjugates. Bioconjug Chem 1991; 2:333–336.

36. Stryer L. Fluorescence spectroscopy of proteins. Science 1968; 162:526–533.

37. Weber G. In: Spectroscopic Approches to Biomolecular Conformation. Chicago, IL: Am Med Assoc, 1970:23–31.

38. Weber G. In: Excited States of Biological Molecules. New York: Wiley, 1976:363–374.

39. Creed D. The photophysics and photochemistry of the near-UV absorbing amino acids. I. Tryptophan and its simple derivatives. Photochem Photobiol 1984; 39:537–562.

40. Haugland RP. In: Excited State of Biopolymers. New York: Plenum, 1983:29–58.

41. Eisinger J, Feuer B, Lamola AA. Intramolecular singlet excitation transfer. Applications to polypeptides. Biochemistry 1969; 8:3908–3915.

42. Shinitzky M, Goldman R. Fluorometric detection of histidine-tryptophan complexes in peptides and proteins. Eur J Biochem 1967; 3:139–144.

43. Edelhoch H, Lippoldt ER. Structural studies on polypeptide hormones. I. Fluorescence. J Biol Chem 1969; 244:3876–3883.

44. Werner TC, Forster LS. The fluorescence of tryptophyl peptides. Photochem Photobiol 1979; 29:905–914.

45. Schiller PW, Natarajan S, Bodanszky M. Determination of the intramolecular tyrosine-tryptophan distance in a 7-peptide related to the C-terminal sequence of cholecystokinin. Int J Pept Protein Res 1978; 12:139–142.

46. Schiller PW. Conformational comparison of (Val5, Trp8)-angiotensin II and (Val4, Trp7)-angiotensin III by fluorescence measurements. Can J Biochem 1979; 57:402–407.
47. Schiller PW, Abraham N, Bellini F, Immer H. In: Peptides: synthesis-structure-function. Rockford, Ill: Pierce Chemical Co, 1981:367–370.
48. Ghiron CA, Bumpus FM, Longworth JW. In: Excited states of biological molecules. New York: Wiley, 1976:363–374.
49. Edelhoch H. In: Biochemical Fluorescence: Concepts, Vol. 2. New York: Dekker, 1976:545–571.
50. Schneider AB, Edelhoch H. Polypeptide hormone interaction. II. Glucagon binding to lysolecithin. J Biol Chem 1972; 247:4986–4991.
51. Dufourcq J, Faucon JF. Intrinsic fluorescence study of lipid-protein interactions in membrane models. Binding of melittin, an amphipathic peptide, to phospholipid vesicles. Biochim Biophys 1977; 467:1–11.
52. Zukin RS, Hartig PR, Koshland DE, Jr. Use of a distant reporter group as evidence for a conformational change in a sensory receptor. Proc Natl Acad Sci 1977; 74:1932–1936.
53. Palladino P, Pedone C, Ragone R, Rossi F, Saviano M, Benedetti E. A simplified model of the binding interaction between stromal cell-derived factor-1 chemokine and CXC chemokine receptor 4. Protein Pept Lett 2003; 10:133–138.
54. Ragone R, De Luca S, Tesauro D, Pedone C, Morelli G. Fluorescence studies on the binding between 1-47 fragment of cholecystokinin receptor CCKA-R(1-47) and nonsulfated cholecystokinin octapeptide CCK8. Biopolymers 2001; 56:47–53.
55. Bradbury AF, Smyth DG, Snell CR. Biosynthetic origin and receptor conformation of methionine enkephalin. Nature 1976; 260:165–166.
56. Bodanszky A, Bodanszky M, Jorpes EJ, Mutt V, Ondetti MA. Molecular architecture of peptide hormones optical rotatory dispersion of cholecystokinin-pancreozymin, bradykinin and 6-glycine bradykinin. Experentia 1970; 26:948–950.
57. Fermandijan S, Morgat J, Fromageot P. Studies of angiotensin-II conformations by circular dichroism. Eur J Biochem 1971; 24:252–258.
58. Blanchard MH, King MV. Evidence of association of glucagon from optical rotatory dispersion and concentration-difference spectra. Biochem Biophys Res Commun 1966; 25:298–303.
59. Giacovazzo C, Monaco HL, Viterbo D, et al. Fundaments of Crystallography. Oxford: Oxford Science Publications, 1992.
60. Ernst RR, Bodenhausen G, Wokaun A. Principles of nuclear magnetic resonance. One and Two Dimensions. Oxford: Clarendon Press, 1987.
61. Oschkinat H, Griesinger C, Kraulis PJ, et al. Three-dimensional NMR spectroscopy of a protein in solution. Nature 1988; 332:374–376.
62. Wüthrich K. NMR of Protein and Nucleic Acids. New York: John Wiley and Sons, 1986.
63. Noggle JH, Schirmer RE. The Nuclear Overhauser Effect—Chemical Applications. New York: Academic Press, 1971.
64. Güntert P, Mumenthaler C, Wüthrich K. Torsion angle dynamics for NMR structure calculation with the new program DYANA. J Mol Biol 1997; 273:283–298.
65. Brooks CL, III, Montgomery Pettitt B, Karplus M. Proteins: A Theoretical Perspective of Dynamics, Structure, and Thermodynamics. New York: John Wiley and Sons, 1988.

66. Mierke DF, Huber T, Kessler H. Coupling constants again: experimental restraints in structure refinement. J Comput Aided Mol Des 1994; 8:29–40.

67. Davis DG, Bax A. Assignment of complex 1H NMR spectra via two-dimensional homonuclear Hartmann-Hahn spectroscopy. J Am Chem Soc 1985; 107:2820–2821.

68. Rance M, Sorensen OW, Bodenhausen B, Wagner G, Ernst RR, Wüthrich K. Improved spectral resolution in COSY1H NMR spectra of proteins via double quantum filtering. Biochem Biophys Res Commun 1983; 117:479–485.

69. Kumar A, Wagner G, Ernst RR, Wüthrich K. Buildup rates of the nuclear overhauser effect measured by two-dimensional proton magnetic resonance spectroscopy: implications for studies of protein conformation. J Am Chem Soc 1981; 103:3654–3658.

70. Reichlin S. Somatostatin. N Engl J Med 1983; 309:1495–1501.

71. Delfs JR, Dichter MA. Effects of somatostatin on mammalian cortical neurons in culture: physiological actions and unusual dose response characteristics. J Neurosci 1983; 3:1176–1188.

72. Iversen LL. Nonopioid neuropeptides in mammalian CNS. Annu Rev Pharmacol Toxicol 1983; 23:1–27.

73. Patel YC, Wheatley T. In vivo and in vitro plasma disappearance and metabolism of somatostatin-28 and somatostatin-14 in the rat. Endocrinology 1983; 112:220–225.

74. Vale W, Rivier J, Ling N, Brown M. Biologic and immunologic activities and applications of somatostatin analogs. Metabolism 1978; 27:1391–1401.

75. Veber DF, Freidinger RM, Perlow DS, et al. A potent cyclic hexapeptide analogue of somatostatin. Nature (London) 1981; 292:55–58.

76. Pohl E, Heine A, Sheldrick GM, et al. Structure of octreotide, a somatostatin analogue. Acta Crystallogr 1995; 51:48–59.

77. Kessler H, Klein M, Wagner K. Peptide conformation. 48. Conformation and biological activity of proline containing cyclic retro-analogues of somatostatin. Int J Pept Protein Res 1988; 31:481–498.

78. Mierke DF, Pattaroni C, Delaet N, et al. Cyclic hexapeptides related to somatostatin. Int J Pept Protein Res 1990; 36:418–432.

79. Melacini G, Zhu Q, Goodman M. Multicongormational NMR analysis of sandostatin (octreotide): equilibrium between beta-sheet and partially helical structures. Biochemistry 1997; 36:1233–1241.

80. Grace CRR, Koerber SC, Erchegyi J, Reubi JC, Rivier J, Riek R. Novel sst4-selective somatostatin agonists. 4. Three-dimensional consensus structure by NMR. J Med Chem 2003; 46:5606–5618.

2

Radiopeptide Targeting for Tumor Therapy: Peptide Receptor Distribution

Jean Claude Reubi

Division of Cell Biology and Experimental Cancer Research, Institute of Pathology, University of Berne, Berne, Switzerland

INTRODUCTION

There are increasing numbers of in vitro studies reporting a high expression of neuropeptide receptors in human cancers. First historical evidence has been given by the high expression of somatostatin receptors in pituitary adenomas (1). Since then, many other human cancers were found to express somatostatin receptors (2). Moreover, peptide receptors such as bombesin receptors, CCK receptors, VIP receptors, substance P receptors, neurotensin (NT) receptors, among others, were found to be overexpressed in several cancers in vitro (2). Based on these results, an increasing number of laboratories have started to develop peptide radioligands suitable for the in vivo targeting of such tumors; current areas of investigations are the somatostatin, bombesin, CCK, and NT field (3). Finally, clinicians have given the proof of principle in vivo that several of these peptide receptors may indeed represent adequate targets to image or even treat human tumors (4–6). In this rapidly growing field, the clinicians, in particular the oncologists and the nuclear physicians, want to know which radioligands they should best use for which type of cancer. This is the aim of the present review.

WHICH TUMORS EXPRESS WHICH PEPTIDE RECEPTOR?

Methodological Considerations

This question can be answered by in vitro methods. The basic principles to search for tumors expressing peptide receptors suitable for targeting are

Table 1 In Vitro Strategy to Select Tumors Expressing Peptide Receptors Suitable for Targeting

Materials and methods	
Use human tumors	Not tumor cell lines
Measure receptor proteins	Not mRNA
Identify ligand binding site	Rather than immunological epitope
Use morphological methods	Not tissue homogenates
Tumor selection is based on	
High density of receptors in tumor	
High receptor ratio tumor: host tissue	
High receptor homogeneity in tumor	
Receptor subtype compatibility with radioligand profile	

summarized in Table 1. One preferably uses human tumors resected from surgery, rather than tumor cell lines, since those may have distinct biological properties. One may preferably measure the receptor proteins rather than the mRNA, since the protein is the true target in the clinical setting. One wishes to identify the ligand binding site rather than an immunological epitope, since in vivo targeting is also based on binding of the radioligand to the receptor in vivo. Finally, the use of a morphological method using tissue sections rather than assays with tissue homogenates is mandatory. There are several possibilities to detect peptide receptors morphologically in tumor tissue sections. One possibility is in vitro receptor autoradiography, which identifies the receptor binding site (protein) that can be pharmacologically characterized and quantitatively assessed (Fig. 1). It is a highly sensitive and specific method. Recently this method has been improved in order to identify peptide receptor subtypes, by using subtype-selective analogs (Fig. 1). One drawback is, however, that in vitro receptor autoradiography does not have a very high resolution. A method analyzing the protein with a higher resolution is receptor immunohistochemistry, which, while dependent on a high quality antibody, can precisely identify membrane-bound receptors in formalin-fixed tissues (Fig. 1). Another possibility is in situ hybridization, which, however, identifies the mRNA and not the protein, and therefore should ideally be combined with a measurement of the receptor protein (Fig. 1).

In Vitro Expression of Peptide Receptors in Cancer

In general, it is not sufficient to evaluate whether a tumor is peptide receptor-positive or -negative. It is also necessary to assess its density, its distribution within the tumor, and its receptor subtype profile. It is well recognized that human tumors have a wide variability of peptide receptor density among individuals, up to 100–1000 times variations. It has been demonstrated that only patients with tumors with particularly high density of receptors should be selected for peptide receptor radiotherapy. Another important criteria for

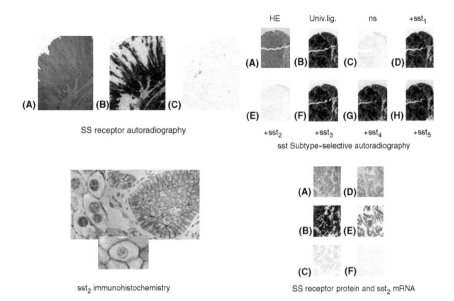

Figure 1 Four different methods to detect somatostatin receptors in vitro. (*Upper left*): Somatostatin receptor autoradiography [(**A**): H+E staining; (**B**): Autoradiogram showing total binding of ^{125}I-Tyr^3-Octreotide; (**C**): nonspecific binding]. (*Upper right*): Subtype-selective autoradiography with (**B**) the universal ligand ^{125}I-LTT-SS-28 in competition with ligands selective for (**D**) sst$_1$, (**E**) sst$_2$, (**F**) sst$_3$, (**G**) sst$_4$ and (**H**) sst$_5$. (*Lower left*): sst$_2$ immunohistochemistry. (*Lower right*): (**A-C**) Combined somatostatin receptor auto-radiography, and (**D-F**) in situ hybridization for sst$_2$ mRNA. *Source*: Adapted from Ref. 7.

selection of a tumor is the homogeneous distribution of receptors within a tumor. Table 2 lists a number of peptide receptors suitable for tumor targeting. Some of those will be discussed in more detail below.

Somatostatin Receptors

Numerous human cancers express somatostatin receptors, often in high density (2). The majority of these tumors express preferentially one of the somatostatin receptor subtypes, the sst$_2$ subtype. The sst$_2$ subtype is the best investigated of the somatostatin receptor subtypes. Moreover, the currently available somatostatin analogs, such as octreotide and lanreotide, have a particularly high affinity for the sst$_2$ subtype. As shown in Table 3, the majority of neuroendocrine tumors express somatostatin receptors, with a predominance of sst$_2$, and include pituitary adenomas (in particular GH- or TSH-producing adenomas), gastroenteropancreatic and lung neuroendocrine tumors, pheochromocytomas, and paraganglio-mas. Also tumors of the nervous system express sst$_2$ receptors, such as medulloblastomas, meningiomas and neuroblastomas. Furthermore, non-neural and non-neuroendocrine tumors also can express sst$_2$ receptors, although in lower

Table 2 Peptide Receptors Suitable for Tumor Targeting

Peptide receptors	Tumor types
Somatostatin receptors	Neuroendocrine tumors, brain tumors
Cholecystokinin-2 receptors	Medullary thyroid carcinomas, small cell lung carcinomas, gastrointestinal stromal tumors
Vasoactive intestinal peptide receptors	Gastrointestinal cancers
Neurotensin receptors	Pancreatic carcinomas, meningiomas
Substance P receptors	Glioblastomas
Neuropeptide Y receptors	Breast carcinomas
Gastrin-releasing peptide receptors	Breast carcinomas, prostate carcinomas, gastrointestinal stromal tumors
Glukagon-like peptide 1 receptors	Insulinomas

incidence or density; those include breast cancer, small cell lung cancer, lymphoma, hepatocellular carcinoma, renal cell carcinoma, and gastric carcinoma. Most of the above mentioned tumors, in particular the neuroendocrine tumors, have been imaged in patients for diagnostic purposes. Moreover, many of

Table 3 Tumors Expressing Somatostatin Receptors

Tumors with predominance of sst_2	Tumors with predominance of other ssts (with or without sst_2)
Pituitary adenomas (GH, TSH)	Selected pituitary adenomas [GH adenomas (sst_5), inactive adenomas (sst_3)]
Gastroenteropancreatic neuroendocrine tumors	Selected gastroenteropancreatic neuroendocrine tumors
Lung neuroendocrine tumors	Selected lung neuroendocrine tumors
Pheochromocytomas	Medullary thyroid carcinomas
Paragangliomas	Prostate carcinomas (sst_1)
Gastric carcinomas	Selected gastric carcinomas
Medulloblastomas	Mesenchymal tumors
Meningiomas	Thyroid carcinomas
Neuroblastomas	
Breast carcinomas	
Small cell lung carcinomas	
Lymphomas	
Hepatocellular carcinomas	
Renal cell carcinomas	
Radioligands of choice: Octreoscan, DOTATOC, DOTATATE	Radioligands of choice: DOTA NOC, DOTA BOC, Pan-Somatostatins

these tumors have been selected for peptide receptor radiotherapy using [90]Yttrium- or [177]Lu -labeled octreotide derivatives.

Table 3 lists also a number of tumors which may, in addition or instead of sst_2, express other somatostatin receptor subtypes, such as sst_1, sst_3, or sst_5. Those include selected pituitary adenomas; some GH-adenomas express preferentially sst_5 and many inactive adenomas have sst_3. Many gastroenteropancreatic and lung neuroendocrine tumors may frequently express multiple somatostatin receptor subtypes, as well as medullary thyroid cancers. Furthermore, prostate cancers often express sst_1 while gastric carcinomas, thyroid carcinomas, and various mesenchymal tumors may express sst_2 as well as other sst receptor subtypes. For those tumors expressing additional sst, the radioligand of choice may have a more universal sst binding profile than the octreotide derivatives, namely having high affinity for sst_2 as well as for other frequently occurring ssts, such as sst_3 or sst_5. Such radioligands include molecules derived from DOTANOC or DOTABOC compounds.

CCK Receptors

Interestingly, CCK receptors, although playing an important role in the gastrointestinal tract, are rarely expressed in gastrointestinal carcinomas, such as gastric cancers, colon cancers, or pancreatic carcinomas, but extremely frequently expressed, as CCK_2 receptor subtype, in a particular endocrine tumor, the medullary thyroid carcinoma (8). CCK_2 receptors have been shown to be well expressed in several other cancers, including some gastroenteropancreatic neuroendocrine tumors, small cell lung cancers, ovarian tumors, (9) and, most interesting, also in gastrointestinal stromal tumors (GIST), where they can be expressed in extremely high density (10). On the basis of these in vitro receptor studies, Behr et al. (5) have selected, as a first choice of tumors, the medullary thyroid carcinoma for in vivo targeting, because of their high incidence of CCK_2 receptors, and have shown extremely promising imaging data and encouraging preliminary PRRT data. The main limiting problem for the development of PRRT using CCK_2 receptors maybe the high and therefore problematic kidney uptake with current CCK analogs.

Gastrin-Releasing Peptide Receptors

Of great potential interest for tumor targeting are gastrin-releasing peptide (GRP) receptors, since they are abundant in most breast and prostate cancers. One should notice that the majority of the samples tested in vitro have only originated from surgically operable tumors; the investigated sample collection therefore consisted predominantly of primaries rather than of metastatic tissues and rarely contained advanced undifferentiated cancers or hormone-insensitive cancers (11,12). Except for a few bone metastases (12), the GRP-R status of the latter tumor group remains largely unknown, having not been investigated for technical reasons. GRP-receptor heterogeneity in breast cancer was frequent and should not be ignored when proposing GRP receptor radiotherapy for those tumors (11).

A further, recent example of tumors that may be extremely attractive for PRRT is GIST, due to an extraordinarily high GRP receptor density (10).

Neurotensin Receptors

A subgroup of ductal pancreatic carcinomas expresses a high density of NT receptors (13). A preliminary in vivo NT receptor scanning study has been able to visualize a faint signal from a tumor with a high density of these receptors (14). These tumors, often consisting of a few, but strongly receptor-positive neoplastic ducts embedded within a receptor-negative surrounding fibrosis (chronic pancreatitis), may be attractive for PRRT, despite the low cellularity of that type of cancer (13). This low cellularity may in part explain the weakness of the in vivo signal. Other tumors expressing NT receptors are meningiomas and Ewing Sarcomas (15).

Vasoactive Intestinal Peptide Receptors

Although a majority of human cancers express vasoactive intestinal peptide (VIP) receptors of the $VPAC_1$ subtype (16), the targeting of $VPAC_1$-receptors for PRRT is unlikely to be of great potential due to the ubiquitous distribution of $VPAC_1$ in most organs (16). Conversely, $VPAC_2$, which is only rarely expressed in normal tissues, may be a target for PRRT in $VPAC_2$-expressing cancers; GIST, with a high $VPAC_2$ receptor density, may be a most attractive example (10). In vivo data using ^{123}I-VIP, as universal ligand targeting $VPAC_1$ and $VPAC_2$, are available as proof of concept that VIP receptor-positive tumors, namely gastrointestinal cancers, can be targeted in vivo in selected cases (17,18).

Neuropeptide Y Receptors

Neuropeptide Y (NPY) receptors have recently been found to be highly expressed in breast cancer, predominantly as Y_1 subtype (19), as well as in a subgroup of ovarian tumors (sex cord stromal tumors) (20) and adrenal tumors (21). More recently, it has been reported that a majority of renal cell carcinomas and nephroblastomas also expressed NPY receptors. This is a new family of peptide receptors for which in vivo scanning studies in human tumors need to be performed.

Glucagon-Like-Peptide 1 Receptors

A very high density of glucagon-like-peptide 1 (GLP-1) receptors was reported in virtually all insulinomas and, at lower density, in gastrinomas (22), suggesting to use radiolabeled GLP-1 analogs for PRRT in these tumors. Whereas rat insulinomas were reported to be targeted in vivo by GLP-1 analogs, such evidence is still missing for human insulinomas.

Corticotropin-Releasing Factor Receptors

Corticotropin-releasing factor (CRF) receptors are expressed in selected human cancers (23). Those with a high density include ACTH-producing pituitary adenomas and paragangliomas (CRF_1) as well as GH-producing and non-functioning pituitary adenomas (CRF_2). They may be attractive PRRT candidates.

NK1 Receptors

Because gliomas have a high density of NK1 receptors (24) that is several fold higher than that of somatostatin receptors, the same topical approach as for somatostatin receptors (25) has been proposed and a pilot study was started in order to evaluate the effect of PRRT in glioblastomas. The study is still in progress, but encouraging preliminary data have been reported (26).

MULTIRECEPTOR TARGETING

The presence of multiple peptide receptors in selected cancers may be the basis for multireceptor radiotherapy (Table 4) using two or more radiotracers concomitantly or specific radiopeptide hybrids. This strategy would have two main advantages. First, two or more radioligands given concomitantly may considerably increase the therapeutic dose to the tumor. Second, some of the problems related to receptor heterogeneity in the tumors may be overcome, as it is likely that in such cases more tumor cells will be targeted with two or more radioligands than would be possible with only one ligand. Such a multireceptor targeting could hopefully prevent or reduce escape from radiotherapy. Figure 2 illustrates a case of a tumor expressing concomitantly 4 peptide receptors: CCK_2, GLP-1, sst_2, and $VPAC_1$ receptors. Tumors of interest for multireceptor targeting may be breast cancers (expressing concomitantly GRP- and NPY receptors), GIST (with GRP-, CCK_2- and $VPAC_2$ receptors) (10,27), and GEP NET (with CCK, GLP-1, sst and $VPAC_1$ receptors).

Table 4 Multireceptor Targeting of Human Tumors

Tissues: human tumors expressing peptide-R concomitantly
  Breast Ca: GRP-R + NPY-R
  GIST: GRP-R + VPAC2 + CCK-R
  GEP NET: CCK-R + GLP1-R + SS-R + VPAC1
Radioligands
  Cocktail of radiopeptides or radiopeptide-hybrids
Advantages
  Brings more radioactivity to the tumor
    allows a more sensitive in vivo detection
    induces a more efficient radiotherapeutic effect
  Brings radioactivity to more tumor cells
    gives a greater chance for a targeting of the whole tumor tissue
Recommendation
  Previous in vitro receptor profile to select adequate tumors

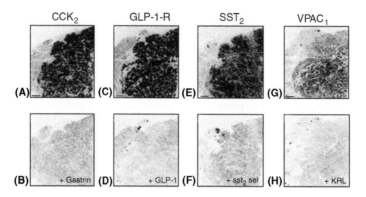

Figure 2 A GEP NET expressing concomitantly 4 peptide receptors: (**A, B**) CCK$_2$ receptors; (**C, D**) GLP-1 receptors; (**E, F**) sst$_2$ receptors; (**G, H**) VPAC$_1$ receptors. (**A, C, E, G**) Total binding. (**B, D, F, H**) nonspecific binding. Such a tumor is suitable for multireceptor targeting. *Source*: Adapted from Ref. 7.

REFERENCES

1. Reubi JC, Landolt AM. High density of somatostatin receptors in pituitary tumors from acromegalic patients. J Clin Endocrinol Metab 1984; 59:1148–1151.
2. Reubi JC. Peptide receptors as molecular targets for cancer diagnosis and therapy. Endocr Rev 2003; 24:389–427.
3. Heppeler A, Froidevaux S, Eberle AN, Maecke HR. Receptor targeting for tumor localization and therapy with radiopeptides. Curr Med Chem 2000; 7:971–994.
4. Krenning EP, Bakker WH, Breeman WAP, et al. Localization of endocrine-related tumors with radioiodinated analogue of somatostatin. Lancet 1989; 1:242–244.
5. Behr TM, Behe MP. Cholecystokinin-B/Gastrin receptor-targeting peptides for staging and therapy of medullary thyroid cancer and other cholecystokinin-B receptor-expressing malignancies. Semin Nucl Med 2002; 32:97–109.
6. Van de Wiele C, Dumont F, Vanden Broecke R, et al. Technetium-99m RP527, a GRP analogue for visualization of GRP receptor-expressing malignancies: a feasibility study. Eur J Nucl Med 2000; 27:1694–1699.
7. Reubi JC. Somatostatin and other peptide receptors as tools for tumor diagnosis and treatment. Neuroendocrinology 2004; 80:51–56.
8. Reubi JC, Waser B. Unexpected high incidence of cholecystokinin B/gastrin receptors in human medullary thyroid carcinomas. Int J Cancer 1996; 67:644–647.
9. Reubi JC, Schaer JC, Waser B. Cholecystokinin (CCK)-A and CCK-B/gastrin receptors in human tumors. Cancer Res 1997; 57:1377–1386.
10. Reubi JC, Korner M, Waser B, Mazzucchelli L, Guillou L. High expression of peptide receptors as a novel target in gastrointestinal stromal tumors. Eur J Nucl Med Mol Imaging 2004; 31:803–810.
11. Gugger M, Reubi JC. GRP receptors in non-neoplastic and neoplastic human breast. Am J Pathol 1999; 155:2067–2076.
12. Markwalder R, Reubi JC. Gastrin-releasing peptide receptors in the human prostate: relation to neoplastic transformation. Cancer Res 1999; 59:1152–1159.

13. Reubi JC, Waser B, Friess H, Büchler MW, Laissue JA. Neurotensin receptors: a new marker for human ductal pancreatic adenocarcinoma. Gut 1998; 42:546–550.
14. Buchegger F, Bonvin F, Kosinski M, et al. Radiolabeled neurotensin analog, (99m)Tc-NT-XI, evaluated in ductal pancreatic adenocarcinoma patients. J Nucl Med 2003; 44:1649–1654.
15. Reubi JC, Waser B, Schaer JC, Laissue JA. Neurotensin receptors in human neoplasms: high incidence in Ewing sarcomas. Int J Cancer 1999; 82:213–218.
16. Reubi JC, Läderach U, Waser B, Gebbers J-O, Robberecht P, Laissue JA. Vasoactive intestinal peptide/pituitary adenylate cyclase-activating peptide receptor subtypes in human tumors and their tissues of origin. Cancer Res 2000; 60:3105–3112.
17. Virgolini I, Raderer M, Kurtaran A, et al. 123-I-vasoactive intestinal peptide (VIP) receptor scanning: update of imaging results in patients with adenocarcinomas and endocrine tumors of the gastrointestinal tract. Nucl Med Biol 1996; 23:685–692.
18. Hessenius C, Bäder M, Meinhold H, et al. Vasoactive intestinal peptide receptor scintigraphy in patients with pancreatic adenocarcinomas or neuroendocrine tumors. Eur J Nucl Med 2000; 27:1684–1693.
19. Reubi JC, Gugger M, Waser B, Schaer JC. Y1-mediated effect of neuropeptide Y in cancer: breast carcinomas as targets. Cancer Res 2001; 61:4636–4641.
20. Korner M, Waser B, Reubi JC. Neuropeptide Y receptor expression in human primary ovarian neoplasms. Lab Invest 2004; 84:71–80.
21. Korner M, Waser B, Reubi JC. High expression of neuropeptide y receptors in tumors of the human adrenal gland and extra-adrenal paraganglia. Clin Cancer Res 2004; 10:8426–8433.
22. Reubi JC, Waser B. Concomitant expression of several peptide receptors in neuroendocrine tumors as molecular basis for in vivo multireceptor tumor targeting. Eur J Nucl Med 2003; 30:781–793.
23. Reubi JC, Waser B, Vale W, Rivier J. Expression of CRF1 and CRF2 receptors in human cancers. J Clin Endocrinol Metab 2003; 88:3312–3320.
24. Hennig IM, Laissue JA, Horisberger U, Reubi JC. Substance P receptors in human primary neoplasms: tumoral and vascular localization. Int J Cancer 1995; 61:786–792.
25. Schumacher T, Hofer S, Eichhorn K, et al. Local injection of the (90)Y-labelled peptidic vector DOTATOC to control gliomas of WHO grades II and III: an extended pilot study. Eur J Nucl Med 2002; 29:486–493.
26. Schumacher T, Eichhorn K, Hofer S, et al. Diffusible brachytherapy (DBT) with radiolabelled substance P in high grade gliomas: first observations. Eur J Nucl Med 2001; 28:1040. OS1305.
27. Reubi JC, Gugger M, Waser B. Coexpressed peptide receptors in breast cancers as molecular basis for in vivo multireceptor tumor targeting. Eur J Nucl Med 2002; 29:855–862.

3

Developments of Radiolabeled Peptides

Ronald E. Weiner

*Department of Diagnostic Imaging and Therapeutics, University
of Connecticut Health Center, Farmington, Connecticut, U.S.A.*

Mathew L. Thakur

*Department of Radiology, Thomas Jefferson University Hospital,
Philadelphia, Pennsylvania, U.S.A.*

INTRODUCTION

In the last two decades, there has been explosive growth in the interest and development of radiolabeled peptides for both diagnostic and therapeutic applications. The foundation of this development was provided some 40 years ago by Merrifield, who developed the ability to easily synthesize pure peptide sequences. Subsequently, this process was automated and methods for their purification and characterization were developed. These developments have made it possible to have large quantities of potentially useful candidate peptides. These new techniques also accelerated the commercial development of these molecules, which provided additional resources to the Nuclear Medicine community. For example, Sandoz (now Novartis, Switzerland) developed Octreotide, an 8-amino acid analog, of Somatostatin, a 14-amino acid endogenous growth hormone (Fig. 1). Somatostatin was shown to have anti-tumor growth effects in cell culture and in animal models, and it was considered to be an effective therapeutic agent. However, it was ineffective in vivo, because Somatostatin has a very rapid blood clearance time ($T_{1/2}$, 2–4 minutes), which prevented significant tumoricsidal effect (1). The analog Octreotide, with its improved circulating $T_{1/2}$ (1.5–2 hours) enhanced delivery of the peptide to the

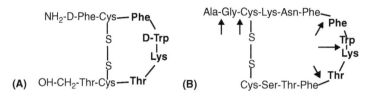

Figure 1 Schematic drawing of (**A**) Octreotide (Sandostatin) and (**B**) Somatostatin. Amino acids in bold are directly involved in Somatostatin receptor binding. Arrows indicate the sites of in vivo enzymatic cleavage. Amino acids are all L-isomers except where noted or an amino alcohol, Thr (CH_2-OH). *Source*: From Refs. 1, 2.

tumor. Encouraged by the greater tumor uptake, Krenning and his colleagues (3) developed OctreoScan (Fig. 2A), Octreotide with an attached chelating moiety, DTPA (diethylenediaminepentaacetic acid). The chelator provided the ability to incorporate a suitable radionuclide with a high stability constant. Krenning and collaborators demonstrated that ^{111}In-labeled DTPA Octreotide (OctreoScan) could accurately localize neuroendocrine tumors (5) and is now widely used for diagnosis and treatment of neuroendocrine disorders (6–8). Thus, OctreoScan became the first labeled peptide approved for human use and was commercialized by Mallinckrodt Imaging (1).

The sequence and target for over 850 endogenous peptides have been well-characterized (9). These peptides offer the investigator a wide array of compounds that can be radiolabeled for a suitable application. Table 1 shows a selected list of peptides, their function, target diseases and receptors that are presently under active investigation. These peptides can be developed as agents for either diagnoses or therapy of disease (mostly cancers), depending on the radionuclide that is attached to the peptide.

The targeted approach, now widely known as Molecular Imaging, to detect or treat disease is not new to the Nuclear Medicine community. This approach accelerated with the development of antibodies to target antigens present on tumors or other cells of interest. The success of this approach yielded a number of

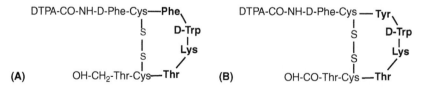

Figure 2 Schematic presentation of (**A**) Pentetreotide (OctreoScan) diethylenetriaminepenta acetic acid (DTPA) and (**B**) [Tyr³] Octreotate-DTPA [tyr replaces phe in position 3]. Amino acids in bold are directly involved in Somatostain receptor binding. Amino acids are all L-isomers except where noted or an amino alcohol, Thr (CH_2-OH). *Source*: From Refs. 2, 4.

Table 1 Peptides, Peptide Function, Target Disease and Cell-Expressing Receptors

Peptide	Function	Target disease or cells	Receptor
Bombesin	CNS & GI tract activity. suppresses feeding in rats	Glioblastomas, SCLC, prostate, breast, gastric, colon and pancreatic CA	GRP-bombesin
CCK/gastrin	Gallbladder contraction/acid secretion	SCLC, GI tumors, pancreatic adenoma and medullary thyroid CA/	CCK 1 & 2
Epidermal growth factor	Growth promoter	Breast CA	Epidermal growth factor
Gastrin releasing peptide	Gastrin secretion	See bombesin	GRP-bombesin
α-MSH	Regulation of skin pigment/CNS	Melanoma cells	Melanocortin 1–5
Neurotensin	GI and cardiac activity, neuro-modulator	Prostate & pancreatic CA	Neurotensin 1–3
Somatostatin & analogs	Growth hormone release inhibiting factor	Neuroendocrine, SCLC, breast CA, monocytes & lymphocytes	Somatostatin 1–5
Substance P	Vasoactive	Glial tumors, astrocytomas, medullary thyroid and breast CA	NK1, NK2, & NK3
VIP	Vasodilator, growth promoter, immunomodulator	nSCLC, breast, colon, pancreatic, prostate, bladder and ovarian CA	VIP 1 & 2
RGD analogs	Endothelial adhesion molecule	Tumor-induced angiogenesis	$\alpha_v\beta_3$ integrin

Abbreviations: CNS, central nervous system; GI, gastrointestinal; SCLC, small cell lung cancer; CA, cancer; nSCLC, non-SCLC; CCK, cholecystokinin; GRP, gastrin releasing peptide; α-MSH, α-melanocyte stimulating hormone; VIP, vasoactive intestinal peptide; RDG, single letter designation for amino acids Arg-Gly-Asp.
Source: From Refs. 10–17.

radiolabeled antibodies that are presently used for both diagnosis and therapy (ProstaScint, Zevalin, Bexxar, CEAscan, MyoScint, NeutroSpec). The approach to find suitable peptides as new diagnostic or therapeutic agents is similar. A chelate needs to be attached to the target-seeking molecule to carry the diagnostic or therapeutic radionuclide. Subsequently sufficient quantities of the molecule need to remain on the target cell to be imaged or treated. Peptides have many advantages over antibodies. Peptides are usually classified as containing less than 50 amino acids, with a molecular weight (MW) of ~5,500 Da.

A peptide with 100 amino acids or more, the string of amino acids is considered as a protein (10,18). This low MW renders peptides low in antigenicity, fast in clearance, and rapid in tissue and tumor penetration (19,20). In contrast, antibodies can be antigenic, may have slow blood clearance, and sluggish tumor penetration. Automated techniques allow peptides to be produced easily and inexpensively (21,22), whereas antibody production is much more complex and hence costly.

Even with these advantages, there are a number of obstacles that have hindered the progress of peptides from being more commonplace in Nuclear Medicine. In contrast to antibodies, endogenous peptides can have physiological effects, which may cause unwanted side effects. For example, vasoactive intestinal peptide (VIP) exerts a wide range of potent physiological effects (Table 1) and was reported to be effective even at pM (1 μg/3000 mL) concentrations (23). To diminish these effects antagonists are preferred. Small peptides can be very sensitive to even slight changes in confirmation. Different metal ions bound to OctreoScan can change the Somatostatin receptor (SSTR) cell affinity constant (K_d) by an order of magnitude (4). Conversion of the terminal amino alcohol of these OctreoScan analogs to regular acid amino acid also has a significantly effect on the SSTR K_d (Fig. 2**B**). While a chelate (300 Da) is tiny in comparison to the MW of an antibody (150 kDa), it is comparable in MW to that of a peptide (<5,500 Da). Thus the coupled chelate can more easily distort the peptide conformation, and can in turn adversely influence target binding (24) or alter in vivo distribution (25). To avoid this problem, chelates are generally placed on peptides so that they will not interfere with binding of the peptides to its biological target. This could be at a certain position away from the receptor-binding site (Fig. 2), or amino acid spacers can be introduced between the parent peptide and a chelating moiety (26–30). Figure 3, a diagram of the first antibody approved for human use, OncoScint, demonstrates the use of a spacer between the chelate and targeting molecule. Most endogenous peptides may have biological

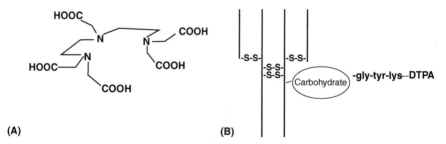

(A) **(B)**

Figure 3 Schematic drawing of (**A**) DPTA and (**B**) monoclonal antibody, OncoScint. DPTA is coupled to the antibody via an amide bond and methylene groups—(CH$_2$) are omitted for clarity. The spacer peptide gly-tyr-lys coupled to carbohydrate of antibody on one end and carboxylic acid of DTPA on the other end. *Source*: From Ref. 31.

$T_{\frac{1}{2}}$'s that are usually too short to be useful as therapeutic or diagnostic vehicles (see above). This is usually, but not always, due to rapid proteolysis in the circulation, which is a way to modulate the in vivo influence of these agents. If it is known where in the sequence the peptide is cleaved in the blood, judicious use of D-amino acids and the end-capping process (modifying the terminal amino acids) can induce resistance to in vivo enzymatic degradation (Fig. 1). Enzymes usually have very defined specificities, e.g., degrading a peptide from either the C or N-termini (exopepidases) or cleaving at the bond between the naturally occurring L-amino acids (endopepidases). For example, proteolysis of ^{111}In-OctreoScan is likely slowed because a D-amino acid replaced an L- in the sequence and both the N and C-terminal amino acids are modified (Fig. 1). Unnatural amino acid or peptide mimetics can also reduce the rate of degradation (Table 2). Also, only the fragment, that is more resistant to proteolysis and binds to the receptor, could be used (Fig. 1). However, using a fragment could reduce the ability of the peptide to bind to a full range of target receptors (section Somatostatin analogs). Lipophilicity or hydrophilicity both contribute to pharmacokinetics and tissue distribution of a given peptide sequence. Lipophilic peptides are generally sequestered by the liver and may be eliminated by hepatobiliary excretion, whereas hydrophilic peptides may be removed by the kidneys. The choice of peptide characteristics usually depends on the targeted anatomic location of a disease. If the object was to detect liver metastases, the peptide should be more hydrophilic to divert it away from the liver to the kidney. Also the radionuclide or attachment site can influence the biodistribution (3). For example, [123]I-[Tyr[3]]-Octreotide (Tyr replaces the 3rd amino acid Phe in the peptide string) where the Tyr is iodinated had significant uptake in the liver and subsequently excretion into the GI. In contrast, ^{111}In-Octreotide where the ^{111}In is bound to a DTPA coupled to the peptide had very little. Lastly, cyclization of peptides can exert restricted conformational mobility and enhance receptor binding or cellular retention (Figs. 4 and 5) (32,33). Thus, there are a large number of iterations that must be considered in modifying the original peptide to be a useful diagnostic or therapeutic agent.

Table 2 Unnatural Amino Acids and Peptide Mimetics Used in Peptide Research

Theroninol	5-Aminovaleric acid
Homo-L-cysteine	Acetylaminoalanine
N-Methyl-phenylalanine	N-Methyl-cysteine
3(β-Naphthyl) alanine	Aminopropyl-L-cystine
PyroGlu (γ-COOH coupled to α-NH$_2$)	Cyclized methionine
Aminobutyric acid	4-NH$_2$-phenylalanine
β-(L 1,2 diaminoproprionic acid)	Serinol
Lysine-amide	Aminobenzoic acid
D-tert-Leucine	

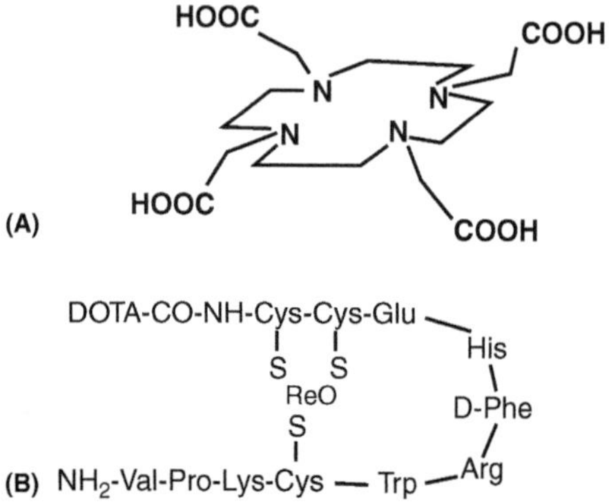

Figure 4 Schematic drawing of the structures of (**A**) 1,4,7,10-tetraazacyclododecane-N, N′,N″,N‴-tetraacetic acid (DOTA) and (**B**) DOTA coupled to Re=O cyclized [Cys^{3,4,10}, D-Phe^7] α-melanocyte-stimulating hormone$_{(3-13)}$. For other details see Figure 1 legend. DOTA is coupled to peptide via an amide bond and methylene groups—(CH$_2$) are omitted for clarity. *Source*: From Ref. 33.

This review will examine specific examples of the problems that have occurred in the development of peptides for specific target cell receptors. We will concentrate on the oncological area since that is the focus of most investigations. The concepts identified in the preceding paragraph will be used as a context for the discussion. Moreover, we will concentrate on those agents used presently, those in clinical trials, and selected agents that pre-clinical (animal) studies have shown to be promising.

BACKGROUND

A number of investigators have demonstrated that ^{111}In-OctreoScan is a highly effective diagnostic agent for neuroendocrine tumors (6,34,35). This effectiveness led to the suggestion that replacing the diagnostic radionuclide with one of the therapeutic characteristics can render OctreoScan or an analog, a useful agent for treatment of cancer. In this paradigm, an analog labeled with a

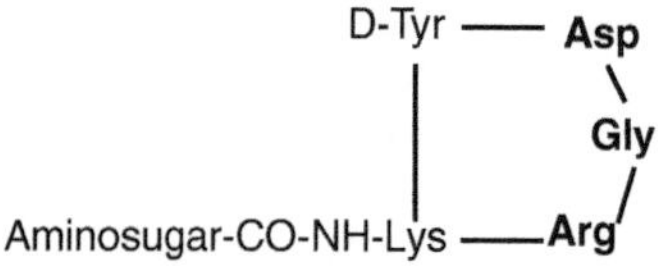

Figure 5 Amino acid sequence of α$_v$β$_3$ antagonist with an amino sugar. Amino acids in bold are directly involved in receptor binding. For other details see Figure 1 legend. Peptide is labeled with ^{123}I at Tyr. *Source*: From Ref. 32.

diagnostic radionuclide could be used to determine the radiation dose, that the therapeutic radionuclide would deliver to the target lesion and normal tissues. These estimates would facilitate maximizing the tumor dose while minimizing the absorbed dose to normal healthy organs. This approach has been applied to neuroendocrine disease with some success (36,37) and now is the dominate paradigm in the development of a wide variety of peptides applicable for other neoplasms. In each case, the peptide is designed to achieve the dual roles of diagnostic and therapeutic agent.

To develop a peptide for diagnostic applications, tumor physiology usually plays a secondary role. As long as the peptide binds to the target cells with high affinity and remains there long enough to be imaged, i.e., a high enough target to background ratio (T/B), is sufficient. This may require a few hours or days depending on tumor concentration and blood background. In contrast, how the peptide-radionuclide combination localizes in the tumor is critical in the choice of the peptide and therapeutic radionuclide. In the introduction we have already detailed the problems the peptide can confront in the blood stream. Once the peptide reaches the tumor, a small peptide can easily diffuse into the tumor mass if the tumor mass is well vascularized. It can then bind, via the receptor, uniformly to cells that are distributed throughout the mass. If peptide-radionuclide complex is bound to the cell surface, it may or may not be internalized. Even if internalized, the radionuclide may be exocytosed rapidly and washed away from the tumor. Even if the radionuclide remains intracellular, does it interact with critical cell components, i.e., DNA? A double strand DNA break (Auger electron "hit") is the most lethal to the cell (38,39). Receptor internalization rates may also play an important role. If the rates are high for a particular receptor then more therapeutic nuclide can be carried into the cell. This would enhance the killing effect of the radionuclide.

Most therapeutic radionuclides presently under investigation are electron (β or Auger) emitters. The short range in tissue of these radiations may minimize damage to nearby normal tissue. If a radionuclide is used with a high maximum β particle range, then cell killing could take place with the nuclide on the cell's surface or at the tumor's periphery. The tumor need not be well vascularized or the peptide receptor complex need not be internalized. A nuclide with this range allows for the possibility of so-called "crossfire." Cells can be irradiated in the nearby vicinity or near a necrotic central zone. However, this long range could increase the toxicity by irradiation of normal cells. For example, ^{90}Y, a high-energy β emitter (maximum 2.3 MeV), has a maximum range of this particle of 11,000 μm in tissue, or about ~ 550 cells [cell diameter $\approx$ 20 μm (40)]. Yttrium-90 does not decay with emission of a γ photon for high resolution imaging and cannot be used to estimate radiation dosimetry. Yttrium does have a positron emitting radioisotope, ^{86}Y ($T_{1/2} = 14.7$ hours, 35% β^+ and assorted γ's). Yttrium-86 could be used initially for imaging and subsequent radiation dosimetry and then the molecule loaded with ^{90}Y for treatment. At the present time, ^{86}Y is not available commercially. Indium-111, which can be used for imaging and has a short penetration Auger electrons (0.5–25 keV) is an alternative (41–44). The average path range of Auger electrons is less than a cell diameter, [0.02–10 µm] (45). Nuclear localization is essential for its therapeutic effect. This means that ^{111}In can potentially be used for therapeutic applications only if an agent containing the nuclide could be internalized in the target cell. This would allow the Auger electrons to interact with critical cellular components, particularly the DNA, while causing minimal toxicity to normal cells (39). Lu-177 has been touted as a compromise between ^{90}Y and [111]In (46). It has an intermediate energy maximum β, 0.497 MeV (78%), conversion electrons, 48 to 143 keV, and a γ photon (0.208 MeV) that can be used for patient imaging, although with very low abundance (11%). The β particle has a much shorter maximum range in tissue, ∼2,000 µm (100 cells), than [90]Y. Thus, ^{177}Lu can participate in crossfire and is expected to deliver less radiation to normal tissue.

The most commonly used radionuclide in Nuclear Medicine is [99m]Tc. The therapeutic radionuclides discussed above are all +3 metal ions and bind with high affinity to many chelating agents. Many such agents are presently used to chelate ^{111}In and used for imaging. To fit this new paradigm, with a ^{99m}Tc diagnostic agent, a therapeutic radionuclide is needed with chelate binding characteristics similar to [99m]Tc. Rhenium is in the same periodic group as and shares many chemical characteristics with technetium. Of the radioisotopes of Rhenium, [188]Re has a number of attractive characteristics. It is produced from a long-lived (69 d) generator [188]W, which provides a ready supply of [188]Re. This radioisotope has a long range β ($E_{max} = 2.11$ MeV), 10 mm (500 cells in tissue) and could participate in crossfire. [188]Re has a comparatively short $T_{1/2}$ (17 hours) so that any anticipated hemopoetic toxicity could be relatively low. Dosimetry calculations are possible since Re-188 decays with emission of a γ photon, 155 keV, but with low abundance (15%).

SOMATOSTATIN ANALOGS

Somatostatin, 14 amino acid peptide hormone, plays a variety of roles in the human body. Most importantly, it inhibits the release of a wide variety of other hormones including: growth hormone, insulin, glucagon, and gastrin (Fig. 1**B**) (5). Particularly because of this inhibition of growth hormone release, Somatostatin was initially studied as an anti-growth agent on cultured tumor cells and animal tumor models. This led to the development of the Somatostatin analog, Octreotide, as a treatment for neuroendocrine tumors in man. Krenning and co-workers (47) realized the potential of this analog to detect the location of tumors for surgical resection. At that time, iodination of Tyr residues was the most common form of labeling proteins and peptides. Therefore these investigators synthesized an analog where the Phe in Octreotide was replaced by a Tyr (Fig. 6). The [123]I-[Tyr³] Octreotide was a successful clinical imaging agent for neuroendocrine tumors (3). However there were a number of

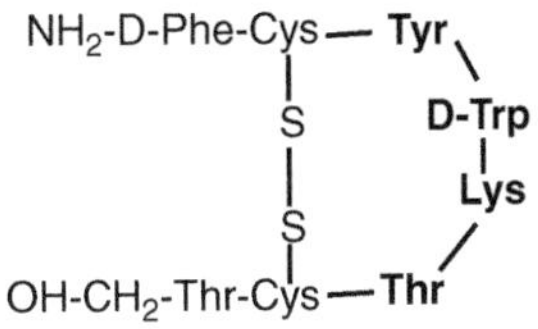

NH$_2$-D-Phe-Cys — Tyr
| \
S   D-Trp
| |
S   Lys
| /
OH-CH$_2$-Thr-Cys — Thr

Figure 6 Schematic presentation of D-Phe^1-Tyr^3-Octreotide.

drawbacks. Probably most important was that in vivo dehalogenation caused significant accumulation of ^{123}I in the liver and intestines, the likely sites for neuroendocrine lesions and hampered lesion visualization. In addition, the isotope was costly and had limited availability because of its short T$_{1/2}$ (13 hours). The development of a procedure to add DTPA chelate to proteins (48) made it possible to radiolabel Octreotide with the longer lived ^{111}In (3).

The overall mechanism of localization of Somatostatin analogs is shown in Figure 7. It was demonstrated that the action of this hormone was associated with a membrane receptor. This receptor, well anchored on the cell surface with seven transmembrane domains, is G-protein, and inhibited the action of cAMP. After ligand binding, the ligand-receptor complex is internalized and the ligand is degraded in a lysosome with the receptor probably recycled to the surface. While it is important that the radionuclide remains tumor-bound for a sufficient time for imaging, the precise details of the internalization mechanism are much more important for therapeutic applications (section Background). Figure 1**B** shows that Somatostatin has four amino acids, Phe-Trp-Lys-Thr, that form the apex of a

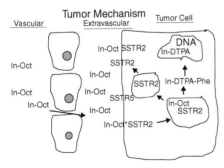

Figure 7 Diagram of proposed mechanism for localization of ^{111}In-OctreoScan (In-Oct) in a neurodocrine tumor. The small peptide easily passes from the blood through endothelial cell layer into the extravascular space, binds Somatostatin receptor subtype 2 (SSTR2) upregulated on the cell's surface, and gets incorporated into intracellular vesicle. The vesicle's contents is transferred to a lysosome where the ^{111}In-OctreoScan is degraded sequentially to In-DTPA-Phe-OH, the SSTR2 is recycled to the surface and In is transported to near the nuclear DNA.

di-cysteine loop. Systematic deletion of these amino acids or replacing each amino acid with an Ala demonstrated that these four are essential for receptor binding. The N-terminal residues are less important. The disulfide bond maintains the critical conformation so that these residues can directly interact with the receptor. Octreotide retained these basic characteristics. However, to improve the tumor uptake, Somatostatin was modified to resist in vivo proteolysis (Fig. 1A). The arrows in Figure 1B show the precise positions of enzymatic hydrolysis of the parent molecule. To develop Octreotide, the basic receptor binding structure was maintained but the peptide was shortened to eliminate the Phe-Phe and Thr-Phe bonds. This would reduce the action of endopepidases. In addition, L-Trp was converted to D-Trp to moderate the catalysis at Trp-Lys. To slow the action of exopepidases, a D-Trp and an amino alcohol were placed at the ends. These modifications appeared to have their desired effect. In patients, ^{111}In-DTPA-Octreotide (^{111}In-OctreoScan) was excreted mainly via the kidneys in contrast to [123]I-[Tyr^3]Octreotide, which had hepatobiliary excretion (see above). The initial clearance rate for ^{111}In-OctreoScan was slower than to [123]I-[Tyr^3]Octreotide. This may have been due to the reduction in the loss of the radionuclide and fewer degradation products (3). Although at 4 hours post injection in the blood the labeled peptide remains mainly intact at later times, a significant ($< 10\%$) amount of hydrolysis is reported. The peptide is excreted intact in the urine. At 24 hours post injection, the agent is distributed in normal liver, thyroid, spleen, kidneys, and bladder, with the kidneys usually more prominent than the other organs. This could interfere with identification of metastatic disease in these organs except the kidneys, which are not likely to be the metastatic target in neuroendocrine disease (5). The renal uptake, however, is a cause of concern in the use of Octreotide analogs in therapeutic applications. More will be discussed about the kidney uptake mechanism later in the section devoted to the therapeutic uses of these analogs. While the amino acid modifications of Somatostatin dramatically increased the blood $T_{1/2}$ and tumor uptake of ^{111}In-OctreoScan, there was a downside. Somatostatin binds to all 5 receptor (SSTR) subtypes with high ($K_d \sim$ nM) (49). In contrast, Octreotide only bound to SSTR2 with high affinity ($IC_{50} = 2$ nM) and to lesser degree SSTR3 ($IC_{50} = 376$ nM) & 5 ($IC_{50} = 299$ nM) (4). There is no binding ($IC_{50} = > 1,000$) to SSTR1 & 4.

Patient data suggest that SSTR2 upregulation plays a critical role in the ^{111}In-OctreoScan localization and that this peptide is an in vivo indicator of SSTR2 expression. There was a strong correlation between a positive image and the presence of SSTR2 as determined by in vitro autoradiography in excised tumor (34). The sensitivity of ^{111}In-OctreoScan in detecting neuroendocrine lesions ranges from 60% to 90% (5,34). Most tumor tissue excised from patients has a high expression of SSTR2 among other subtypes (50–52). However, it was suggested that the lower sensitivity in some lesions may be due to the absence of SSTR2 (53). Forssell-Aronsson et al. (54) have shown that the target to background (T/B) in various neuroendocrine tumors correlated directly with the mRNA assay for SSTR2. In contrast, in a disease where OctreoScan is not as effective, e.g., colon cancer, there is a high density of SSTR3 and only modest density of SSTR2 & 5 (55). OctreoScan can detect primary lesions in both small cell (SCLC) and non-small cell lung cancer (nSCLC) (56–59) but there was not a high correlation with receptor data. Previously, SSTR2 had been detected only in tissues from SCLC patients but not on nSCLC cells (3,57,58). It was argued that lymphocytes, which have a high density of SSTR2, at the tumor site may account for OctreoScan localization in nSCLC. More recent western blot data have demonstrated the presence of a high density of SSTR4 and modest density of subtypes 2,3 and 5 in nSCLC (60). In Hodgkin's and non-Hodgkin's Lymphoma, sensitivity for lesion detection was low but specificity was very high (98–100%), suggesting that SSTR2 may not be expressed on all lesions (61,62). Lastly, SSTR2 also appears to be critical for normal OctreoScan localization (63). Mice, which have a SSTR2 gene deletion, had dramatically lower uptake (83% lower) in normal tissues than wild type mice.

It is well established that OctreoScan analogs are important in the detection of neuroendocrine lesions. Therefore, the most recent thrust of investigations has been to determine which, if any, radiolabeled OctreoScan analogs can be used to treat these diseases. These radiolabeled peptides could fill a therapeutic gap since chemotherapy is largely ineffective in these diseases and non-radioactive analogs have time-limited effectiveness (64). To optimize therapeutic effectiveness, understanding of localization of these analogs was essential. Krenning et al. (3) first demonstrated that the residence $T_{1/2}$ of ^{111}In-OcreoScan in tumors was > 700 hours. It was also demonstrated in vitro that the ^{111}In-OctreoScan was internalized into tumor cells, localized in the cytoplasm and near the nucleus (65). Most recent data further support the nuclear localization of ^{111}In-OctreoScan (66,67). Janson et al. (66) utilized tumor tissue from patients injected with ^{111}In-OctreoScan and showed that the ^{111}In-OctreoScan was first localized on the tumor cell membrane, cytoplasm, and then finally inside the nucleus. In another cell culture study, ^{111}In-OctreoScan was incubated with receptor-positive and receptor-negative cells and then the nuclear cell fraction was isolated (67). The presence of ^{111}In in the nuclear fraction increased as a function of incubation time only for the receptor-positive cells. Thus there is strong mechanistic data supporting the use of ^{111}In-OctreoScan with its short range Auger electrons (see section Background) for therapy. Studies using ^{111}In-OctreoScan for the treatment of patients with refractory neuroendocrine disease are in the phase I/II stage (41–44). Over 85 patients have been treated with a 62–69% response (either stabilizing the disease or reducing tumor size).

The critical organ for all of the OctreoScan analogs in clinical therapeutic trials is the kidney (64). The objective has been to limit the kidney dose to ~25 Gy. It is known from treating patients with external beam radiation that 5–50% of patients in a 5 years follow-up had significant renal toxicity. Thus, there are on-going investigations to determine the mechanism of uptake in order to reduce renal absorbed dose while increasing the tumor dose. This prominent renal uptake is likely due to general peptide and amino acid re-absorption in the renal tubules (68). This phenomena was first demonstrated when radiolabeled antibody fragments, Fab or Fab'$_2$, were used for tumor treatment (69). Most recent autoradiography of kidney sections from patients demonstrates primarily cortical localization (70). This suggests that localization of radio-labeled peptides in the renal tubules is likely. The high absorbed dose due to these fragments was ameliorated by the infusion of an amino acid mixture. It was subsequently demonstrated that kidney uptake with ^{111}In-OctreoScan could be reduced with a similar infusion (71). Further studies in animals and humans showed that a mixture of positively charged amino acids, Lys, and Arg, was most effective (72,73). While the exact mechanism is not fully understood, this data imply that ^{111}In-OctreoScan is reabsorbed by a negatively charged carrier-based process. In general, after peptides/proteins bind the carrier; these molecules are internalized into intracellular vesicle (endosome), which releases the contents to lysosome for ultimate degradation (74). It is likely that ^{111}In-OctreoScan follows this pathway (Fig. 8). Maleate (72) and cholchicine, (75) which are known to inhibit this endocytic process, substantially reduce ^{111}In-OctreoScan kidney uptake. These labeled metabolites then become trapped in the lysosomes of the renal tubule cells with little loss of the ^{111}In from these cells (76,77). When these metabolites are extracted from liver, kidney, tumor or other organs, the most common are ^{111}In-DTPA-Phe-Cys-OH and ^{111}In-DTPA-Phe-OH (78). If the extraction is done at a later time, more of these species are formed. Extractions done at 24 hours post injection showed little intact OctreoScan left. Thus, there appears to be no efficient means to transport this complex out of the lysosomes

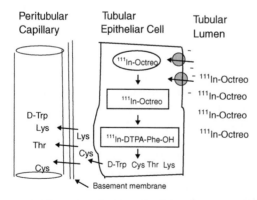

Figure 8 Diagram of the proposed mechanism for the localization of ^{111}In-OctreoScan (In-Oct) in kidney tubules. Peptide is transported from the tubule lumen via a negatively charged carrier molecule into an endocytic vesicle in tubular epithelial cell. The vesicle's contents are transferred to a lysosome where the ^{111}In-OctreoScan is degraded sequentially. The ^{111}In-DTPA-Phe-OH remains in the lysosome while the individual amino acids are transported into the peritubular capillary.

and then out of the cells. Investigators are trying to develop alternate chelate coupling strategies that would facilitate more rapid radionuclide exocytosis (79). However, the simplest way to reduce the kidney dose is to reduce initial transport into the tubular epithelium. De Jong and co-workers (72) showed in rats that altering renal pH can inhibit reabsorbtion. The most practical method of reducing the influx is the infusion of positively charged mixture of amino acids. This approach has been shown to be effective with a number of different OctreoScan analogs. Amino acid infusion reduced the absorbed dose in patients from 20–40% (36,37,73,80).

There have been a variety of OctreoScan analogs tested in clinical trials using both amino acids modifications of the basic OctreoScan sequence and different radionuclides. These different analogs provide additional insights on the localization mechanism. Otte et al. (81,82) were first to treat patients with 1,4,7,10-tetraazacyclododecane-N,N′,N″,N‴-tetraacetic acid (DOTA) coupled to D-Phe^1-Tyr^3-Octreotide (DOTATOC) and labeled with ^{90}Y. DOTA has a high affinity for both ^{111}In and ^{90}Y (log $K_{ML} = 29$). The advantage of DOTA is that the ^{111}In labeled derivative can be used to detect lesions and the nuclide can be replaced with ^{90}Y for therapy. In contrast, ^{90}Y is not tightly bound to DTPA and is eluted from the DTPA in vivo. Neither the addition of the DOTA moiety or the ^{90}Y affected the in vitro cell affinity, which was comparable to the affinity of DTPA-Octreotide (4). ^{111}In-DOTATOC was directly compared to ^{111}In-OctreoScan. ^{111}In-DOTATOC had the same diagnostic precision but was cleared faster from the blood and other tissues (81). Thus, exchange Phe^3 for Tyr^3 did not interfere with SSTR binding and the more hydrophilic Tyr stimulated faster renal uptake. In the treated patients, there was no observed acute renal but delayed renal toxicity did develop (83). The most common toxicity (grade III and IV) was hematological. In contrast, in clinical studies with ^{111}In-OctreoScan, even though the kidney received the highest absorbed dose, that had little effect on kidney function (42,43,84). Animal studies have also suggested there is little tissue damage using histological techniques (85). Theoretical considerations support the lesser toxicity of ^{111}In, an Auger emitter, compared to ^{90}Y, a high energy β emitter (section Background).

Kwekkeboom and colleagues (86) have initiated the use of ^{177}Lu-DOTA-Octreotate. Octreotate is identical to Octreotide except that the C-terminal threonine amino alcohol is replaced by threonine (Fig. 2**B**). This analog DOTA-Octreotate (DOTATATE) has a 9-fold higher affinity for SSTR2 than DOTATOC, which was not influenced by metal ion binding (86). This suggests that tumor uptake might be increased but also shows that minimal changes in the peptide can have profound effects. Animal studies demonstrated that this analog was particularly effective in treating small (<1 cm^2) SSTR receptor positive tumors (87). In patients, ^{177}Lu- DOTATATE was directly compared to ^{111}In-OctreoScan (46). ^{177}Lu-DOTATATE had similar blood clearance but significantly lower urinary excretion. Localization in the tumor was estimated to be 3- to 4-fold higher for ^{177}Lu-DOTATATE, which appeared to correlated with

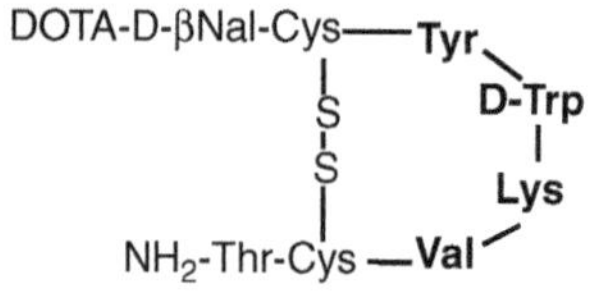

```
DOTA-D-βNal-Cys——Tyr
                |    \
                S     D-Trp
                |      |
                S     Lys
                |    /
   NH₂-Thr-Cys —Val
```

Figure 9 Schematic presentation of Lanreotide. Amino acids in bold are directly involved in receptor binding. Amino acids are all L-isomers except where noted. DOTA is coupled to the peptide via a peptide bond. *Abbreviation*: D-βNal, β-naphthyl alanine. *Source*: From Ref. 87.

the higher affinity for the SSTR2. Uptake in liver, kidneys, and spleen was comparable between the two peptides, even though spleen contains a high concentration of SSTR2. The organ-absorbed dose is generally intermediate between ^{111}In-OctreoScan and ^{90}Y-DOTATOC.

DOTA has been coupled (60,88,89) to Lanreotide (DOTALAN), an Octreotide analog (Fig. 9). Lanreotide appeared to bind SSTR3 and 4 in addition to subtypes 2 and 5 with high affinity ($K_d \sim 4$–10 nM) (89). However, Reubi and co-workers (4) have not been able to confirm a high affinity of DOTALAN for SSTR3 and 4. DOTA coupling to Lanreotide does not interfere with receptor binding since SSTR2 binding affinity remains high ($K_d \sim$ nM). Even though this analog appears quite different than OctreoScan (cf. Fig. 2A and Fig. 9), the substitutions when analyzed demonstrate a high degree homology. In the receptor binding region, Tyr is exchanged for a more hydrophobic Phe and Val for Thr, with Val slightly more hydrophobic. In the amino terminal region, considered less important for receptor binding, a β-napthyl alanine (relatively hydrophobic) is substituted for another hydrophobic residue Phe. Thus, Lanreotide shares many of OctreoScan's in vivo characteristics. This derivative rapidly clears from circulation by urinary excretion with only 3% of the ID left after 2 hours. At 4 hours, a total of 21% of the ID is the urine, which rises to 62% at 72 hours. The peptide remains intact up to 24 hours in the urine but after that only metabolic products are detected. On a normal early image, the liver, spleen, bladder, and kidney are prominent.

^{99m}Tc-NeoTect

NeoTect was developed as ^{99m}Tc-based Somatostatin analog for detection of lung cancer and not for therapy (Fig. 10A). It had been previously shown that ^{111}In-OctreoScan could detect both SCLC and nSCLC with high sensitivity. To be able to incorporate a ^{99m}Tc and the subsequently required reducing conditions, Pearson et al. (91) synthesized an analog that eliminated the disulfide bond in the receptor loop. The receptor loop was kept via a cyclic hexapeptide sequence (compare Fig. 2B and Fig. 10A). Also, a Thr was changed to a Val, making the loop slightly more hydrophobic. End capping in the form of N-MePhe and amide

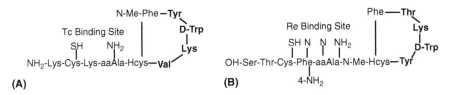

Figure 10 Schematic presentation of (**A**) NeoTect (P829) and (**B**) P-2045. Amino acids in bold are directly involved in receptor binding. Amino acids are all L-isomers except where noted. Unusual amino acids; *Abbreviations*: Hcys, homo-L-cys; N-Me-Hcy, N-methyl-homo-L-cys; N-Me-Phe, N-methyl-Phe; aaAla, acetylaminoAla 4-NH₂-Phe; Lys-NH₂, Lys-amide; Ser-OH, amino alcohol. *Source*: From Refs. 89, 90.

Lys was added to slow exopepidase attack. A ^{99m}Tc binding peptide sequence, acetyl amino-Ala-Lys-Cys, was incorporated in the tail away from the receptor binding loop. NeoTect has retained the high affinity ($K_d \sim 2$ nM) for SSTR subtypes 2 and 5, but also subtype 3 (92). In a rat tumor model, ^{99m}Tc-NeoTect had higher uptake compared to ^{111}In-OctreoScan (4.8 vs. 2.8% ID/g) (93). However, the blood or muscle washout for NeoTect was not nearly as fast. An injected dose of Octreotide reduced the tumor uptake 86% at 90 minutes in this model. This demonstrated specificity for SSTR2. NeoTect had an animal biodistribution comparable to OctreoScan but with more activity in the GI tract. At 1 hour post injection (PI), very little (5%) of this peptide was excreted in the GI tract. In contrast, 30% was found in the kidneys and 20% excreted into the bladder. This biodistribution was similar to what was seen in patients. This agent localizes in the kidney, spleen, bladder, thyroid, and bone. Blood clearance $T_{1/2}$ was very short with $t_\alpha = 4$ minutes. NeoTect was relatively resistant to proteolysis. At 4 hours PI, 70–80% of the activity in blood and 61% of radioactivity excreted in urine are still bound to NeoTect. Protein binding was minimal, only 10–20%. The kidneys are the critical organs. In the initial studies, there were a high number of false positives, 17% in inflammations. Both lymphocytes and monocytes express SSTR. It was likely that NeoTect was binding to these cells in the inflammation.

Re-P-2054

This peptide is a NeoTect analog (Fig. 10**B**). It was developed as a treatment for lung cancer since NeoTect has a high sensitivity and specificity for lung cancer detection. There is very little data in the literature about the localization mechanism for this peptide. However, it is most likely that the localization is similar to NeoTect and the other Somatostatin analogs. Figure 10 shows that the receptor binding sequence is reversed compared to NeoTect and the Val is changed back to Thr, which is originally present on OctreoScan and [Tyr³]Octreotate (Fig. 2). Even though the binding sequence is reversed, this analog has high affinity for SSTR 2, 3, and 5. The metal ion binding sequence is positioned away from the binding site, similar to other analogs. It also contains two unusual amino acids, e.g., 4-amino Phe and acetyl amino Ala. This peptide does fit the new paradigm. This peptide binds both ^{99m}Tc and ^{188}Re (therapeutic radionuclide) with high affinity. The ^{99m}Tc-P-2054 would be used to insure that the malignant lesions take up the activity and non-malignant lesions do not. Since NeoTect localizes in most lesions, the main concern for a therapeutic agent with similar binding characteristics would be uptake in false positive sites, e.g., inflammations. A pilot study for P-2045 was recently presented with 7 nSCLC patients (94). There were 4/7 mild adverse events. Uptake was demonstrated in the lung tumors for both ^{99m}Tc and ^{188}Re. As with most of the other peptides, the kidney absorbed dose was a limiting factor. This was a promising start. However, apparently further data were not as supportive since Berlex dropped this project.

CHOLECYSTOKININ-B/GASTRIN

Compounds that are directed at the Cholecystokinin-B (CCK-B)/gastrin receptor are furthest along in development, second only to SSTRs targeted molecules. There have been some preliminary clinical trials which have demonstrated the proof of concept (95–98). Receptors are found in the GI mucosa and brain. CCK and gastrin are involved in regulating various functions in the GI tract (Table 1). CCK can act as a growth factor for normal and malignant cells (99). The actions of CCK are mediated by two receptors, CCK-A and CCK-B. CCK binds to each of these receptors with high affinity. In contrast, gastrin has a high affinity for only the CCK-B. Using receptor autoradiography, Reubi and co-workers (99) have demonstrated a high incidence (90%) of CCK-B receptors (CCK-BR) in medullary thyroid cancers (MTC) but not in differentiated thyroid cancers. CCK-BR were also upregulated in other uncommon cancers (Table 1). In normal tissues, CCK-B are expressed in GI mucosa and brain, and CCK-A receptors (CCK-AR) in gallbladder, pancreas, and brain.

With CCK receptors, as with many other targets, investigators are still trying to determine which peptide analog is the best. Generally, fragments are used which retain receptor binding characteristics but would not be expected to act as growth stimulants. Human gastrin-I (Fig. 11**B**), a shortened version of big gastrin (Fig. 11**A**), has selectivity for CCK-B/gastrin receptor with an affinity ∼0.1 nM range while its affinity for CCK-A receptor is ∼1 mM (100). A further shortened version of big gastrin, minigastrin retained the affinity and selectively for CCK-BR (Fig. 11**C**) (97). An alternative class of molecules is based on CCK, a 33 amino acid peptide (Fig. 12**A**). It has a sulfated (SO$_3$H) Tyr, which is necessary for its a high affinity for both CCK-AR and -BR. A fragment, CCK$_{(26–33)}$, called CCK8, also has a high affinity for both receptors since this truncated molecule includes the sulfated Tyr^{26} and the C-terminal amino acids required for receptor binding, Trp-Met-Asp-Phe-HN$_2$ (Fig. 12**B**). The focus of most investigators has been the nonsulfated analogs of this fragment CCK8 since it has a high affinity for only CCK-BR and not CCK-AR.

pGlu-Leu-Gly-Pro-Gln-Gly-Pro-Pro-His-Leu-Val-
Ala-Asp-Pro-Ser-Lys-Lys-Gln-Gly-Pro-Trp-Leu-
Glu-Glu-Glu-Glu-Glu-Ala-Tyr-Gly-**Trp-Met-**
(A) **Asp-Phe-NH$_2$**

pGlu-Gly-Pro-Trp-Leu-Glu-Glu-Glu-Glu-Glu-Ala-
(B) Tyr-Gly-**Trp-Met-Asp-Phe-NH$_2$**

Leu-Glu-Glu-Glu-Glu-Glu-Ala-Tyr-Gly-**Trp-Met-**
(C) **Asp-Phe-NH$_2$**

DTPA-D-Glu-Leu-Glu-Glu-Glu-Glu-Glu-Ala-Tyr-Gly-
(D) **Trp-Met-Asp-Phe-NH$_2$**

Figure 11 Amino acid sequence of (**A**) Big gastrin, (**B**) Human gastrin-I, (**C**) Minigastrin, and (**D**) DTPA^0-D-Glu^1-minigastrin. Amino acids in bold are directly involved in receptor binding and are all L-isomers except where noted. N-terminal of amino acid sequence is at left and C-terminal is converted to amide [NH$_2$]. *Source*: From Ref. 97.

A wide variety of CCK and gastrin derivatives conjugated with ^{131}I, ^{111}In and ^{90}Y have been studied in pilot experiments to detect and treat MTC (95–97,101). Initial work was performed with [^{131}I-Tyr^{12}] human gastrin-I because this endogenous peptide contained a Tyr that could be easily labeled with iodine and was commercially available (96). High tumor uptake and uptake was observed in gallbladder, stomach, kidneys, and pancreas, 1 hour PI in a nude mouse model of MTC. Only tumor, stomach, and pancreas uptake could be blocked with non-radioactive peptide, suggesting receptor-based uptake in these

Lys-(Ala,Gly-Pro,Ser)-Arg-Val-(Ile, Mer, Ser)-
Lys-Asn-(Asn, Gln, His Leu, Leu, Pro, Ser, Ser)
Arg-Ile-(Asp, Ser)-Arg-Asp-Tyr[SO$_3$H]-Met-
(A) Gly-**Trp-Met-Asp-Phe-NH$_2$**

Asp-Tyr[SO$_3$H]-Met-Gly-**Trp-Met-Asp-**
(B) **Phe-NH$_2$**

DTPA-D-Asp-Tyr-Nle-Gly-**Trp-Nle-Asp-Phe-**
(C) **NH$_2$**

DTPA-D-Glu-Gly-Asp-Tyr-Met-Gly-**Trp-Met-**
(D) **Asp-Phe-NH$_2$**

Figure 12 Amino acid sequence of (**A**) sulfated CCK (**B**) sulfated CCK$_{(26–33)}$ [CCK8], (**C**) nonsulfated DTPA-[D-Asp^{26}, Nle^{28,31}]-CCK8 and (**D**) nonsulfated DTPA^0-D-Glu^1-Gly^2-CCK8. Amino acids in bold are directly involved in receptor binding and are all L-isomers except where noted. N-terminal of amino acid sequence is at left and C-terminal is converted to amide [NH$_2$]. *Source*: From Refs. 101, 102.

organs. The peptide was also tested in a few patients and localization was seen in possible metastatic sites. Subsequently Behr et al. (97) tested more iodinated gastrin or CCK analogs in in vitro and in vivo MTC models. The cell binding studies showed that labeled analogs retained a high affinity ($IC_{50} \sim 1$–10 nM) for CCK-BR. The IC_{50} of gastrin fragment I, 1–14 (Fig. 11**A**) was substantially reduced (>0.1 mM) compared to C-terminal fragment 11–17 (10 nM). This demonstrated the essential nature of this sequence. The Met in the sequence could be converted to a Leu or Nle without loss of receptor affinity. Serum stability of most analogs was several hours, however, peptides with a cyclized N-terminal pyroGlu had $T_{1/2} > 24$ hours. HPLC analysis showed that a substitution of the D-Leu at position 1 in minigastrin (Fig. 11**C**) considerably improved the serum stability ($T_{1/2} = 8$ hours versus 45 minutes @ 37°C). Peptides that had high in vitro affinity showed high in vivo uptake in CCK-BR expressing tissues including the tumor. However, there was rapid washout from these tissues ($>50\%$ decline @ 5 hours PI) but washout for other tissue was even faster ($>50\%$ decline @ 1 hours PI). Because preliminary experiments (96) suggested that ^{131}I-Gastrin-I could diagnose patient medullary thyroid disease, this derivative was tested in this animal model. There was significant ($P < 0.03$) retardation of tumor growth compared to untreated controls, with ^{131}I-C-terminal fragment 11–17 (97). Only hemopoetic toxicity (blood cell nadirs) was detected, which recovered. While this peptide was not optimal, this data provided encouragement. Minigastrin (Fig. 11**C**) had the lower kidney uptake compared to gastrin-I but maintained high affinity for the CCK-BR. Even though tested in an animal model, minigastrin with long anionic sequence [Glu_5^{2-6}] would likely have low tubular cell incorporation in patients (Fig. 8).

DTPA was coupled to [D-Leu^1] and minigastrin to label this analogue with several radionuclides (97). In a few patients, this derivative showed uptake in known lesions, liver (modest), and kidneys. The long Glu sequence did not appear to reduce kidney uptake. There should be low liver uptake since the liver does not have a high expression of CCK-BR. The liver uptake might be due to loss of the ^{111}In to blood protein, transferrin, and subsequent transport to the liver. To overcome this problem, Behr and colleagues developed an open chain chelator DTPA-D-Glu (95). When this chelate was coupled to minigastrin, the complex, DTPA^0-D-Glu^1-minigastrin (Fig. 11**D**) had improved stability for a variety of metal ions including ^{90}Y, ^{111}In, ^{67}Ga, and [153]Sm. When DTPA is usually coupled to a peptide there is a loss of one of the carboxylic groups to the peptide bond. This leaves only four to coordinate with the metal ion. In this case, the γ carboxylic acid from the Glu provides a fifth group for coordination to the metal ion. All the five carboxylic groups are coordinated to Indium in the crystal structure of ^{111}In-DTPA (103). The therapeutic effectiveness of these metal peptide complexes were studied in a nude mouse model of MTC. Again, the kidneys were the dose-limiting organ. Minigastrin analogs labeled with Auger emitters were more therapeutically effective ($p < 0.01$) than those labeled with β emitters. At the maximum tolerated dose (MTD), even though the GI tract has many CCK-BR, no toxicity was observed with the β labeled analogs. In contrast, the animals receiving Auger labeled peptides at their MTD demonstrated hemorrhagic gastritis. Next ^{111}In-DTPA^0-D-Glu^1-minigastrin was tested in normal volunteers. There was mild nausea which resolved and uptake was restricted to stomach with its high concentration of CCK-BR and the kidneys. There was much less uptake in the liver or spleen. Then this derivative was evaluated as a diagnostic agent in 75 patients in preparation for therapeutic trials (95). There was expected uptake in the stomach and the main route of excretion was the kidney. Little or no uptake was observed in the liver or spleen. Patient based-sensitivity (detecting lesions only detected by other imaging modalities) appeared to be high (92%). Eight MTC patients were treated with ^{90}Y-DTPA^0-D-Glu^1-minigastrin. While the response to the disease was good, 6/8, there was considerable nephrotoxicity.

Other groups have attempted to use CCK analogs for the diagnosis and treatment of MTC (98,101,102). Reubi et al. (104) tested DOTA and DTPA derivatives of a nonsulfated CCK8 analog, [D-Asp^{26}, Nle^{28,31}] CCK$_{26-33}$ (Fig. 12C). These derivatives had ~1–3 nM and > 100 nM affinity for CCK-BR and -AR, respectively. De Jong and co-workers (98) determined that ^{111}In-DOTA^0-CCK8 was specifically internalized in a CCK-BR positive tumor cell line. In rat tumor model, ^{111}In-DOTA^0-[D-Asp^{26}, Nle^{28,31}] CCK8 [CCK8 (Asp, Nle)] and ^{111}In-DTPA^0-CCK8 (Asp, Nle) showed similar uptake. There was high kidney localization (~10-fold of liver) at 24 hours PI, whereas other tissues including stomach washed out rapidly (~50% reduction at 4 hours PI). Tumor uptake was more stable (~20% reduction at 4 hours PI). Uptake appeared to be specific, since injection of non-radioactive peptide did reduce ^{111}In-DOTA^0-CCK8 (Asp, Nle) uptake both in the stomach and tumor of the rats. However, in a comparison with ^{125}I-CCK10, the DOTA derivative had much lower uptake in all tissues (5-fold less in the stomach) except kidney. One MTC patient was injected with ^{111}In-DTPA^0-CCK8 (Asp, Nle) and showed lesion and stomach localization but high liver uptake. This derivative was studied in 6 more MTC patients (102). Similar results were observed with activity appearing in the GI tract at 24 and 48 hours PI. Some known lesions were missed and uptake was generally low. This was explained by HPLC analysis of the patients' serum and urine. At 1 hour PI, little agent remained intact and suggested that this derivative was rapidly degraded in vivo. Aloj et al. (101) have examined the stability of the ^{111}In-DTPA^0-D-Glu^1-Gly^2-CCK8 (nonsulfated) in a variety of in vitro and in vivo models (Fig. 12D). This analog bound to CCK-BR positive cells with a high affinity (~20 nM) and many sites ($1.6–4.7 \times 10^6$ sites/cell). It was internalized into the cells. Non-radioactive peptide could displace < 10% of this derivative from the cells if the cold peptide was added after 1 hour incubated at 37°C with the radioactive one. Kidney uptake was the highest in a CCK-BR positive mouse model. Over a 6 hours period, tumor and stomach uptake was similar while most other tissues washed out. Blood clearance was extremely rapid. HPLC showed that while incubating ^{111}In-DTPA^0-D-Glu^1-Gly^2-CCK8 with mouse serum produced no effect, samples recovered from the animals showed at 30 minutes PI showed almost no remaining original peptide. Incubation of liver and kidney tissue homogenates with the labeled peptide demonstrated similar rapid degradation. The ^{111}In did not appear to be transchelated to other proteins or molecules. Thus the poor in vivo character of this peptide appeared due to rapid tissue accretion, action by a variety of pepidases, and return of the labeled fragments to the blood. This animal model seemed to be a better predictor of the human results than the rat model use by de Jong et al. (98). Even though there was good tumor uptake it probably would have been prudent to analyze the blood and urine to assay for any degradation. This analysis might have provided clues for the eventual uptake response in humans.

These results with the CCK analogs probably rule these out for use in MTC and other diseases where CCK-BR is upregulated. The approach of Behr and co-workers (95), using analogs of gastrin, are likely to lead to more useful diagnostic and therapeutic radiopharmaceuticals. Refinements are still necessary to moderate the nephrotoxicity. The next set of experiments should determine whether this peptide follows the general mechanism of peptide uptake in the kidney. If so, maybe a mixture of amino acid could moderate the kidney uptake.

BOMBESIN

Bombesin (BBN), a 14-amino acid peptide (Fig. 13A), originally isolated from frog skin, has a high affinity for gastrin releasing peptide receptor (GRPR). Bombesin belongs to a peptide family, which includes GRP, a 27-amino acid (Fig. 13B) and Neuromedin B, a 10-amino acid peptide (Fig. 13C) derived from pig tissue. These neuropeptides/growth factors have receptors that are normally present in the CNS, GI tract, and pancreas. Bombesin, as well as its related peptides, stimulates the muscles of the GI tract, pancreatic enzymes and GI hormone secretion, and proliferation of rat andrenocortical cells. GRPR are overexpressed in a variety of cancers and their activation stimulates both cell growth and proliferation (Table 1). Bombesin agonists also appear to function as paracrine/autocrine growth stimulators for tumor cells in culture (24,108). Studies with these receptors as targets have been performed mostly in cultured cells or with animal models and limited human studies. A number of groups are examining different analogs (24,107–110).

The peptide sequence of BBN contains no Cys residues that could be cross-linked to constrain the secondary structure. However, in solution, NMR and molecular modeling suggests that residues, Asn^6-Met^{14}, form an α-helix under conditions which enhance receptor binding (111). Thus, the C-terminal portion of BBN is likely responsible for receptor binding. The N-terminal part of the peptide remains linear. Small modifications of the last two C-terminal residues, Leu^{13}-Met^{14}, may be responsible for determining whether an analog is an antagonist or agonist.

(A) pGlu-Gln-Arg-Leu-Gly-Asn-Gln-**Trp-Ala-**
Val-Gly-His-Leu-Met-NH$_2$

(B) Ala-Pro-Val-Ser-Val-Gly-Gly-Thr-Val-Leu-Ala-
Lys-Met-Tyr-Pro-Arg-Leu-Gly-Asn-His-**Trp-**
Ala-Val-Gly-His-Leu-Met-NH$_2$

(C) Gly-Asn-Leu-**Trp-Ala-Thr-Gly-His-Phe-**
Met-NH$_2$

(D) DTPA-Pro-Gln-Arg-Tyr-Gly-Asn-Gln-**Trp-**
Ala-Val-Gly-His-Leu-Met-NH$_2$

Figure 13 Amino acid sequence of (**A**) Bombesin, (**B**) Gastrin Releasing Peptide and (**C**) Neuromedin B and [DTPA, Pro^1, Tyr^4]bombesin. Amino acids in bold are directly involved in receptor binding, and are all L-isomers, pGlu = pyroGlu where γ-COOH is coupled to α-NH$_2$. N-terminal of amino acid sequence is at left and C-terminal is converted to amide [NH$_2$]. *Source*: From Refs. 10, 105, 106.

A receptor antagonist would be preferred for diagnostic/therapeutic agent. Antibody antagonists for GRPR have had modest treatment success in patients with SCLC. However, when tested in model systems (108), only BBN agonists, not antagonists, were internalized after receptor binding. The agonist gave higher specific uptake and higher T/B ratio than the antagonist.

Investigators have been able to produce a wide variety of analogs, which retain their receptor affinity when labeled with either ^{125}I, ^{99m}Tc [N$_2$S$_2$, peptidic chelate, or dithiaphosphine (P$_2$S$_2$)], ^{111}In/^{90}Y (DOTA), or ^{111}In (DTPA). Many of the initial studies have been performed with BBN fragments. Rogers et al. (112) iodinated bombesin fragments, BBN$_{(7-13)}$ NH$_2$ via a N-succinimidyl ester of metaiodobenzoate coupled to the N-terminal amine, and used intrinsically labeled Tyr^4-bombesin as a control. In cultured cells, internalization rates were similar but loss of ^{125}I from the cells was much higher with Tyr^4-bombesin. This rapid loss of ^{125}I from intracellular peptide catabolism is a common occurrence. Similar rapid label exocytosis has been observed when iodinated antibodies were internalized in cultured tumor cells (113). Baidoo et al. (24) coupled two types of a ^{99m}Tc chelate, diaminodithiol (N$_2$S$_2$), to the ε-amino group of [Lys^3]bombesin. These two N$_2$S$_2$ derivatives produced a neutral Tc(V)oxo core and a positively charged chelate. Syn and anti-isomers of these chelates could be separated on the HPLC. Thus, each isomer could be tested separately with high specific activity. Unlabeled material could also be removed by HPLC. The labeled material actually had a higher affinity (K$_i$ = 3.5–7.4 nM) for the GRPR than the un-conjugated (K$_i$ = 21 nM) and conjugated unlabeled (K$_i$ = 18–21 nM). In normal mice, the derivative with neutral core was rapidly taken up by the liver and then excreted into to the intestines. The intestines contained 40–60% of the injected dose at 15 minutes PI and > 90% at 3 hours PI. This compared to ∼20% at 15 minutes and ∼25% for the derivative with the positively charged chelate.

It is tempting to conclude that only a small change in the charge on the chelate dramatically influenced the biodistribution. However, it is not known if any of these peptides are intact after 3 hours PI. HPLC analysis of the complex in blood from mice would have been very useful. It is possible that these two derivatives experienced different rates of in vivo catabolism and that was the reason for the differential liver uptake. The two different chelates had many structural differences, which could have altered the molecule enhancing attack by pepidases. To remove the chelate structure farther from the main peptide, a 5 CH_2 spacer, 5-amino valeric acid, was added between the P_2S_2 chelate and to the amino terminus of $BBN_{(7-14)}$ (114). This should reduce the influence of the chelate function on the peptide's conformation. When [188]Re was bound to the analog, it had an affinity comparable to bombesin in a competitive cell binding assay. In normal mice, the ^{99m}Tc-P_2S_2 analog had high transport through the liver into the intestines, $\sim$30% in intestines at 4 hours PI, high urinary output 57% at the same time, and good pancreatic uptake. The specific pancreatic washed out rather rapidly. In a 3.5 hours time interval, there was a 65% reduction of the activity. Uptake was also studied using [188]Re bound to this analog (114). The [188]Re analog appeared identical in structure to the ^{99m}Tc labeled compound and retained in a mouse model GRPR targeting. However in either of these studies there was no HPLC analysis of the blood. The stability in blood of these fragments is still unknown. In the most recent study, these investigators (115) changed the chelate to a peptidic N_3S and tested the addition of 0 to 11 carbon spacers between the chelate and the same $BBN_{(7-14)}$ analog. Molecules with spacers, 3, 5, and 8, retained high affinity and specificity for the GRPR. Biodistribution in normal mice showed that uptake in GRPR-positive tissue was maximized with a 3 carbon interval. The uptake in this tissue as a function of carbon intervals was almost bell-shaped. Washout through the liver was the inverse with the 3 carbon being the 2nd lowest. GRPR-positive tissue washout with the 5 carbon and the N_3S chelate was similar ($\sim$70% in 3.5 hours) to the washout observed with the P_2S_2 analog. The number of carbons clearly influences the three dimensional structure of this linear peptide. With 0 or 11 carbons the affinity is directly affected. For 3, 5, and 8 carbons the influence on the structure may be more subtle. The biodistribution data suggest that the internalization rate for GRPR and "normal" tissue uptake was affected. These carbons could also influence in vivo catabolism by slowing or speeding attack by pepidase in the blood or in tissue. However neither urine nor blood was analyzed for the presence of intact peptide. These data also imply that at least in these animal models there are intracellular process that readily exocytose the [99m]Tc.

Breeman and co-workers (105,107,116) studied ^{111}In DTPA conjugated bombesin analogs. The high affinity antagonist, e.g., [DTPA, Tyr^5, D-Phe^6]$BBN_{(5-13)}$ HNEt (Et=ethyl), and agonist, [DTPA, Pro^1, Tyr^4]BBN (Fig. 13D), among them had the highest affinity in vitro but only the agonist internalized into receptor-positive cells. In a rat animal model, the agonist had much higher specific uptake in both tumor and pancreas and lower in receptor-negative tissue, such as lung, liver, and blood. Even though it might be expected (Table 1), there also appeared to be a little pharmacological effect on the rats for up to 100 μg of [Tyr^4]BBN injected. In a subsequent study, Breeman et al. (107) used high concentrations [Tyr^3]BBN injected into the rats to demonstrate that uptake in receptor-positive tissue (tumor and pancreas) was specific. If the [Tyr^3]BBN was given 30 minutes after injection of [^{111}In-DTPA-Pro^1, Tyr^4]BBN, radioactivity uptake in these tissue was not effected. This demonstrated rapid BBN-mediated tissue uptake by this derivative and suggested that the peptide was not significantly degraded within this time frame. High kidney localization was not effected by [Tyr^3]BBN injections. There was rapid excretion with > 50% of the activity in urine within 5 hours PI. About 50% of output in the urine was peptide bound up to 48 hours PI. Although it was not determined whether this was intact or degraded peptide, HPLC analysis of the agent in blood was also not performed. It is still unknown how stable this peptide is in the blood. Radionuclide washout from the BBN-positive tissues was slow (21% loss during 4 to 24 hours PI) suggesting that [^{111}In-DTPA-Pro^1, Tyr^4]BBN could be used for diagnosis. In the latest study, Breeman et al. (105) tested this peptide along with [^{111}In-DOTA-Pro^1, Tyr^4]BBN in two different GRPR-positive cell lines. Both analogs had high affinity but the DTPA derivative was internalized 4-fold greater. In normal rats, the DOTA derivative has slightly higher uptake in GRPR-positive tissue but higher uptake in liver. Uptake in other tissues was comparable. In this case, a slight change in the chelate structure did not markedly influence the biodistribution as it did with the P$_2$S$_2$ analog (see above).

Hoffman et al. (108) have shed more light on the loss of activity from the cells. They tested the effect of the number of carbons between the chelate DOTA and BBN$_{(7-14)}$ fragment on tumor uptake. As seen with the ^{99m}Tc analog, 3, 5, and 8 carbon spacers did not affect GRPR affinity. Pancreatic uptake for the different ^{111}In-DOTA analogs peaked at 5 carbons. Different from the ^{99m}Tc analog, washout through liver increased as the number of carbons was increased. Most interestingly, with an 8 CH$_2$ ^{111}In-DOTA analog there was considerably slower washout from the tissue as a function of time. In 3.5 hours, there was a 40% loss in activity in the pancreas compared to 65–70% seen with the ^{99m}Tc derivatives. The caveat is that these are different mouse models. It is unlikely that different models could cause such a difference. It is more likely that it related to the labile nature of ^{99m}Tc-chelate complexes because this was seen with work comparing ^{99m}Tc and ^{111}In labeled antibodies over a wide variety of model systems (113). These investigators also provided data with the same peptide BBN analog [DOTA-8-aminooctanoic acid (Aoc)-BBN$_{(7-14)}$] in the same animal model and just with two different radionuclides, ^{177}Lu and ^{111}In. Table 3 shows the loss of tissue/organ activity as a function of time PI. Both of these derivatives had high affinities for GRPR (IC$_{50}$ ∼1 nM) and similar urinary washout rates, 68% at 1 hour PI. Even though the values appear quite different, the uptake for lung pancreas and tumor was not significant between the two isotopes. Liver uptake was significantly different. In contrast, tissue washout had striking

Table 3 Comparison of ^{177}Lu Versus ^{111}In Labeled DOTA-8-Aoc-BBN$_{(7-14)}$ Washout in Tumor Bearing SCID Mouse Tissue

| Tissue/organ | ^{177}Lu | | | ^{111}In | | |
| | Time post injection | | | | | |
	1 hour	4 hours	24 hours	1 hour	4 hours	24 hours
Lung	100(0.18)[a]	100[b]	−94	100(0.50)	50	82
Liver	100(0.3)	56	90	100(1.34)	−7	72
Pancreas	100(39)	42	87	100(19)	11	64
Tumor	100(4.22)	28	64	100(3.63)	51	57

[a] Values in parentheses are absolute % ID/g value.
[b] % Reduction in %ID/g assuming 1 hour value is 100%.
Source: From Refs. 108, 115.

differences between the two isotopes with ostensible similar structures. In lung, a tissue that has little GRPR-dependence, for ^{177}Lu there was little washout and actually increased at 24 hours PI, whereas ^{111}In activity was substantially reduced. With the other tissues in all cases there was considerable loss of activity (57–90%) for each isotope at 24 hours PI. However, there was considerable variability at the 4 hours time point. In the tissue that has high GRPR dependence, pancreas, ^{111}In activity only declined 11% versus 42% for ^{177}Lu. In liver and tumor with moderate GRPR-dependence, the early washout was not consistent. For liver there was very little loss for ^{111}In and 56% decline for ^{177}Lu. This was the reverse for the tumor. There was a large decline (51%) for ^{111}In and a small one for ^{177}Lu. These data suggest that processes to expel the radionuclides are tissue-dependent. This information could be extremely important if the investigators could tailor the rapid loss to the background tissue while promoting longer retention for GRPR tumors.

Taken together, the data from the in vitro and in vivo models show that the chelated BBN analogs are internalized and readily take up GRPR-known positive (but not tested) tissue. Excretion is mostly urinary but a significant amount of activity is taken up by the liver and particularly with ^{99m}Tc activity excreted into the GI tract. Usually ^{99m}Tc forms much more labile chelate complexes than ^{111}In or ^{177}Lu. It is likely that all the BBN analogs are rapidly incorporated in receptor endosome transferred to a lysosome for degradation. Once the peptide is in the lysosome, the exocytosis of the radionuclide from the cell is tissue- and radionuclide-dependent. This mechanism follows closely the mechanism of OctreoScan (Fig. 7). Also, a CH_2 spacer of various lengths was inserted between the chelates and peptide moiety. The number of CH_2 groups influenced the peptide's biodistribution and affinity for GRPR. The stability of any of these peptides in the plasma has not been studied.

A phase I study in humans has been performed with a BBN analog, RP-527, mainly to determine toxicity. RP-527 is a $BBN_{(7-14)}$ fragment coupled at the N terminal with a 5 carbon linker group and ^{99m}Tc-binding peptide sequence (109,117). Initial images in humans showed that animal models appear to be a good predictor of the human biodistribution. Only bladder and liver activity were observed. Most other tissues had low uptake including pancreas. As time progressed, activity was excreted into the GI tract. Activity was rapidly excreted into the urine, ~60% and only 4% in the feces at 48 hours PI. Unexpectedly, breasts in women and testes in men were also visualized. The tumors of patients with prostate cancer were not visualized. However, tumors of patients with breast cancer were. Thus, data from animals, although not perfect, should be able to help refine BBN derivatives to provide a successful diagnostic/therapeutic agent.

ALPHA MELANOCYTE STIMULATING HORMONE

Five melanocortin receptors (MC1R–MC5R) have been identified and are involved in pigmentation (MC1R), feeding behavior and obesity (MC3R and MC4R), and exocrine gland functions (MC5R) (17). Alpha melanocyte stimulating hormone (α-MSH; α-melanocortin) (Fig. 14A) is one of three endogenous MSHs (β and γ), which bind to these receptors and affects the pigmentation in peripheral tissue, especially the skin (120). MC1R are present on human and murine melanoma cell lines. While the murine melanoma cells and mice are useful models, there are significant differences compared to human melanoma cells (121). In murine melanoma cells, α-MSH has an excellent $K_d = 0.3$–1.0 nM, for these receptors with modest number of receptors/cell (5,000–20,000). In contrast, in human cells, the K_d for α-MSH is 5-fold higher with a 10-fold lower receptor density (500–2000). MC1R

(A) Ac-Ser-Tyr-Ser-Met-Glu-His-Phe-Arg-Trp-
Gly-Lys-Pro-Val-NH$_2$

(B) Ac-Ser-Tyr-Ser-Nle-Glu-His-D-Phe-Arg-Trp-
Gly-Lys-Pro-Val-NH$_2$

(C) Ac-Nle-Asp-His-D-Phe-Arg-Trp-Lys-
DTPA-Lys-Trp-Arg-D-Phe-His-Asp-Nle-
Ac

(D) DOTA-βAla-Nle-Asp-His-D-Phe-Arg-Trp-Lys-
NH$_2$

Figure 14 Amino acid sequence of (**A**) α-Melanocyte Stimulating Hormone, (**B**) [Nle^4-D-Phe^7] α-MSH (**C**) DTPA-bis-{[Nle^4, Asp^5, D-Phe^7, Lys^{10}(bis DHP)] α-MSH$_{(4-10)}$ and (**D**) DOTA-{[βAla^3-Nle^4, Asp^5, D-Phe^7, Lys^{10}] α-MSH$_{(3-10)}$. Amino acids are all L-isomers except where noted, Ac-Ser = acetylated (CH$_3$-CO-) serine. N-terminal of amino acid sequence is at left and C-terminal is converted to amide [NH$_2$]. *Source*: From Refs. 118, 119.

were identified in $> 80\%$ of tumor samples from melanoma patients (122). Both the N-terminal acetyl and carboxamide groups are important for potency (Fig. 14A). The amino acid sequence His^6 to Trp^9 is involved in receptor binding while the other residues appear to modulate this activity. If D-Phe is exchanged for L-Phe[7], there is an increase in resistance to in vivo proteolytic degradation without affecting the biological activity. The oxidation of Met^4 causes a substantial loss of biological activity, which can be averted by substituting a Nle in this position. This analog $[Nle^4, D\text{-}Phe^7]$ α-MSH (NDP) (Fig. 14B) has a much higher affinity for MC1R than the parent compound (123). The iodinated derivative $[^{125}I\text{-}Tyr^2]$ NDP is internalized in murine melanoma cells (124). If the α-MSH is cyclized via a disulfide bond $[Cys^{4,10}, D\text{-}Phe^7]$ α-MSH, this molecule is also resistant to in vivo proteolysis and retains high affinity for MC1R (125).

Radiolabeled α-MSH peptide analogs have been studied for more than a decade for melanoma lesion detection (33,118,119,124,126). The first analog synthesized contained a single DTPA coupled to two identical peptide segments of α-MSH. This derivative, labeled with ^{111}In, $^{111}In\text{-}DTPA\text{-}[Nle^4, Asp^5, D\text{-}Phe^7, Lys^{10}]$ α-$MSH_{(4-10)}$ (Fig. 14C), had high tumor uptake compared to normal tissues at 24 hours PI and was competitively inhibited by an injection of a 200-molar excess of α-MSH. Uptake by other tissues, e.g., brain, liver, kidney, and skin, was not affected by the excess α-MSH (118). In patients, it also appeared effective, detecting 41 of 46 known lesions very early after injection (4 hours PI). However, this analog had high kidney and liver uptake. This made lesion identification in the liver, a known metastatic site, difficult (126). To reduce the tissue background, a DTPA coupled to a single $[Nle^4, Asp^5, D\text{-}Phe^7, Lys^{10}]$ α-$MSH_{(4-10)}$ was tested in a mouse melanoma model (127). Liver and kidney activity were reduced but tumor uptake by the monomer ($0.64\%ID/g$) was also substantially reduced compared to the dimer (128).

To add ^{99m}Tc for diagnosis and ^{188}Re for therapy, Chen and co-workers (128) added Cys-containing peptidic chelators to the N-terminal of the α-MSH analog, NDP. Unfortunately, in a mouse melanoma model, activity washed out very rapidly from the tumor and other tissues. Tumor activity declined 70–75% within 4 hours PI. The likely reason for the rapid tissue loss is that ^{99m}Tc chelates are generally very labile. However, it was surprising that the ^{188}Re also washed out since this isotope usually forms much more stable chelates. However, facile proteolysis of these analogs can not be excluded. No HPLC analysis was performed on the urine or blood from these animals to determine if these analogs were still intact. To eliminate the confounding aspect of ^{99m}Tc chelate lability, these investigators added a chelate, DOTA, that has high stability for a wide variety of potential diagnostic or therapeutic radionuclides to the N-terminal (33). This analog DOTA- $[Cys^{3,4,10}, D\text{-}Phe^7]$ α-$MSH_{(3-13)}$ [DOTA-ReCCMSH] is cyclized via a ReO that coordinates Cys^4 and Cys^{10} (Fig. 4). This derivative was compared to a number of analogs, including a linearized version without Re, DOTA-CCMSH. The cyclization or DOTA conjugation did not affect receptor binding. Both analogs had a high affinity for the MC1R, $IC_{50} = 1.2$ nM [cyclized], and 4.9 [linear]. This compared to $IC_{50} = 0.21$ nM for the NDP analog. When tested in a melanoma animal model, tumor concentration for the different derivatives did not follow their affinity profile. The biodistribution of ^{111}In-DOTA-ReCCMSH showed very rapid clearance from the blood, low liver, modest kidney, and the highest tumor uptake. In comparison, ^{111}In-DOTA-CCMSH also had rapid blood washout (higher absolute uptake), highest liver, highest kidney, and lowest tumor uptake. Tumor uptake by ^{111}In-DOTA-NDP was significantly different than ^{111}In-DOTA-ReCCMSH until 24 hours PI, when it was significantly lower. Tumor concentration for DOTA-ReCCMSH remained constant for at least 4 hours but dropped by 50% at 24 hours. This pattern of activity loss from the tumor was followed by the other analogs. The most striking aspect of DOTA-ReCCMSH was the washout from normal tissues compared to the other analogs. For example, blood activity was 1.57%ID/g at 30 minutes PI which declined to 0.07% at 2 hours PI (96% reduction). In contrast, ^{111}In-DOTA-NDP started out lower at 30 minutes, 0.56% but was 0.22% at 2 hours (60% reduction). This pattern was observed for many other normal tissues, including heart, liver, spleen, pancreas, and muscle. Thus, the target to background (T/B) ratios (blood, muscle, lung, and liver) was very high for DOTA-ReCCMSH and ranged from 7–600 to 1. Tumor uptake appeared to be specific. A co-injection of NDP reduced by more than an order of magnitude the tumor uptake of DOTA-ReCCMSH. It would be expected that the higher affinity NDP should easily be able to displace ^{111}In-DOTA-ReCCMSH. Excretion was mostly urinary for all analogs (60–80%), with very little (1–2%) activity in the GI tract. To properly interpret this data, it is essential to know the in vivo stability of all these analogs. No analysis was performed on the urine, or blood to determine whether at any time any of these peptides were intact. These investigators suggest that free sulfhydryls in ^{111}In-DOTA-CCMSH and ^{111}In-DOTA-[Cyc^{4,10}, D-Phe^{7}]α-MSH (4–13) is the reason for the increased kidney uptake. Since these residues would be negatively charged in the urine this explanation would be inconsistent with the present theory of renal tubular uptake (Fig. 8). A decrease, not an increase in kidney uptake, would be expected. Rapid proteolysis, which could decrease receptor interaction and increase uptake by normal tissues or kidney excretion, would be a more likely explanation. Once the analog localized in normal tissue there was usually a slow loss of the ^{111}In label from intracellular catabolism. The data strongly suggests that the cyclic nature of the ^{111}In-DOTA-ReCCMSH profoundly affected background tissue retention. While tumor uptake and retention was influenced, there is a more substantial effect on the washout from normal tissue. This may give some insight into the intracellular processing for normal tissue. Peptides taken up less specific mechanisms, e.g., pinocytosis, and might be more easily exocytosed, if the molecule was resistant to proteolysis (cyclic in this case). If susceptible to proteolysis, the molecular fragment containing the radionuclide would be shunted to the cytoplasm or lysosomes where it would be less easily exocytosed. In the next series of experiments, Chen and collaborators (129) coupled an iodine binding molecule (iodobenzoate [IBA] to their cyclic peptide via an acetylated L- or D-Lys at the N-terminal and also converted Lys^{11} to Arg^{11} to give Ac-D(L)-Lys(^{125}I-IBA)-ReCCMSH (Arg^{11}). The conversion of Lys for Arg in this position increased the tumor and decreased kidney uptake (130). The objective was to add an ^{18}F or ^{123}I, for diagnosis or ^{131}I for therapy. In cultured cells, there was good uptake and internalization (129). However, ~50% of the activity washed out of the cells within the first 4 hours. The K_d values for these derivatives were very high ~10 pM and comparable to literature values. When studied in the mouse melanoma model, uptake and washout for tumor were similar to the ^{111}In-DOTA analog discussed above. The major difference was that the uptake of this iodinated analog was split (~50/50) between liver and kidney and not all urinary. Excretion was also split between GI tract (10%, 4 hours PI) and urinary (56%, 4 hours PI). However, at 24 hours PI the tumor to kidney ratio was substantially better for the ^{125}I analog (6.6) versus the ^{111}In derivative (1.4). The catabolism of these analogs was examined. A small amount of the Ac-L-Lys remained up to 24 hours PI. In contrast, considerably more of the D-Lys analog was present at 24 hours but clearly there was a large amount of catabolism as early as 30 minutes PI. The addition of the hydrophobic benzoic acid shifted the excretion mode from kidney to a mixture. Unfortunately, we can not directly compare the catabolism of these cyclic derivatives to the ^{111}In-DOTA cyclic analog. However, this data does suggest that they are more resistant than the linear version but still have a moderate rate of proteolysis. This moderate rate may affect the washout from the normal tissues.

Froidevaux and co-workers (119,131) also tested α-MSH analogs with a DOTA attached. However, these investigators did analyze, using HPLC, the urine of animals injected with a few of the ^{111}In labeled derivatives. They determined that DOTA coupled to NDP was fully catabolized within 4 hours PI. In contrast, a unique analog, DOTA is coupled to N-terminal of an α-MSH analog DOTA-[βAla^3, Nle^4, Asp^5, D-Phe^7] α-MSH$_{(3-10)}$ [DOTA-MSH$_{oct}$], was intact at 4 hours PI but at 24 hours was fully catabolized. When tested in cell culture the addition of DOTA did reduce (~7-fold) the affinity, of MSH$_{oct}$ for MC1R which was more than 30-fold lower than that affinity (IC$_{50}$) of DOTA-NDP. Even with the lower affinity, tumor uptake in the mouse model was still ~70% of DOTA-NDP uptake. This could be explained by improved stability of DOTA-MSH$_{oct}$. The downside of the improved stability was higher (70%) kidney uptake at 4 hours PI. Both analogs washed (~50% reduction) out at 24 hours PI. Kidney uptake was higher than tumor and remained much higher than tumor for both analogs up to 48 hours PI. This would make it unlikely that this analog could be used as a therapeutic agent. Kidney uptake was not effected by an injection of non-radioactive α-MSH, whereas tumor uptake was substantially reduced. Other background tissues were low. Autoradiographs demonstrated high uniform uptake in target tissue and low uptake in normal skin. This supports the notion that small peptides can easily penetrate into the tumors and also suggests that DOTA-MSH$_{oct}$ is specific. Kidney activity was distributed uniformly only in the cortex of the kidney, which would be consistent with tubular uptake (Fig. 8).

These investigators also tested a derivative where the DOTA was coupled at different position on the amino acid chain. It was attached to amino group of a Lys, [Nle^4, Asp^5, D-Phe^7, Lys^{11} (DOTA)] α-MSH$_{(4-11)}$ [DOTA-NAPamide]. Similar to DOTA-MSH$_{oct}$, the addition of the DOTA did cause a reduction (5-fold) of cell binding affinity but it was ~7-fold higher than DOTA-MSH$_{oct}$. This time the affinity increase was reflected in a substantial increase in specific tumor uptake by DOTA-NAPamide in a mouse model. Also, kidney uptake was significantly reduced (60%, P <0.001 1 versus 4 hours PI) but kidney uptake was not higher than tumor uptake at 4 hours PI. As with the other peptides, activity washed out rather rapidly from tumor (~70% at 24 hours PI). At 24 hours PI, kidney and tumor uptake were comparable. Kidney uptake could be reduced (64%) by infusion of L-Lys. No analysis was performed on the stability of this new conjugate. It might be cautiously assumed that DOTA-NAPamide was intact up to 4 hours PI.

For MC1R as the target, we are in the very early stages of development. As yet we are not yet anywhere near able to test any of these analogs in humans. The thrust of the research should concentrate on therapeutic aspects since a competing technology, PET imaging, is extremely effective for melanoma detection (132). In contrast, there is a lack of therapeutic options since chemotherapy is generally ineffective. For further development, it is essential to understand the localization mechanism in these models. The data presented above confirms a number of aspects of this mechanism (see Introduction). There was generally good tumor uptake by these peptides but also rapid loss of activity as a function of time. Kidney uptake was high, which was comparable to tumor concentration at the later times. Kidney uptake and retention would likely limit the use of these analogs as a therapeutic peptide. Kidney uptake could not be reduced by adding increased non-radioactive peptide concentration. However, the addition of positively charged amino acids substantially reduced uptake. This fits into the model of general kidney localization for peptides (Fig. 8). For certain α-MSH analogs, the addition of the chelate to the peptide did reduce affinity of the peptide for the MC1R. While affinity for the receptor is important, the tumor uptake profile for the analogs did not follow the affinity profile. More important for both tumor and kidney uptake was the in vivo stability of these MC1R targeting molecules. There is some information emerging about the effects of proteolysis. For these peptides, cyclization appeared to resist catabolism but there is still substantial peptide breakdown even at 30 minutes PI. The linear peptides were much less resistant. The increased resistance to proteolysis of DOTA-ReCCMSH in vivo could partially explain greater tumor and less kidney uptake compared to the linearized peptides. This allowed more of the DOTA-ReCCMSH to interact with the MC1R and less interaction with non-specific processes, e.g., kidney and normal cells. The differences in tissue washout for different analogs could be possibly attributed to the radionuclide and proteolytic resistance. Rapid activity loss was expected with the ^{99m}Tc/^{188}Re experiments because of the chelate lability. In contrast, there was less loss with the more stable ^{111}In-based derivatives. The cyclic targeting molecule DOTA-ReCCMSH had much faster loss from the normal tissue which gave great T/B ratios. The cyclic peptides were resistant enough to be rapidly incorporated intracellularly. It is possible that once incorporated in normal cells, this resistance enhanced exocytosis. That is, peptides taken up non-specifically, e.g., pinocytosis, might not be shunted to the lysosomes. Lysosomes do readily send their contents to the cytoplasm where the radionuclide could be released from the cell (133,134). Peptides that are taken up specifically get incorporated into an endosome that eventually fuses into a lysosome. Once in the lysosome the chelate peptide complex is degraded and the contents are slowly transferred to the cytoplasm. Much more information is needed about this washout process for both normal and tumor cells.

$\alpha_v\beta_3$ ANTAGONISTS

The general strategy to target tumors has been to target specific receptors or antigens upregulated on the tumor cell's surface. An alternative would be to target a general process that is utilized by all tumors. This potentially could provide a universal targeting agent. Adhesion molecules may be this target. These molecules play a critical role in cell traffic, allowing cells to bind to specific vascular sites within the body. Four families of these molecules have been identified: integrins, selectins, cadherins, and immunoglobulin super family (e.g., intercellular adhesion molecules). Adhesion molecules are particularly important in metastatic invasion by tumor cells and tumor-induced angiogenesis. Angiogenesis, the sprouting of new blood vessels from pre-existing ones, is a complex process including endothelial and other cells and a variety of soluble factors. This process requires degradation of the basement membranes surrounding exiting vessels, migration of endothelial cells into the interstitial space, endothelial proliferation, and maturation of nascent blood vessels (135). Integrins, hetreodimeric (α and β subunits), transmembrane glycoproteins, are well-documented participants in tumor invasion and angiogenesis. The extracellular portion of the subunits is globular with a stalk inserted in the membrane, and ligand binding is divalent cation-dependent. One integrin, $\alpha_v\beta_3$, has been widely studied as a target since it is not readily detected on normal vessels but is upregulated on angiogenic vessels (136). It is found predominately on endothelial cells but also on platelets, vascular smooth muscle cells, monocytes, macrophages, osteoclasts, and some B-cells (137). Antagonists to $\alpha_v\beta_3$ can bind to tumor cells, block tumor-associated angiogenesis, and can cause tumor regression (138). These antagonists also caused apoptosis in actively proliferating vascular cells and not in pre-existing ones. This integrin $\alpha_v\beta_3$, as well as others, has an RGD (single letter designation for amino acids, Arg-Gly-Asp) binding site and binds a number of blood proteins including fibrinogen, fibrinonectin, vonWillebrand factor, vitronectin, and thrombospondin. Thus, molecules with this common motif, RGD, bind to integrins with different affinities. It is likely that the three-dimensional structure surrounding the RGD sequence is the reason for these differences (106). In vitro studies have demonstrated that a cyclic RGD sequence with less mobility has a higher potency for a particular integrin. A restricted conformation can more easily fit into the binding site. Data suggest that the binding pocket for $\alpha_v\beta_3$ is narrower and less flexible than the pocket for $\alpha_{IIb}\beta_3$ (139). Thus, cyclic pentapeptides versus hexapeptides are preferred. Also, D-Phe in the 4th position gives the sharpest γ turn by allowing stronger hydrogen bonding between the Asp^3 and Gly^2 (Fig. 5). While other peptide-bound integrins are internalized into the cell, there is little data to determine if this is the case for $\alpha_v\beta_3$ and endothelial or tumor cells.

The $\alpha_v\beta_3$ expression was demonstrated in a small number of prostate, breast, and lung cancer tissue samples using autoradiography with an ^{125}I labeled peptide, c(RGDyK[DTPA]). The lower case indicates a D-amino acid. In this peptide, a DTPA is coupled to the Lys (Fig. 15). This expression was confirmed by immunohistochemical staining (140). This peptide appeared to be internalized with a receptor-like saturation in two different cultured cell types, rat pancreatic CA20948 and Bon carcinoid cells. However, only two concentrations were used and no K_d was determined. The presence of the $\alpha_v\beta_3$ receptor was confirmed only in the Bon cell type. In many of the in vivo and in vitro experiments, the expression of $\alpha_v\beta_3$ is unknown and has not been tested. In subsequent discussions, it can be assumed that $\alpha_v\beta_3$ expression was not tested unless otherwise specified. In in vivo blocking experiments using the ^{111}In labeled analog in a rat CA20948 model, the kidney was one of the few organs where uptake was not reduced with the co-injection of non-radioactive peptide. Kidney uptake was the highest with liver concentration second. To decrease the hydrophobicity and increase kidney excretion of the RGD peptide,

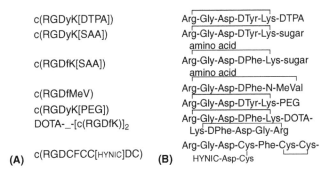

Figure 15 Peptide Ligands for $\alpha_V\beta_3$ Receptors. Amino acid sequence using (**A**) single letter designation and (**B**) the corresponding three letter abbreviations for the amino acids where the lower case letter indicates a D instead of an L amino acid. All peptides are cyclic where the Arg is usually coupled to terminal amino acid either Val or Lys via a peptide bond (solid line). The exception is the cysteine containing peptide where disulfide bonds (solid lines) are used to constrain the three dimensional structure. Chelates or other additional groups are usually attached to the ε-amino group of Lys. *Source*: From Refs. 32, 138, 140–143.

Haubner and co-workers (32) added a sugar amino acid (SAA), 3-acetamido-2,6 anhydro-3-deoxy-β-D-glycero-D-gulo-heptonic acid, to the peptide (Fig. 5). This peptide, c[RGDyK(SAA)], labeled with ^{125}I, had good selectivity. The IC_{50}, competing with vitronectin, was ~100-fold smaller for a $\alpha_v\beta_5$ target compared to $\alpha_v\beta_3$. However, results in tumor models were modest with low tumor to background values (2.5–16 to 1) and rapid washout (4 hours PI) of the label from the tumor. Tumor activity in two different animal models, both had high $\alpha_v\beta_3$, expression was comparable to kidney and liver at 4 hours PI. Activity was transported out of the liver and concentrated in the intestine. Expected thyroid uptake was very high. The non-radioactive sugar peptide reduced tumor uptake to 15% of the control, suggesting specificity. More recently, this group coupled a ^{18}F to D-Phe on the peptide where the D-Tyr was converted to D-Phe (Fig. 5) (144). Catabolism of the peptide was studied in normal mice. At 2 hours PI, extraction efficiency varied among tissue. The highest was kidney (93%) and the lowest was liver (60%). A high fraction, 75–87%, of the extracted material was the intact peptide. The peptide in both tumor and blood was mainly intact (>86%). In normal rabbits, this peptide was rapidly excreted with little activity in either kidney or liver.

Other groups have also labeled RGD analogs with positron emitters, ^{18}F or [64]Cu. Ogawa et al. (141) fluorinated the Phe ring on a cyclic RGD peptide, c(RGDfMeV) where Phe replaced Tyr (Fig. 15). This derivative, being much more hydrophobic, had high liver uptake (40–46%/organ at 5 minutes PI) and low tumor (U87MG) uptake (0.9–1%). All activity was rapidly reduced by >50% at 60 minutes PI, except for intestine, which increased. Peptide catabolism was not studied and control (scrambled) peptides were not used. Non-radioactive peptide injected 60 minutes after the radiolabeled one significantly affected (22–50% reduction) normal organs spleen (28%), pancreas (23%), heart (37%), and lung (47%), and tumor only 53%. This suggests that some of the activity may have already been fixed in the tissue. Another group, Chen et al. (145), coupled a ^{18}F-benzoate group to the Lys of c(RGDyK) (Fig. 15). Similar results in vivo were observed. Comparable uptake in tumor (U87MG), liver, and kidney was rapidly reduced by >50% at 2 hours PI. The benzyl group promoted liver uptake and GI washout. Blocking experiments were performed with co-injections and reduced tumor ~7-fold. Knight and co-workers (146) labeled Bitistatin with ^{64}Cu via a DOTA moiety and compared this to a ^{125}I labeled analog. This high MW (>5 kDa) disintegrin binds to $\alpha_v\beta_3$. The addition of the DOTA did not effect in vitro affinity of bitistatin. In cultured cells (EMT-6), there was little difference between the labeled peptide and non-specific binding. In animals (EMT-6 tumor), the different radiolabels gave disparate results. Kidney uptake was >10-fold for the ^{64}Cu analog and tumor uptake 4-fold lower. Tumor uptake, although low (1–1.5%ID/g), was stable over 6 hours with the ^{64}Cu derivative. In contrast, for the ^{125}I analog, uptake peaked at 2 hours. Thus, as we have seen with other peptides, how tissues and cells handle a particular radionuclide plays a critical part in the localization process.

To improve uptake, Chen et al. (142) added to monomethoxy poly(ethylene glycol) [PEG] at the ε-amino group of the Lys of c(RGDyK) and iodinated the Tyr. The addition of PEG to proteins and antibodies is known to increase the blood $T_{1/2}$ of these molecules. An increase in the blood $T_{1/2}$ should give the peptide more access to the tumor. However, while over a 2 hours period, tumor uptake did not decline, it was slightly lower than the control, un-PEG analog. Kidney uptake was low and lower than tumor. This was not the case for the control. The PEG peptide excretion was shifted to GI since intestinal activity increased as a function of time. Non radioactive peptide blocked uptake. As an alternative strategy, Janssen and co-workers (138) used a dimeric peptide containing two RGD sequences to improve uptake. These investigators coupled a DOTA or hydrazino nicotinamide (HYNIC) chelator at the ε amino of the Lys group (Fig. 15). This peptide, DOTA/HYNIC-ε-[c(RGDfK)]$_2$, was tested in $\alpha_v\beta_3$ expressing tumored (NIH:OVCAR-3) mice over a 24 hours interval. For the ^{111}In analog, the T/B (blood) ratios were high (75–100 to 1) and tumor washout for an RGD peptide analogs was relatively slow. The tumor activity peaked at 2 hours but had only a ~20% decline at 8 hours and a further 46% decline at 24 hours PI. However, uptake in tumor, spleen, kidney, and liver were comparable (4–6%ID/g at 8 hours PI). In contrast, the ^{99m}Tc labeled peptide showed very high kidney uptake 13%ID/g at 1 hour PI which declined to 6% at 8 hours. The tumor uptake and washout was similar to the ^{111}In analog. At 24 hours PI, there was a ~50% decline in tumor concentration compared to the 1 hour value. Blocking experiments, i.e., co-injection of non-radioactive peptide, suggested that this peptide had a high degree of specificity since tumor uptake was reduced 26-fold. Kidney uptake was not effected but other organs, spleen, and liver were. This implied liver and spleen expressed $\alpha_v\beta_3$ while the kidney did not. Using an ^{111}In labeled DOTA RGKfD analog, only kidney uptake and washout was observed. This supported the notion that the dimeric peptide was highly specific and that kidney excretion was a general peptide process. These investigators also tested the therapeutic potential of this peptide using the ^{90}Y labeled analog. They showed a significant (p <0.05) increase in median survival of these animals compared to a scrambled peptide. In the initial time (0–6 weeks), the difference between the tumor volume of the ^{90}Y-RGDfK analog was much less than the ^{90}Y-RGKfD analog. At greater than 6 weeks, the difference in tumor volumes between the two peptides was much smaller. This implied that even the control peptide had some effect, which is surprising since there was little tumor uptake for this peptide. Toxicity appeared modest at the MTD. Even kidney function (creatine, BUN) did not appear to be affected. The relatively high kidney uptake would likely be a limitation if this peptide was used in patients.

Su and co-workers (143,147) have perform a number of basic experiments using cultured endothelial cells. They prepared a ^{99m}Tc labeled RGD peptide, c(RGDCFCC[HYNIC]DC), cyclized with 2 Cys bonds. The ^{99m}Tc was bound to a HYNIC group coupled to a Cys. A scrambled peptide c(RGDFCC[HYNIC]DC) was used as a control. These peptides were incubated with purified $\alpha_v\beta_3$ and demonstrated only modest affinity of the RGD peptide ~ 7 µM but no detectable binding of the RGE. When tested with endothelial cells, there was high uptake by the RGD peptide (5–28-fold greater than control) but specific activity had little influence on uptake. Specific target-based uptake which should show saturation was linear. This linear relationship between bound and free peptide and adding non-radioactive RDG peptide to the incubation medium suggested a 50% decrease in binding at ~ 10 nM. These investigators suggest that $\alpha_v\beta_3$ may not be a good target with a limited number of sites on tumor cells and modest affinity. In a typical experiment, they estimate that only one labeled molecule would be bound to 1,000 tumor cells and that any other binding would be nonspecific. This may explain the low absolute binding and easy washout that many investigators have experienced. However, it was argued that an alternative reason was problems with this particular peptide. The labeling with HYNIC may have reduced the affinity or there was particularly low expression of $\alpha_v\beta_3$ in this model system (148). Expression was not tested in this model.

It is difficult to compare different models to understand the localization mechanism. This is particularly true for this receptor system because many of the in vivo models have not been tested for expression $\alpha_v\beta_3$ and very few basic experiments have been performed in cultured cells. The internalization process has been very sparsely studied. Also, in vivo blocking experiments where non-radioactive peptide is co-injected have been used to test for specificity. The assumption is that the receptor is saturated at higher peptide concentrations. However, this uptake could be a type of carrier mediated process and not necessarily specific interaction with $\alpha_v\beta_3$. A scrambled peptide is the best way to test specificity and unfortunately relatively few investigators have used this approach.

Considering these caveats, what can we decipher about the mechanism? This peptide/receptor system shares many of the characteristics observed in the other previously discussed systems. Most of the peptides had a relatively high affinity for $\alpha_v\beta_3$. However it is impossible to compare peptides from different investigators since only IC_{50} was presented. This value is specific activity dependent and can only be compared within the same system. Most peptides were usually a 100-fold better than vitronectin, which has a high affinity for $\alpha_v\beta_3$. Even with this high affinity, in most models, there was low absolute tumor uptake, ~ 1–6%ID/g at 4 hours PI (32,138,141,143,145,146). This might be explained by in vivo catabolism. Catabolism was examined in normal mice but not in any of these animal models. Modest tumor to blood ratios were obtained because blood clearance was more rapid. There is also relatively rapid radiolabel washout from the tumors. Although many investigators tested their model system only for short (1–4 hours) time periods. This washout was radionuclide dependent. Even with ^{111}In which is usually the most stable there was 50% washout at 24 hours (138). With other radionuclides, e.g., ^{125}I, ^{18}F, ^{64}Cu or ^{99m}Tc, there was more rapid tumor and tissue washout (32,141,143,145,146). Adding hydrophilic or hydrophobic groups did shift the biodistribution either toward or away from the kidney (32,141,145). The kidney does not express $\alpha_v\beta_3$ and uptake is confined to general peptide localization. Other organs besides the tumor, e.g., spleen and liver, appeared to express $\alpha_v\beta_3$. While the potential exists that peptides targeting $\alpha_v\beta_3$ could be used to detect or treat lung, prostate, or colorectal cancer, we have a very long way to go before testing in humans can begin.

CONCLUSION

There has been an exponential growth in the development of radiolabeled peptides for diagnostic and therapeutic applications. Peptides have many advantages including fast clearance, rapid tissue penetration, and low antigenicity, and can be produced easily and inexpensively. In contrast, peptides have problems with in vivo catabolism, unwanted physiological effects, and chelate attachment. ^{111}In-OctreoScan, the first peptide approved for human use has become the diagnostic gold standard for neuroendocrine tumors. This effectiveness led to the approach of replacing the diagnostic radionuclide with a therapeutic nuclide; then OctreoScan or an analog could be used for treatment. This approach has been applied to neuroendocrine disease with some success and now is the dominant paradigm in the development of a wide variety of peptides. How the peptide-radionuclide combination localizes in the tumor is critical in the choice of the peptide and therapeutic radionuclide. The mechanism of ^{111}In-OctreoScan, characterized the best, starts with a peptide modified to resist blood proteolysis. Then ^{111}In-OctreoScan binds to upregulated SSTRs, internalized, and finally the radionuclide is translated to the nucleus. Thus, ^{111}In, with a short therapeutic range in tissue, can be used for therapy along with ^{90}Y with a longer range. Alterations of the amino acid in the peptide string can modify the biodistribution and different radionuclides can alter the affinity constant for the receptor. Kidney uptake, which is dose limiting, appears to incorporate ^{111}In-OctreoScan by a negatively charged carrier-based process. After the peptide binds, it is internalized into a vesicle, vesicle contents released to a lysosome and then become trapped in these renal tubule lysosomes. NeoTect, an approved, ^{99m}Tc-labeled, SSTR-binding analog, used for lung cancer detection, spawned the development, of [188]Re-P-2054 for treatment. There is little information about the localization mechanism. Most of the data on other peptide/receptor systems has been in the oncology realm and are not as well characterized as ^{111}In-OctreoScan. In general, for all these systems, tumor uptake is modest for high affinity peptide analogs but tumor and tissue washout is rapid. Tumor uptake could be low because of in vivo catabolism, which was not usually studied. Alternatively, receptor expression could be low. Many models used were known to express the receptor but were not tested. Tumor and other tissue washout was radionuclide-dependent with ^{125}I, ^{18}F, ^{64}Cu, or ^{99m}Tc much less stable than [111]In. Moderate tumor to blood ratios were achieved because of more rapid blood clearance. Kidney and tumor concentrations were comparable at latter times (4–8 hours PI). Kidney uptake followed the general peptide mechanism described for OctreoScan. Kidney uptake and retention would likely limit the therapeutic use of these analogs. With other peptides CCK-BR targeting molecules are furthest along in development. $DTPA^0$-D-Glu^1-minigastrin bound a wide range of diagnostic and therapeutic radionuclides with good stability. However, its blood stability or ability to internalize has not been studied. This peptide was moderately effective in diagnosing and treating patients with MTC. Kidney localization and toxicity would limit its effectiveness. CCK analogs with high specificity for CCK-BR were internalized in tumor cells but were rapidly degraded in blood. This explains the low to moderate tumor uptake with rapid washout. The C-terminal sequence $BBN_{(7-13)}$ coupled with a variety of different chelates targeted the GRPR. Also, a CH_2 spacer of various lengths was inserted between the chelates and peptide moiety. These analogs were readily taken up by GRPR-positive (known but not tested) tissue and internalized in cultured cells. Excretion was mostly urinary but a significant amount of activity was taken up by the liver. More ^{99m}Tc activity was excreted into the GI tract than ^{111}In because ^{99m}Tc forms much more labile chelate complexes. The number of CH_2 groups influenced the peptide's biodistribution and affinity for GRPR. The peptides, stability in the plasma was not studied. For melanocortin receptor (MC1R) as the target, there was good tumor uptake in animal models of melanoma and internalization in cultured cells by alpha melanocyte stimulating hormone (α-MSH) analogs. While affinity for the receptor is important, the tumor uptake profile for the analogs did not follow the affinity profile. Cyclized peptides, e.g., DOTA- $[Cys^{3,4,10}, D$-$Phe^7]$ α-$MSH_{(3-13)}$, were more resistant to in vivo catabolism than linear ones, e.g., DOTA-$[\beta Ala^3, Nle^4, Asp^5, D$-$Phe^7]$ α-$MSH_{(3-10)}$, but there is still substantial cyclized peptide breakdown even at 30 minutes PI. The integrin $\alpha_v\beta_3$ has been widely studied as a universal tumor target since it is directly involved in the formation of new tumor blood vessels. This integrin has a RGD binding sequence. The low absolute tumor uptake might be related to either low amount of internalization or in vivo catabolism. Neither has been carefully examined. Adding hydrophilic or hydrophobic groups did shift the biodistribution either toward or away from the kidney. Other organs besides the tumor, e.g., spleen and liver, appeared to express $\alpha_v\beta_3$. Taken together, much more basic information needs to be clarified in these model systems before the potential of peptides in Oncology can be realized.

REFERENCES

1. Froidevaux S, Eberle AN. Somatostatin analogs and radiopeptides in cancer therapy. Biopolymers 2002; 66:161–183.
2. OctreoScan Package Insert. St Louis (MO): Mallinckrodt, 2000. http://imaging. mallinckrodt.com/Attachments/PackageInserts/Octreoscan%20PI.pdf accessed 3/9/06.
3. Krenning EP, Kwekkeboom DJ, Bakker WH, et al. Somatostatin receptor scintigraphy with $[^{111}In$-DTPA-D-$Phe^1]$ and $[^{123}I$-$Tyr^3]$-octreotide: the Rotterdam experience with more than 1000 patients. Eur J Nucl Med 1993; 20:716–731.

4. Reubi JC, Schär JC, Waser B, et al. Affinity profiles for human somatostatin receptor subtypes SST1-SST5 of somatostatin radiotracers selected for scintigraphic and radiotherapeutic use. Eur J Nucl Med 2000; 27:273–282.

5. Lamberts SWJ, Krenning E, Reubi J-C. The role of somatostatin and its analogs in the diagnosis and treatment of tumors. Endocr Rev 1991; 12:450–482.

6. Kwekkeboom DJ, Krenning EP, de Jong M. Peptide receptor imaging and therapy. J Nucl Med 2000; 41:1704–1713.

7. Kwekkeboom DJ, Krenning EJ, de Jong M, et al. Somatostatin receptor scintigraphy. In: Sandler MP, Coleman RE, Wackers F, eds. Diagnostic Nuclear Medicine. 4th ed. Baltimore: Lippincott, Williams & Wilkins, 2003:735–746.

8. Balon HR, Goldsmith SJ, Siegel BA, et al. Procedure guideline for somatostatin receptor scintigraphy with ^{111}In-pentetreotide. J Nucl Med 2001; 42:1134–1138.

9. McAfee JG, Neumann RD. Radiolabeled peptides and other ligands for receptors overexpressed in tumor cells for imaging neoplasms. Nucl Med Biol 1996; 23:673–676.

10. Okarvi SM. Recent developments in ^{99}Tc^{m}-labelled peptide-based radiopharmaceuticals. An overview. Nucl Med Commun 1999; 20:1093–1112.

11. Reubi JC. Neuropeptide receptors in health and disease: the molecular basis for in vivo imaging. J Nucl Med 1995; 36:1825–1835.

12. Reubi JC. Regulatory peptide receptors as molecular targets for cancer diagnosis and therapy. Q J Nucl Med 1997; 41:63–70.

13. Heasly LE. Autocrine and paracrine signaling through neuropeptide receptors in human cancer. Oncogene 2001; 20:1563–1569.

14. Moody TW, Chan D, Fahrenkrug J, Jensen RT. Neuropeptides as autocrine growth factors in cancer cells. Curr Pharm Des 2003; 9:495–509.

15. Hennig IM, Laissue JA, Horisberger U, Reubi JC. Substance-preceptors in human primary neoplasms: tumoral and vascular localization. Int J Cancer 1995; 61:786–792.

16. Hua C, Shu XK, Lei C. Pancreatoblastoma. A histochemical and immunohistochemical ananlysis. J Clin Pathol 1996; 49:952–954.

17. Koikov LN, Ebetino FH, Solinsky MG, Cross-Doersen D, Knittel JJ. Subnanomolar hMC1R agonists by end-capping of the melanocortin tetrapeptide His-D-Phe-Trp-NH$_2$. Med Chem Lett 2003; 13:2647–2650.

18. McGilvery RW. Biochemistry. 3rd ed. A Functional Approach. Philadelphia: W.B. Saunders, 1983.

19. Fujimori K, Covell DG, Fletcher JE, Weinstein JN. A modeling analysis of monoclonal antibody percolation through tumors: a binding-site barrier. J Nucl Med 1990; 31:1191–1198.

20. Jain RK. Transport of molecules in the tumor interstitium: a review. Cancer Res 1987; 47:3039–3051.

21. Dean RT, James JL, Lees RS, Vallabhajosula S, Goldsmith SJ. Peptides in biomedical sciences: principles and practice. In: Martin-Comin J, Thakur ML, Piera C, Roca M, Lomena F, eds. Radiolabeled Blood Elements. New York: Plenum Press, 1994:195–199.

22. Thakur ML, Kolan HR, Rifat S, et al. Vapreotide labeled with Tc-99m for imaging tumors: preparation and preliminary evaluation. Int J Oncol 1996; 9:445–451.

23. Virgolini I, Kurtaran A, Raderer M, et al. Vasoactive intestinal peptide receptor scintigraphy. J Nucl Med 1995; 36:1732–1739.

24. Baidoo KE, Lin K-S, Zhan Y, Finley P, Scheffel U, Wagner HN, Jr. Design, synthesis, and initial evaluation of high-affinity technetium bombesin analogues. Bioconjug Chem 1998; 10:218–225.

25. Qu T, Wang Y, Zhu Z, Rusckowski M, Hnatowich DJ. Different chelators and different peptides together influence the in vivo properties of [99]Tc[m]. Nucl Med Commun 2001; 22:203–215.

26. Pallela VR, Thakur ML, Consigny PS, Rao PS, Vasileva-Belinkolavska D. Imaging thromboembolism with Tc-99m-labeled thrombospondin receptor analogs TP-1201 and TP-1300. Thromb Res 1993; 93:191–202.

27. Pallela VR, Thakur ML, Chakder S, Rattan S. ^{99m}Tc-labeled vasoactive intestinal peptide receptor agonist: functional studies. J Nucl Med 1999; 40:352–360.

28. Thakur ML, Marcus CS, Saeed S, et al. ^{99m}Tc-labeled vasoactive intestinal peptide analog for rapid localization of tumors in humans. J Nucl Med 2000; 41:107–110.

29. Rao PS, Pallela VR, Vassileva-Belnikolavska D, Jungkind D, Thakur ML. A receptor specific peptide for imaging infection and inflammation. Nucl Med Commun 2000; 21:1063–1070.

30. Rao PS, Thakur ML, Pallela V, et al. [99m]Tc labeled VIP analog: evaluation for imaging colorectal cancer. Nucl Med Biol 2001; 28:445–450.

31. OncoScint, 1992. Package Insert. Princeton, NJ: Cytogen, 1992. http://www.biopharma.com/sample entries/256.html accessed 3/9/06.

32. Haubner R, Wester H-J, Burkhart F, et al. Glycosylated RGD-containing peptides: tracer for tumor targeting and angiogenesis imaging with improved biokinetics. J Nucl Med 2001; 42:326–336.

33. Chen JQ, Cheng Z, Owen NK, et al. Evaluation of an ^{111}In-DOTA-Rhenium cyclized α-MSH analog: a novel cyclic-peptide analog with improved tumor-targeting properties. J Nucl Med 2001; 42:1847–1855.

34. Krenning EP, Kwekkeboom DJ, Pauwels S, Kvols LK, Reubi JC. Somatostatin receptor scintigraphy. Nucl Med Ann 1995;1–50.

35. van Eijck CH, de Jong M, Breeman WA, Slooter GD, Marquet RL, Krenning EP. Somatostatin receptor imaging and therapy of pancreatic endocrine tumors. Ann Oncol 1999; 10:1777–1781.

36. Jamar F, Barone R, Mathieu I, et al. [86]Y-DOTA[0]-D-Phe[1]-Tyr[3]-octreotide (SMT487)—a phase 1 clinical study: pharmacokinetics, biodistribution and renal protective effect of different regimens of amino acid co-infusion. Eur J Nucl Med 2003; 30:510–518.

37. Paganelli G, Bodei L, Junak DH, et al. ^{90}Y-DOTA-D-Phe[1]-Tyr[3]-Octreotide in therapy of neuroendocrine malignancies. Biopolymers 2002; 66:393–398.

38. Pouget J-P, Mather SJ. General aspects of the cellular response to low- and high-LET radiation. Eur J Nucl Med 2001; 28:541–561.

39. Thakur ML, Coss R, Howell R, et al. Role of lipid soluble complexes in targeted tumor therapy. J Nucl Med 2003; 44:1293–1300.

40. O'Donoghue JA, Bardies M, Wheldon TE. Relationships between tumor size and curability for uniformly targeted therapy with beta-emitting radionuclides. J Nucl Med 1995; 36:1902–1909.

41. Buscombe JR, Caplin ME, Hilson AJW. Long-term efficacy of high-activity ^{111}In-pentetreotide therapy in patients with disseminated neuroendocrine tumors. J Nucl Med 2003; 44:1–6.

42. De Jong M, Breeman WAP, Bernard HF, et al. Therapy of neuroendocrine tumors with radiolabeled somatostatin-analogues. Q J Nucl Med 1999; 43:356–366.
43. McCarthy KE, Woltering EA, Anthony LB. In situ radiotherapy with ^{111}In-pentetreotide. state of the art and perspectives. Q J Nucl Med 2000; 44:88–95.
44. Argiris A, Peccerillo K, Murren JR, Cornelius E, Modlin IM. Phase I/II trial with ^{111}In-pentetreotide in patients with advanced malignancies (abstract). Dig Dis Week 2000;2748.
45. Silvester J. Consequences of Indium-111 decay in vivo: calculated absorbed radiation dose to cells labeled by Indium-111 oxine. J Lab Comp Radiopharm 1978; 19:196–197.
46. Kwekkeboom DJ, Bakker WH, Kooij PPM, et al. [^{177}Lu-DOTA^0,Tyr^3]octreotate: comparison with [^{111}In-DTPA^0]octreotide in patients. Eur J Nucl Med 2001; 28:1319–1325.
47. Krenning EP, Bakker WH, Breeman WA, et al. Localization of endocrine-related tumors with radioiodinated analogue of somatostatin. Lancet 1989; 4:242–244.
48. Hnatowich DJ, Layne WW, Childs RL. The preparation and labeling of DTPA-coupled albumin. Int J Appl Radiat Isot 1982; 33:327–332.
49. Breeman WAP, van Hagen PM, Kwekkeboom DJ, Visser TJ, Krenning EP. Somatostatin receptor scintigraphy using [^{111}In-DTPA^0]RC-160 in humans: a comparison with [^{111}In-DTPA^0]octreotide. Eur J Nucl Med 1998; 25:182–186.
50. Reubi JC, Schär J-C, Waser B, Mengod G. Expression and localization of Somatostatin receptor STR1, SSTR2, and SSTR3 messanger RNAs in primary human tumors using in situ hybridization. Cancer Res 1994; 54:3455–3459.
51. Nilsson O, Kölby L, Wängberg B, et al. Comparative studies on the expression of somatostatin receptor subtypes, outcome of octreotide scintigraphy and response to octreotide treatment in patients with carcinoid tumors. Br J Cancer 1998; 77:632–637.
52. Reubi JC, Waser B. Concomitant expression of several peptide receptors in neuroendocrine tumors: molecular basis for in vivo multireceptor tumor targeting. Eur J Nucl Med 2003; 30:781–793.
53. Kvols LK. Somatostatin-receptor imaging of human malignancies: a new era in the localization, staging, and treatment of tumors. Gastroenterology 1993; 105:1909–1914.
54. Forssell-Aronsson EB, Nilsson O, Benjegård SA, et al. ^{111}In-DTPA-D-Phe^1-octreotide binding and somatostatin receptor subtypes in thyroid tumors. J Nucl Med 2000; 41:636–642.
55. Virgolini I, Pangerl T, Bischof C, Smith-Jones P. Peck-radosavljevic M. Somatostatin receptor subtype expression in human tissue: a prediction for diagnosis and treatment of cancer? Eur J Clin Invest 1997; 27:645–647.
56. Kirsch CM, von Pawel J, Grau I, Tatsch K. Indium-111 pentetreotide in the diagnostic work-up of patients with bronchogenic carcinoma. Eur J Nucl Med 1994; 21:1318–1325.
57. O'Byrne KJ, Halmos G, Pinski J, et al. Somatostatin receptor expression in lung cancer. Eur J Cancer 1994; 30A:1682–1687.
58. Kwekkeboom DJ, Kho GS, Lamberts SWJ, Reubi JC, Laissue JA, Krenning EP. The value of Octreotide scintigraphy in patients with lung cancer. Eur J Nucl Med 1994; 21:1106–1113.

59. Bombardieri E, Crippa F, Cataldo I, et al. Somatostatin receptor imaging of small cell lung cancer (SCLC) by means of ^{111}In-DTPA octreotide scintigraphy. Eur J Cancer 1995; 31A:184–188.

60. Traub T, Petkov V, Ofluoglu S, et al. ^{111}In-DOTA-lanreotide scintigraphy in patients with tumors of the lung. J Nucl Med 2001; 42:1309–1315.

61. Lipp RW, Silly H, Ranner G, et al. Radiolabeled octreotide for the demonstration of somatostatin receptors in malignant lymphoma and lymphadenopathy. J Nucl Med 1995; 36:13–18.

62. Lugtenburg PJ, Löwenberg B, Valkema R, et al. Somatostatin receptor scintigraphy in the initial staging of low-grade non-Hodgkin's lymphomas. J Nucl Med 2001; 42:222–229.

63. Hofland LJ, Lamberts SWJ, van Hagen M, et al. Crucial role for somatostatin receptor Subtype 2 in determining the uptake of [^{111}In-DTPA-D-Phe[1]]octreotide in somatostatin receptor-positive organs. J Nucl Med 2003; 44:1315–1321.

64. Weiner RE, Thakur ML. Radiolabeled peptides in oncology: role in diagnosis and treatment. Bio Drugs 2005; 19:145–163.

65. Andersson P, Forssell-Aronsson E, Johanson V, et al. Internalization of Indium-111 into human neuroendocrine tumor cells after incubation with Indium-111-DTPA-D-Phe[1]-octreotide. J Nucl Med 1996; 37:2002–2006.

66. Janson ET, Westlin JE, Ohrvall U, Oberg K, Lukinius A. Nuclear localization of ^{111}In after intravenous injection of [^{111}In-DTPA-D-Phe[1]]-octreotide in patients with neuroendocrine tumors. J Nucl Med 2000; 41:1514–1518.

67. Hornick CA, Anthony CT, Hughey S, Gebhardt BM, Espenan GD, Woltering EA. Progressive nuclear translocation of somatostatin analogs. J Nucl Med 2000; 41:1256–1263.

68. Sumpio BE, Maack T. Kinetics, competition, and selectively of tubular absorption of proteins. Am J Physiol 1982; 243:F379–F392.

69. Lang L, Jagoda E, Wu C, et al. Factors influencing the in vivo pharmacokinetics of peptides and antibody fragments: the pharmacokinetics of two PET-labeled low molecular weight proteins. Q J Nucl Med 1997; 41:53–61.

70. de Jong M, Valkema R, van Gameren A, et al. Inhomogeneous localization of radioactivity in the human kidney after injection of [^{111}In-DTPA]octerotide. J Nucl Med 2004; 45:1168–1171.

71. Hammond PJ, Wade AF, Gwilliam ME, et al. Amino acid infusion blocks renal tubular uptake of an Indium-labeled Somatostatin analogue. Br J Cancer 1994; 67:1437–1439.

72. de Jong M, Rolleman EJ, Bernard BF, et al. Inhibition of renal uptake of Indium-111-DTPA-octerotide in vivo. J Nucl Med 1996; 37:1388–1392.

73. Rolleman EJ, Valkema R, de Jong M, Kooij PPM, Krenning EP. Safe and effective inhibition of renal uptake of radiolabelled octreotide by a combination of lysine and arginine. Eur J Nucl Med 2003; 30:9–15.

74. Christensen EI, Nielsen S. Structural and functional features of protein handling in the kidney proximal tubule. Semin Nephrol 1991; 11:414–439.

75. Rolleman EJ, Krenning, van Gameren A, Bernard BF, de Jong M. Uptake of ^{111}In-DTPA[0]]octreoide in the rat kidney is inhibited by colchicine and not by fructose. J Nucl Med 2004; 45:709–713.

76. Duncan JR, Welch MJ. Intracellular metabolism of Indium-111-DTPA-labeled receptor targeted proteins. J Nucl Med 1993; 34:1728–1738.

77. Duncan JR, Stephenson MT, Wu HP, Anderson CJ. Indium-111-diethylenetria-triaminepentaacetic acid-octreotide is delivered in vivo to pancreatic, tumor cell, renal, and hepatocyte lysosomes. Cancer Res 1997; 57:659–671.

78. Bass LA, Lanahan MV, Duncan JR, et al. Identification of the soluble in vivo metabolites of Indium-111-diethylenetriaminepentaacetic acid-D-Phe[1]-octreotide. Bioconjug Chem 1998; 9:192–200.

79. Whetstone PA, Akizawa H, Meares CF. Evaluation of cleavable (Tyr[3])-octreoate derivatives for longer intracellular probe residence. Bioconjug Chem 2004; 15:647–657.

80. Waldherr C, Pless M, Maecke H, Schumacher E, Nitzsche, Mueller J. Improvement of life quality in patients with advanced neuroendocrine tumors after treatment with 200 MCI/M^2 ^{90}Y-DOTATOC (abstr). J Nucl Med 2001; 42:37.

81. Otte A, Jermann E, Béhé M, et al. DOTATOC: a powerful new tool for receptor-mediated radionuclide therapy. Eur J Nucl Med 1997; 24:792–795.

82. Otte A, Mueller-Brand J, Dellas S, Nitzsche EU, Hermann R, Maecke HR. Yttrium-90-labelled somatostatin-analogue for cancer treatment. Lancet 1998; 351:417–418.

83. Otte A, Hermann R, Heppeler A, et al. Yttrium-90 DOTATOC: First clinical results. Eur J Nucl Med 1999; 26:1439–1447.

84. Modlin IM, Kidd M, Hinoue T, Lye KD, Murren J, Argiris A. Molecular strategies and 111in-labelled somatostatin analogues in defining the management of neuroendocrine tumor disease: a new paradigm for surgical management. Surgeon 2003; 1:137–143.

85. Krenning BJ, Konings IR, Norenberg JP, De Jong M, Kvols LK, Kusewitt DF. Long-term histological organ damage in animals following peptide receptor radionuclide therapy (PRRT) with high doses of ^{90}Y- and ^{111}In-labeled [DOTA^0,Tyr^3]octreotide (DOTATOC) (abstract). J Nucl Med 2001; 42:37.

86. Kwekkeboom DJ, Bakker WH, Kam BL, et al. Treatment of patients with gastroenteropancreatic (GEP) tumors with the novel radiolabelled somatostatin analogue [^{177}Lu-DOTA^0,Tyr^3]octreotate. Eur J Nucl Med 2003; 30:417–422.

87. de Jong M, Breeman WAP, Bernard BF, et al. [^{177}Lu-DOTA^0,Tyr^3]octreotate for somatostatin receptor-targeted radionuclide therapy. Int J Cancer 2001; 92:628–633.

88. Virgolini I, Szilvasi I, Kurtaran A, et al. Indium-111-DOTA-lanreotide: biodistribution, safety and radiation absorbed dose in tumor patients. J Nucl Med 1998; 39:1928–1936.

89. Smith-Jones PM, Bischof C, Leimer M, et al. DOTA-lanreotide: a novel somatostatin analog for tumor diagnosis and therapy. Endocrinology 1999; 140:5136–5148.

90. NeoTect, Package insert. Londonderry (NH): Diatide, 1999. http://www.fda.gov/oder/foi/label/1992/210121b1.pdf accessed 3/9/06.

91. Pearson DA, Lister-James J, McBride WJ, et al. Thrombus imaging using technetium-99m-labeled high-potency GPIIb/IIIa receptor antagonists. Chemistry and initial biological studies. J Med Chem 1996; 39:1372–1382.

92. Virgolini I, Leimer M, Handmaker H, et al. Somatostatin receptor subtype specificity and in vivo binding of a novel tumor tracer. ^{99m}Tc-P829. Cancer Res 1998; 58:1850–1859.

93. Vallabhajosula S, Moyer BR, Lister-James J, et al. Preclinical evaluation of technetium-99m-labeled somatostatin receptor-binding peptides. J Nucl Med 1996; 37:1016–1022.

94. Magram MY, Edelman MJ, Forero A, et al. A novel Rhenium-188 labelled somatostatin receptor (SSTR) targeting peptide, P2045, as potential targeted therapy for lung cancer (abstract). J Nucl Med 2003; 44:137.

95. Béhé M, Behr TM. Cholecystokinin-B (CCK-B)/gastrin receptor targeting peptides for staging and therapy of medullary thyroid cancer and other CCK-B receptor expressing malignancies. Biopolymers 2002; 66:399–418.

96. Behr TM, Jenner N, Radetzky S. Targeting of cholecystokinin-B/gastrin receptors in vivo: Preclinical and initial clinical evaluation of the diagnostic and therapeutic potential of radiolabelled gastrin. Eur J Nucl Med 1998; 25:424–430.

97. Behr TM, Jenner N, Béhé M, et al. Radiolabeled peptides for targeting cholecystokinin-B/gastrin receptor-expressing tumors. J Nucl Med 1999; 40:1029–1044.

98. de Jong M, Bakker WH, Bernard BF, et al. Preclinical and initial clinical evaluation of ^{111}In-labeled nonsulfated CCK_8 analog: a peptide for CCK-B receptor-targeted scintigraphy and radionuclide therapy. J Nucl Med 1999; 40:2081–2087.

99. Reubi JC, Schär J-C, Waser B. Cholecystokinin (CCK)- A and CCK-B/gastrin receptors in human tumors. Cancer Res 1997; 57:1377–1386.

100. Jensen RT, Qian JM, Lin JT, Mantey SA, Pisegna JR, Wank SA. Distinguishing multiple CCK receptor subtypes. Studies with guinea pig chief cells and transfected human CCK receptors. Ann NY Acad Sci 1994; 713:88–106.

101. Aloj L, Caraco C, Panico M, et al. In vitro and in vivo evaluation of ^{111}In-DTPAGlu-G-CCK8 for cholecystokinin-B receptor imaging. J Nucl Med 2004; 45:485–494.

102. Kwekkeboom DJ, Bakker WH, Kooij PPM, et al. Cholecystokinin receptor imaging using an octapeptide DTPA-CCK analogue in patients with medullary thyroid carcinoma. Eur J Nucl Med 2000; 27:1312–1317.

103. Mäcke HR, Riesen A, Ritter W. The molecular structure of Indium-DTPA. J Nucl Med 1989; 30:1235–1239.

104. Reubi JC, Waser B, Schaer JC, et al. Unsulfated DTPA-and DOTA-CCK analogs as specific high-affinity ligands for CCK-B receptor-expressing human and rat tissues in vitro and in vivo. Eur J Nucl Med 1998; 25:481–490.

105. Breeman WAP, de Jong M, Erion JL, et al. Preclinical comparison of ^{111}In-Labeled DTPA-or DOTA-bombesin analogs for receptor-targeted scintigraphy and radionuclide therapy. J Nucl Med 2002; 43:1650–1656.

106. Knight LC. Radiolabeled peptides for tumor imaging. In: Welch M, Redvanly C, eds. Handbook of Radiopharmaceuticals: Radiochemistry and Applications. West Sussex, U.K.: John Wiley Publishers, 2003:643–684.

107. Breeman WAP, de Jong M, Bernard BF, et al. Preclinical evaluation of [^{111}In-DTPA-Pro^1, Tyr^4] -bombesin, a new radioligand for bombesin-receptor scintigraphy. Int J Cancer 1999; 83:657–663.

108. Hoffman TJ, Gali H, Smith CJ, et al. Novel series of ^{111}In-labeled bombesin analogs as potential radiopharmaceuticals for specific targeting of gastrin releasing peptide receptors expressed on human prostate cancer cells. J Nucl Med 2003; 44:823–831.

109. Van de Wiele C, Dumont F, Dierckx RA, et al. Biodistribution and dosimetry of ^{99m}Tc-RP527, a gastrin-releasing peptide (GRP) agonist for the visualization of GRP receptor-expressing malignancies. J Nucl Med 2001; 42:1722–1727.

110. Karra SR, Schibli R, Gali H, et al. ^{99m}Tc-labeling and in vivo studies of a bombesin analog with a novel water-soluble dithiadiphosphine-based bifunctional chelating agent. Bioconjugate Chem 1999; 10:254–260.

111. Condamine E, Chapdeleine G, Demarcy L, et al. Biological activity and three-dimensional structure of an agonist analog of bombesin. J Pept Res 1998; 51:55–64.

112. Rogers BE, Rosenfeld ME, Khazaeli MB, et al. Localization of iodine-125-mIP-Des-Met14-bombesin (7-13)NH$_2$ in ovarian carcinoma induced to express the gastrin releasing peptide receptor by adenoviral vector-mediated gene transfer. J Nucl Med 1997; 38:1221–1229.

113. Hnatowich DJ. Antibody radiolabeling, problems and promises. Nucl Med Biol 1990; 17:49–55.

114. Gali H, Hoffman TJ, Sieckman GL, Owen NK, Katti KV, Volkert WA. Synthesis, characterization, and labeling with ^{99m}Tc/^{188}Re of peptide conjugates containing a dithiabisphosphine chelating agent. Bioconjug Chem 2001; 12:354–363.

115. Smith CJ, Gali H, Sieckman GL, Higginbotham C, Volkert WA, Hoffman TJ. Radiochemical investigations of ^{99m}Tc-N$_3$S-X-BBN[7-14]NH$_2$: an in vitro/in vivo structure-activity relationship study where X = 0-, 3-, 5-, 8-, and 11-carbon tethering moieties. Bioconjug Chem 2003; 14:93–102.

115a. Smith CJ, Gali H, Sieckman GL, et al. Radiochemical investigations of ^{177}Lu-DOTA-8Aoc-BBN[7-14]NH$_2$: an in vitro/in vivo assessment of the targeted ability of this new radioparhamceutical for PC3 human prosate cancer cells. Nuc Med Biol 2003; 30:101–109.

116. Breeman WAP, Hofland LJ, de Jong M, et al. Evaluation of radiolabeled bombesin analogs for receptor-targeted scintigraphy and radiotherapy. Int J Cancer 1999; 81:658–665.

117. Van de Wiele C, Dumont F, Broecke RV, et al. Technetium-99m RP527, a GRP analog for visualization of GRP receptor-expressing malignancies: a feasibility study. Eur J Nucl Med 2000; 27:1694–1699.

118. Bard DR, Knight CG, Page-Thomas DP. A chelating derivative of alpha-melanocyte stimulating hormones as a potential imaging agent for malignant melanoma. Br J Cancer 1990; 62:919–922.

119. Froidevaux S, Calame-Christe M, Tanner H, Sumanovski L, Eberle AN. A novel DOTA-α-melanocyte-stimulating hormone analog for metastatic melanoma diagnosis. J Nucl Med 2002; 43:1699–1706.

120. Kadekaro AL, Kanto H, Kavangh R, Abdel-Malek ZA. Significance of the melanocortin 1 receptor in regulating human melanocyte pigmentation proliferation and survival. Ann N Y Acad Sci 2003; 994:359–365.

121. Siegrist W, Solca F, Stutz S, et al. Characterization of receptors for alpha-melanocyte-stimulating hormone on human melanoma cells. Cancer Res 1989; 49:6352–6358.

122. Tatro JB, Entwistle ML, Lester BR, Reichlin S. Melanotropin receptors of murine melanoma characterized in cultured cells and demonstrated in experimental tumors in situ. Cancer Res 1990; 50:1237–1242.

123. Hruby VJ, Sharma SD, Toth K, et al. Design, synthesis, and conformation of super potent and prolonged acting melanotropins. Ann N Y Acad Sci 1993; 680:51–63.

124. Adams G, Olivier GW, Branch SK, Moss SH, Notarianni LJ, Pouton CW. Evidence for the ingernalization of [^{125}I-Tyr^2, Nle^4, D-Phe^7] alpha-MSH following binding to the MSH receptor of B16 murine melanoma cells. Ann N Y Acad Sci 1993; 680:440–441.

125. Cody WL, Mahoney M, Knittel JJ, Hruby VJ, Castrucci AM, Hadley ME. Cyclic melanotropins. 9. 7-D-Phenylalanine analogues of the active-site sequence. J Med Chem 1985; 28:583–588.

126. Wraight EP, Bard DR, Maughan TS, Knight CG, Page-Thomas DP. The use of a chelating derivative of alpha melanocyte stimulating hormone for the clinical imaging of malignant melanoma. Br J Cancer 1992; 65:112–118.

127. Bagutti C, Stolz B, Albert R, Bruns C, Pless J, Eberie AN. [^{111}In]DTPA-labeled analogues of alpha-melanocyte-stimulating hormones for melanoma targeting: receptor binding in vitro and in vivo. Int J Cancer 1994; 58:749–755.

128. Chen JQ, Giblin MF, Wang N, Jurisson SS, Quinn TP. In vivo evaluation of ^{99m}Tc/^{188}Re-labeled linear alpha-melanocyte stimulating hormone analogs for specific melanoma targeting. Nucl Med Biol 1999; 26:687–693.

129. Cheng Z, Chen J, Quinn TP, Jurisson SS. Radioiodination of Rhenium cyclized α-melanocyte-stimulating hormone resulting in enhanced radioactivity localization and retention in melanoma. Cancer Res 2004; 64:1411–1418.

130. Miao Y, Owen NK, Whitener D, Gallazzi F, Hoffman TJ, Quinn TP. In vivo evaluation of ^{188}Re-labeled alpha-melanocyte stimulating hormone peptide analogs for melanoma therapy. Int J Cancer 2002; 101:480–487.

131. Froidevaux S, Calame-Christe M, Schuhmacher J, et al. A gallium-labeled novel DOTA-α-melanocyte-stimulating hormone analog for PET imaging of melanoma metastatic. J Nucl Med 2004; 45:116–123.

132. Gambhir SS, Czernin J, Schwimmer J, Silverman DHS, Coleman RE, Phelps ME. A tabulated summary of the FDG PET literature. J Nucl Med 2001; 42:1S–93S.

133. Mukherjee S, Ghosh RN, Maxifield FR. Endocytosis. Physiol Rev 1997; 77:759–803.

134. Authier F, Posner BI, Bergeron JJM. Endosomal proteolysis of internalized proteins. FEBS Lett 1996; 389:55–60.

135. Leikens S, De Clercq E, Neyts J. Angiogensis regulators and clinical applications. Biochem Biopharmacol 2001; 61:253–270.

136. Brooks PC, Cheresh DA. Requirement of vascular integrin alpha$_v$beta$_3$ for angiogenesis. Science 1994; 264:569–571.

137. Shattil SJ, Gao J, Kashiwagi H. Not just another pretty face regulation of platelet function at the cytoplasmic face of integrin alpha IIbbeta 3. Thromb Haemost 1997; 74:220–225.

138. Janssen ML, Oyen WJ, Dijkgraaf I, et al. Tumor targeting with radiolabeled α$_v$β$_3$ integrin binding peptides in a nude mouse model. Cancer Res 2002; 62:6146–6151.

139. Pfaff M, Tangemann K, Muller B, et al. Selective recognition of cyclic RGD peptides of NMR defined conformation by α$_{II}$β$_3$, α$_V$β$_3$ and α$_5$β$_1$ integrins. J Biol Chem 1994; 269:20233–20238.

140. van Hagen PM, Breeman WAP, Bernard HF, et al. Evaluation of a radiolabeled cyclic DTPA-RGD analogue for tumor imaging and radionuclide therapy. Int J Cancer 2000; 90:186–198.

141. Ogawa M, Kentaro H, Oishi S, et al. Direct electrophilic radiofluorination of a cyclic RGD peptide for in vivo $\alpha_V\beta_3$ integrin related tumor imaging. Nucl Med Biol 2003; 30:1–9.

142. Chen X, Park R, Shahinian AH, Bading JR, Conti PS. Pharmacokinetics and tumor retention of ^{125}I-labeled RGD peptide are improved by PEGylation. Nucl Med Biol 2004; 31:11–19.

143. Su ZF, He J, Rusckowski M, Hnatowich DJ. In vitro cell studies of Technetium-99m labeled RGD-HYNIC peptide, a comparison of tricine and EDDA as co-ligands. Nucl Med Biol 2003; 30:141–149.

144. Haubner R, Kuhnast B, Mang C, et al. [18F]Galacto-RGD: synthesis, radiolabeling, metabolic stability and radiation dose estimates. Bioconjug Chem 2004; 15:61–69.

145. Chen X, Park R, Shahinian AH, et al. 18F-labeled RGD peptide: initial evaluation for imaging brain tumor angiogenesis. Nucl Med Biol 2004; 31:179–189.

146. McQuade P, Knight LC, Welch MJ. Evaluation of ^{64}Cu-and[125]I-radiolabeled as potential agents for targeting $\alpha_V\beta_3$ integrins in tumor angiogenesis. Bioconjug Chem 2004; 15:988–996.

147. Su ZF, Liu G, Gupta S, Zhu Z, Rusckowski M, Hnatowich DJ. In vitro and in vivo evaluation of a Technetium-99m-labeled cyclic RGD peptide as a specific marker of $\alpha_V\beta_3$ integrin for tumor imaging. Bioconjug Chem 2002; 13:561–570.

148. Haubner R, Weber W. Comment on "In vitro and in vivo evaluation of a Technetium-99m-labeled cyclic RGD peptide as a specific marker of $\alpha_V\beta_3$ integrin for tumor imaging". Bioconjug Chem 2003; 14:274.

4

The Labeling of Peptides with Positron-Emitting Radionuclides: The Importance of PET in Cancer Diagnosis

Stefano Papi, Nicoletta Urbano, Esteban R. Obenaus,
and Marco Chinol

Division of Nuclear Medicine, European Institute of Oncology, Milan, Italy

INTRODUCTION

The impressive developments in technology, with advancements in computer processing capabilities during the past 15 years, have positively affected almost all medical specialities, allowing more efficient processing of vast amounts of imaging data.

In this regard Positron Emission Tomography (PET) represents, among the available imaging techniques, the standard of excellence. The high sensitivity and very good spatial resolution of PET scanners have revolutionized the field of Nuclear Medicine and provided a new leading tool in oncologic, cardiac, and neurologic imaging.

Nowadays, PET plays an important role in the evaluation of malignant disease where it allows the in-vivo visualization of tissue function, representing, therefore, an important tool for the development of anticancer strategies. It is widely used in the diagnosis and staging of primary tumors, detection of subclinical disease, and recurrence and assessment of therapy response. Moreover, it offers the capability to determine the quantitative uptake kinetics for intra-individual therapy planning and control. PET can visualize very small metastatic lesions, including tumor growth in regional lymph nodes, with better resolution and lower radioactivity dose than that normally required for planar or Single Photon Emission Computed Tomography (SPECT) gamma-camera imaging.

With these promising advantages, the application of positron-labeled bioactive peptides has emerged as a useful and dynamic field in nuclear oncology (1–6). The fast blood clearance makes the radiolabeled peptides useful carriers to be used with short-lived positron emitters. Peptides-based PET tracers involve not only somatostatin (SS) analogs, which have already gained considerable impact on diagnostic nuclear medicine and Peptide Receptor-mediated Radionuclide Therapy (PRRT) during the last ten years, but also bombesin (BN), gastrin-releasing peptide (GRP), vasoactive intestinal peptide (VIP) analogs, and recently, cyclic peptides which are playing an important role in development and application of anti-angiogenic therapies (7) and new drugs (8). The α_v-integrins ($\alpha_v\beta_3$, $\alpha_v\beta_5$) could be attractive for antiangiogenic treatment of malignant gliomas (9) that remain largely incurable despite intensive multimodality treatments. Besides their use as PET imaging agents, these peptides might be a tool for research on individual receptor status and for optimal fine tuning of PRRT.

THE DIFFERENT POSITRON-EMITTING RADIOISOTOPES

The first step in a development of a PET radiopharmaceutical is, apart from the choice of the target molecule, the choice of the most suitable radioisotope for the intended use. Several parameters have to be taken into account: the half-life, the availability and mode(s) of production, the types of emissions and, last but not least, some considerations on the energy of the positron which reflect into radioprotection issues and in its intrinsic spatial resolution. All the physical and chemical properties of the chosen radionuclide will drive the radiolabeling/purification strategies in the next steps. Table 1 lists the most common positron-emitters employed in the labeling of bioactive peptides.

Fluorine-18 (^{18}F)

[18]F ($T_{1/2} = 109.7$ minutes, $E\beta^+_{max} = 634$ KeV, 96.7% abundance) represents the ideal radionuclide for PET (10) because of its physico-chemical properties. Fluorine is the element with the highest electronegativity, resulting in a very small radius and, in fact, it can substitute hydrogen atoms without steric hindrance. Provided that changing H for F does not alter too much the electronic distribution of the molecule, usually fluorinated molecules are not affected in their biological properties, especially if their molecular weight is relatively high. In other cases, as in [18F]-2-fluoro-2-deoxyglucose ([18F]-FDG), insertion of ^{18}F is the key feature to trap the radiopharmaceutical inside the cell and thus to achieve the diagnostic signal. Moreover, the low β^+ energy results in optimal image resolution and the high abundance of positron decay generates high signals

Table 1   Physical properties of positron-emitting radioisotopes employed in the labeling of peptides. ^{86}Y and ^{124}I have more than 50 γ emissions: only the main lines are listed

Positron emitter	Production modes	$T_{1/2}$ (h)	Main β^+_{max} Energy (keV)	Abundance (%)	Main γ Energy (keV)	Abundance (%)	Intrinsic spatial resol. loss (mm)
^{18}F	^{18}O(p,n)^{18}F ^{20}Ne(d,α)^{18}F	1.83	634	96.7	–	–	0.7
^{68}Ga	^{68}Ge/^{68}Ga Generator	1.13	1899 822	87.9 1.2	–	–	2.4
^{66}Ga	^{66}Zn(p,n)^{66}Ga	9.50	4200 924	56.0 3.7	–	–	–
^{64}Cu	^{64}Ni(p,n)^{64}Cu ^{64}Ni(d,2n)^{64}Cu	12.70	653	17.4	–	–	0.7
^{86}Y	^{86}Sr(p,n)^{86}Y ^{nat}Rb(^{3}He,2n)^{86}Y	14.70	1221 1545 2021	12.5 5.6 3.6	443 628 646 703 777 1077 1153 1854 1921	16.9 32.6 9.2 15.4 22.4 82.5 30.5 17.2 20.8	1.8
^{124}I	^{124}Te(p,n)^{124}I ^{124}Te(d,2n)^{124}I ^{125}Te(p,2n)^{124}I	100.2	1535 2138	11.2 11.2	603 723 1691	62.9 10.1 10.6	2.3
^{110m}In	^{110}Cd(p,n)^{110m}In ^{110}Sn/^{110m}In Generator	1.15	2260	62.0	–	–	–

with low amount of radioactivity. The ease of production of ^{18}F makes it very attractive, nevertheless, a medical cyclotron is needed, although its half life allows remote supply of ^{18}F to a satellite lab. ^{18}F can be obtained with different nuclear reactions, but it is usually produced by ^{18}O(p,n)^{18}F nuclear reaction, bombarding enriched ^{18}O-water with protons to give [^{18}F]-fluoride. Theoretically, if 100% of conversion is obtained, [^{18}F]-Fluoride should have an intrinsic specific activity of about 1710Ci/μmole but, due to the decay and the saturation yield of the cyclotron, usually much lower amounts of [^{18}F]-Fluoride are produced in a 2mL target, generally not more than 4-5Ci. Another method is to produce gaseous [^{18}F]-F$_2$ (with the ^{20}Ne(d,α)^{18}F reaction), suitable for aromatic electrophilic substitutions, but in this case it is not possible to achieve high specific activity in the labeling and there is a theoretical 50% yield limitation due to the diatomic nature of [^{18}F]-F$_2$. A more convenient method for electrophilic substitutions has been using [^{18}F]acetyl-hypofluorite, but recently linking ^{18}F to aromatic ring is accomplished through aromatic nucleophilic substitutions.

Gallium-68 (^{68}Ga)

^{68}Ga ($T_{1/2} = 68$ minutes, $\beta^+ = 89\%$, $E\beta^+_{max} = 1,92$ MeV, EC $= 11\%$) is a radionuclide of great practical interest for clinical PET (11). It is produced by physical decay from the parent ^{68}Ge, via different ^{68}Ge/^{68}Ga generators, commercially available or home-made. ^{68}Ga-radiopharmaceuticals can be thus developed without the need of an in-site cyclotron. Its short half-life allows application of suitable activities while maintaining an acceptable radiation dose to the patient. Moreover, its established metallic chemistry allows it to be stably bound to the carrier peptide sequence via a suitable bifunctional chelator (usually DOTA, DTPA). The major problems with ^{68}Ga are its chemical form and purity when eluted from the generators: in fact, for a successful labeling of peptides in nanomolar amounts, a high specific activity, concentration, and (radio)chemical purity are mandatory. For this reason, several efforts have been devoted to develop generators producing ^{68}Ga in high concentration and without chemical interfering species (i.e., chelators used for milking). ^{68}Ge breakthrough is, because of its long half life (270 days), a critical issue to ensure safety of the final radiopharmaceutical. The latest ^{68}Ge/^{68}Ga generators implement the formation of a tetrachloro complex $[^{68}GaCl_4]^-$ in strong hydrochloric acid: this can be retained onto an anion exchange cartridge, whereas all the metallic impurities (from the stationary phase and the same ^{68}Ge) are eluted in waste. The $[^{68}GaCl_4]^-$ complex is then destroyed with a small amount of water to give the free $^{68}Ga^{3+}$, eluted into the reaction vessel. This method allows both for purification and concentration of $^{68}Ga^{3+}$, thus ready for the labeling reaction of DOTA-peptides.

^{68}Ga-DOTATOC is a promising PET tracer for imaging neuroendocrine tumors (12–15) and their metastases (15), which may become of paramount importance for staging and therapy decisions. It allows quantitative assessment of tracer accumulation within tissues, which may be used for dosimetry and prediction of the efficiency of the ^{90}Y-DOTATOC therapy. Another specific advantage is low kidney accumulation. Generator-produced ^{68}Ga and the development of small chelator-coupled peptides with affinity to receptors over-expressed on a variety of human tumors may open a new generation of kit-formulated PET radiopharmaceuticals similar to routinely used ^{99m}Tc-based radiopharmaceuticals (11,16).

Other ^{68}Ga-radiopeptides have been also developed and pre-clinically tested for the targeting of melanocortin 1 receptor in melanoma treatment (17), and the BN receptor in patients with prostate cancer (18,19).

Gallium-66 (^{66}Ga)

More accurate PET-based quantitative evaluation of SS receptors in neuro-endocrine tumors were obtained with positron-emitting radiogallium isotopes (20–22). Among them, ^{66}Ga ($T_{1/2} = 9.5$ hours, $\beta^+ = 56\%$, $E\beta^+_{max} = 4.2$ MeV), is produced carrier-free by the cyclotron nuclear reaction $^{66}Zn(p,n)^{66}$Ga and, along with the isotope ^{68}Ga, shares the same metallic chemistry. Although its half life would be favourable for long term studies, the high positron energy is a drawback from the clinical point of view because of image resolution loss. Moreover, handling high energy positron emitters like ^{66}Ga requires care and safety by the radiochemist, whereas the development of (semi)automated synthesis modules would be appreciable. ^{66}Ga was also useful for therapy (21,22) due to its energetic positron emission, but the high radiation dose to the kidneys limits its use.

Copper-64 (^{64}Cu)

An attractive radionuclide readily produced on a medical cyclotron (23,24) is ^{64}Cu ($T_{1/2} = 12.7$ hours, EC $= 41\%$, E$\beta^-_{max} = 0.573$ MeV (40%), E$\beta^+_{max} = 0.656$ MeV (17.4%) and E$\gamma = 1.34$ MeV (0.5%). Due to its physical properties, it has shown its versatility in both PET imaging (4,25–27) and therapy (28,29) because of its favorable β^- particle emissions (30) as well as Auger electrons emissions (31) by its electron capture decay. Therefore, ^{64}Cu as efficient as ^{67}Cu for tumor treatment (32) results as an interesting radionuclides for combined PET/PRRT. The metallic properties of ^{64}Cu are somewhat similar to ^{68}Ga but to achieve high radiochemical stability of the complex, depending on the ionic radius, and the valence number of the radioisotope, different macrocyclic chelators (DOTA, TETA) or, better, cross-bridged ones (CB-TE2A, H$_2$CB-TE2A, H$_2$CB-DO2A) have been employed (33,34). These ligands have been shown to form Cu(II) complexes (35,36) with superior kinetic stability and improved biological behaviour compared to their nonbridged analogs (37,38).

Different ^{64}Cu-SS analogs were evaluated in animal models (28–30) and in patients with neuroendocrine tumors (4). Overexpression of the gastrin-releasing peptides receptor (GRPR) in a variety of neoplasms, such as breast, prostate, pancreatic, and small cell lung cancers, prompted the development of ^{64}Cu-labeled GRP analogs for PET imaging of GRPR-positive tumors. Recently, ^{64}Cu has been also used to label BN analogs for the detection of GRPR-positive tumors in a mouse model of human prostate cancer (26,39), VIP analogs in preclinical PET imaging studies of oncogene receptors overexpressed in breast and other cancers (40) and cyclic RGD peptide for PET imaging of α_v-integrin expression in breast cancer (8,41).

Yttrium-86 (^{86}Y)

^{90}Y is a pure β^- emitter widely used for therapeutic radiopharmaceuticals. Unfortunately, lacking of γ lines, it is not suitable for imaging; therefore dosimetric studies are conventionally carried out using the same molecule labeled with ^{111}In. Some concerns may arise on the assumption that no effect is played by ^{111}In for ^{90}Y substitution as regards to the biodistribution properties. Thanks to the advancements in nuclear technology, it is nowadays possible to utilize a β^+ analogue with the same coordination chemistry of ^{90}Y: its isotope ^{86}Y, which has been historically considered as a surrogate to mimic ^{90}Y in radiopharmaceuticals for dosimetric purposes. In fact, being the same element, it may be assumed that biodistribution will not be affected by the isotope change. ^{86}Y ($T_{1/2} = 14.7$ hours, $E\beta^+_{max} = 1.2$ MeV) can be produced in a cyclotron, as evidenced in 1993 by Rösch (42) and co-workers: they studied the nuclear data relevant to the production of ^{86}Y for medical purposes. Two nuclear reactions and relative excitation functions were studied: ^{86}Sr(p,xn)^{86,86m,85,85m}Y and ^{nat}Rb(^{3}He,xn)^{87,87m,86,86m,85,85m}Y. Their conclusion was that the ^{86}Sr pathway is favoured, using a medium-sized cyclotron and highest purity target, giving an integral thick target yield of 10.8mCi/µAh when the proton energy range is 14–10 MeV. Major impurities are ^{85,85m}Y raising from the ^{86}Sr(p,2n) reaction at high incident energy. Other impurities less relevant are ^{87,87m,88}Y and they depend on the isotopic abundance of ^{87}Sr and ^{88}Sr in the enriched ^{86}Sr target. Moreover, they developed an ion chromatographic method for purification of the irradiated target from other metals using α-hydroxyisobutyrate, thus to obtain carrier-free ^{86}Y ready for medical applications. ^{86}Y production requires high purity starting ^{86}Sr target, some fine tuning, and purification steps, but it is possible to achieve enough activity for labeling DOTA-derivatized ligands in carrier-free form.

In the treatment of patients with neuroendocrine tumors by ^{90}Y-DOTATOC and ^{90}Y-DOTA-peptide analogs, accurate pretherapeutic dosimetry would allow for individual planning of the optimal therapeutic strategy. The positron-emitting isotope ^{86}Y was used as surrogate of its isotope ^{90}Y (43,44) for DOTA-peptide analogs labeling (45–47). These PET tracers, chemically identical to the therapeutic agents, resulted the most authentic quantitative approach to measure the pharmacokinetics of ^{90}Y-DOTA-peptide analogs.

Iodine-124 (^{124}I)

The relatively long half-life of ^{124}I ($T_{1/2} = 100.2$ hours, $E\beta^+_{max} = 2.13$ MeV (23%), $E\gamma = 0.6$–1.69 MeV) that allows the in-vivo detection and quantification of longer-term biological processes, is suitable for labeling not only peptides but also monoclonal antibodies. This cyclotron-generated radionuclide can be prepared in advance and the traditional radioiodine labeling techniques can be carefully applied. However, the relatively low positron emission rate (23%) and several high-energy gamma emissions (0.60–1.69 MeV) could be unfavourable. Despite this fact, Iodine-124 is still considered an interesting radiohalogen for PET radiopharmaceuticals (48,49).

Indium-110m (^{110m}In)

Last but not least, ^{110m}In ($T_{1/2} = 69$ minutes, $E\beta^+_{max} = 2.26$ MeV (62%), $E\gamma = 0.658$ MeV) show similar characteristics to its analogue ^{111}In, widely used in

SPECT examinations. ^{110m}In can be produced either from a ^{110}Sn/^{110m}In generator or using the ^{110}Cd(p,n)^{110m}In nuclear reaction on low-energy cyclotrons. Because of its short half-life, ^{110m}In is suitable for the labeling of low molecular weight peptides with fast kinetics such as octreotide. Moreover, the availability of commercial kit ready for labeling with ^{110m}In makes it a potential tool for better temporal and spatial resolution than ^{111}In-octreotide SPECT (50).

LABELING REACTIONS WITH β$^+$ EMITTERS

Labeling with ^{18}F

Insertion of a ^{18}F halogen atom can only be obtained with a covalent C-F bond, stable to defluorination. In the glucose analogue [^{18}F]-FDG, the most common positron-emitting radiopharmaceutical approved for clinical use, fluorine is directly bond on the second carbon atom. It is taken up by cells with abnormal metabolism due to either increased need for or an inefficient glucose metabolism, such as cancer. In neuroendocrine tumors [^{18}F]-FDG has failed presumably due to the generally high differentiation grade and low anaerobic glycolysis of these tumors (51). For this reason, several groups are facing the task to develop new [^{18}F]-fluorinated molecules, especially peptides, which may become useful for cancer diagnosis. Taking the experience from [^{18}F]-FDG synthesis, [^{18}F]-fluoride is routinely used for labeling biomolecules using aliphatic/aromatic nucleophilic substitutions (S_N^1–S_N^2 reactions). The idea is to react a nucleophilic ^{18}F-fluoride atom with an electrophilic precursor, functionalized with a good leaving group. The nucleophilic behaviour of ^{18}F-fluoride is usually enhanced through a drying process and using phase-transfer catalysts like Kryptofix K222. Because of peptide chemical complexity, to drive the selectivity of the fluorination reaction it is often necessary to protect other potential functional groups and/or to prepare an intermediate fluorinated prosthetic group, which would be subsequently bound to the peptidic sequence. Initially this approach led to time-consuming ^{18}F-labeling approaches, requiring multi-step syntheses with low overall radiochemical yield (RCY) and, thus, limited applications. Octreotide and its derivatives are among the molecules most studied because of their great interest in neuroendocrine tumor imaging and it represents a model compound to test different fluorination techniques. Improvements in this field often have been obtained using octreotide derivatives and subsequently transferred to other molecules.

Over the past two decades, several fluorinated precursors have been developed. In 1987 Kilbourn published the synthesis of two [^{18}F]-reagents to label proteins, methyl 3-[^{18}F]fluoro-5-nitrobenzimidate and 4-[^{18}F]fluoro-phenacylbromide ([^{18}F]FPB), starting from 3,5-dinitrobenzonitrile and 4-nitro-benzonitrile respectively (52). The reagents can be prepared in moderate yields (30-50% EOB) in 50–70 minutes. This preliminary good result was anyway affected by 2–4 hours synthesis time and by the presence of competing species during the coupling to the proteins, resulting in pseudo-low specific activity that, when working with trace receptor amount, is one of the major issues. Vaidyanathan and Zalutsky introduced in 1992 (53) another precursor for labeling proteins, N-succinimidyl-4-[^{18}F]fluorobenzoate ([^{18}F]SFB). Starting from 4-formyl-N,N,N-trimethilanilinium triflate, they first obtained [^{18}F]fluoro-benzaldehyde, then it was oxidized to [^{18}F]fluorobenzoic acid and activated with N-hydroxysuccinimide (NHS)/dicyclohexylcarbodiimide (DCC) system. Although synthesis time was 100 minutes and overall RCY 25% decay corrected, [^{18}F]SFB was one of the first useful precursors for labeling peptides like octreotide. Two years later, the same group (54) improved the preparation of [^{18}F]SFB using disuccinimidyl carbonate (DSC) in place of NHS/DCC: by this method they shortened total reaction time by 45 minutes. Wester and colleagues published in 1996 another method (55) to obtain [^{18}F]SFB, starting from ethyl-N, N, N-trimethylammonium benzoate: the difficult oxidation step was replaced with a more convenient saponification to give [^{18}F]fluorobenzoic acid. Moreover, they used TSTU (a tetramethyluronium tetrafluoroborate salt) as activator for coupling NHS to [^{18}F]fluorobenzoic acid, because of its faster reactivity and ease of byproducts purification. In this way, he was able to prepare SFB in less time (35′) and with RCY ranging 50–60%. Synthesis of [^{18}F]fluorobenzoic acid ([^{18}F]FBA) is presented in Figure 1, whereas the different synthetic strategies to obtain [^{18}F]SFB are depicted in Figure 2.

The first [^{18}F]-octreotide analog appeared in 1994 by Guhlke et al. (56), using the activated 4-nitrophenyl ester of [^{18}F]fluoropropionic acid in two steps: acylation of N-terminal Phe and deprotection of Boc-Lys-Octreotide. They prepared 2-[^{18}F]fluoropropionyl-D-Phe^1-octreotide in 70% RCY after 30 minutes; moreover, using hydroxybenzotriazol catalysis, RCY was >90% in only 5 minutes (Fig. 3).

Downer in 1997 studied the reactivity of [^{18}F]fluorophenacylbromide ([^{18}F]FPB) for radiolabeling peptides (57), but their data suggested that octreotide was not a suitable target for labeling with [^{18}F]FPB. The same year Wester studied the pharmacokinetics of 2-[^{18}F]fluoropropionyl-D-Phe^1-octreo-tide; although tumor uptake was rapid, the short tumor residence time and its hepatobiliary excretion imposed further developments, to obtain a more

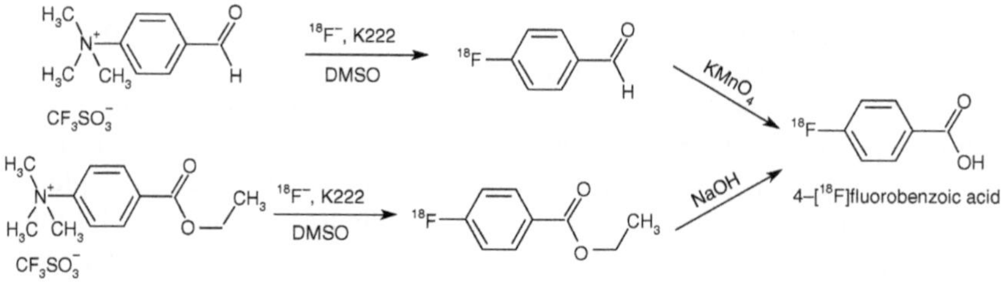

Figure 1 Synthesis of [^{18}F]fluorobenzoic acid ([^{18}F]FBA).

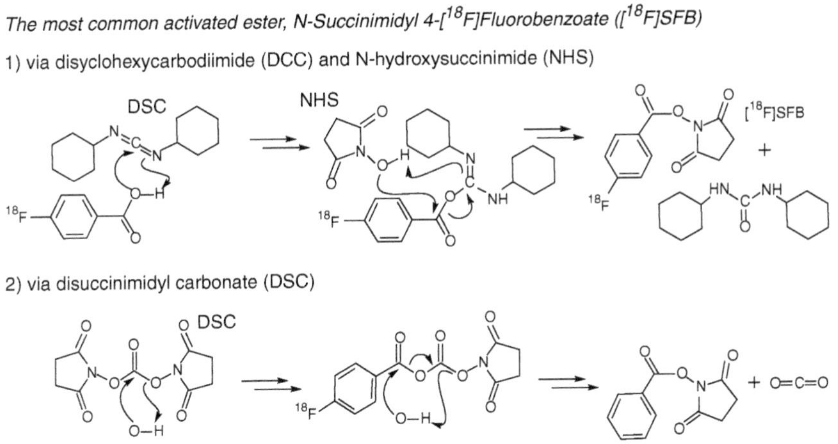
The most common activated ester, N-Succinimidyl 4-[18F]Fluorobenzoate ([18F]SFB)
1) via disyclohexycarbodiimide (DCC) and N-hydroxysuccinimide (NHS)
DSC
NHS
[18F]SFB
2) via disuccinimidyl carbonate (DSC)
DSC
+ O=C=O

Figure 2 Pathways of activation of 4-[^{18}F]fluorobenzoic acid ([^{18}F]FBA) for peptide coupling: from [^{18}F]FBA to [^{18}F]SFB.

hydrophilic derivative (58). In 2001 Okarvi (59) published an extensive overview of the progress in [^{18}F]-labeling of peptide radiopharmaceuticals; among the different methods cited, he enlightened the importance of [^{18}F]SFB obtained via TSTU; nevertheless, the [^{18}F]fluorobenzoyl- and [^{18}F]fluoropropionyl-octreotide so far studied showed unfavourable biological properties, claiming an improvement in pharmacokinetic behaviour of [^{18}F]-octreotide analogs. In 2002 Southcliffe-Goulden and colleagues (60) published a rapid solid phase synthesis and fluorination method of linear peptides, using [^{18}F]fluorobenzoic acid and HATU/DIPEA for coupling (Fig. 4). They achieved 80–90% RCY (decay corrected), with a radiochemical purity greater than 95% in an overall synthesis time of 20 minutes; however tumor uptake of these [^{18}F]fluorobenzoyl-peptides was still not selective.

The same year an interesting paper appeared by Schottelius et al. (61), showing that the pharmacokinetic of radioiodinated TOC can be improved when conjugated to carbohydrates. This approach gave to the biomolecule a more hydrophilic behaviour and partially overcame the liver uptake problem

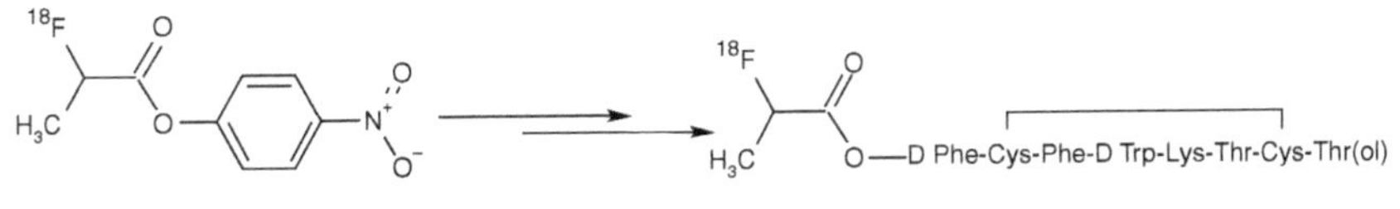
D Phe-Cys-Phe-D Trp-Lys-Thr-Cys-Thr(ol)

Figure 3 Synthesis of 2-[^{18}F]fluoropropionyl-D-Phe[1]-octreotide.

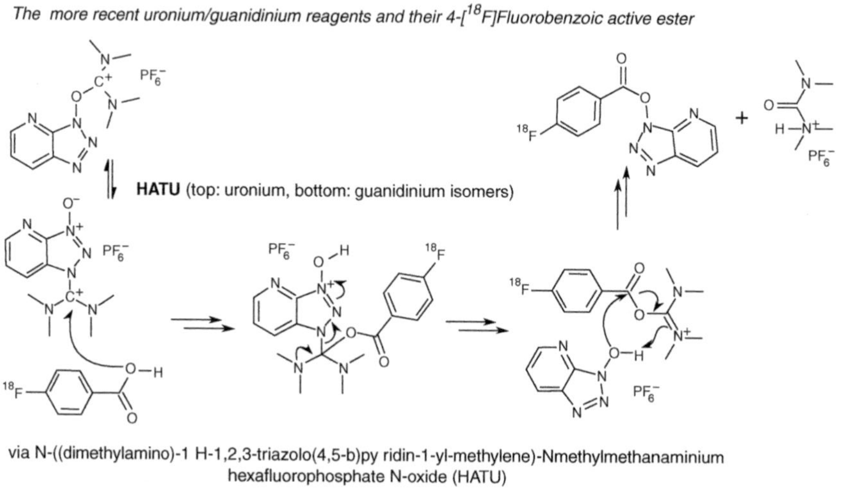

The *more recent uronium/guanidinium reagents and their 4-[18F]Fluorobenzoic active ester*

HATU (top: uronium, bottom: guanidinium isomers)

via N-((dimethylamino)-1 H-1,2,3-triazolo(4,5-b)py ridin-1-yl-methylene)-Nmethylmethanaminium hexafluorophosphate N-oxide (HATU)

Figure 4   Activation of [^{18}F]FBA via HATU.

previously encountered. In 2003 the same group published also (5) the synthesis of a novel ^{18}F labeled carbohydrated SS analogue ([^{18}F]FP-Gluc-TOCA), starting from the already described 4-nitrophenyl [^{18}F]fluoropropionate. [^{18}F]FP-Gluc-TOCA was completed in 3 hours with 20-30% yield (Fig. 5). The binding was specific and affinity for sstr was very high for subtype 2 (2.8nM), while LogP was rather low (-1.7). The idea was to use not a direct fluoropropionic moyety on D-Phe, but a trivalent Lys bridge between TOCA, Gluc, and FP, the latter being attached to Nε of Lys.

^{18}F-fluorothiols have also been proposed by Glaser in 2004 (62) as an alternative approach for chemoselective labeling of peptides. Their work showed the possibility to use fluorothiol derivatives as synthons for labeling

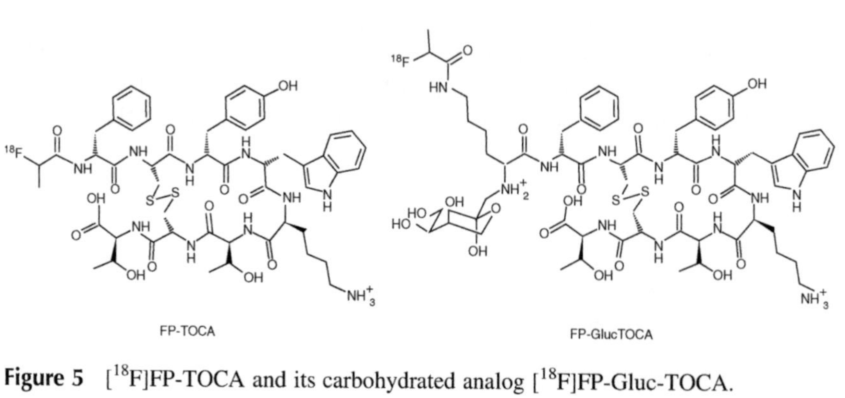

FP-TOCA   FP-GlucTOCA

Figure 5   [^{18}F]FP-TOCA and its carbohydrated analog [^{18}F]FP-Gluc-TOCA.

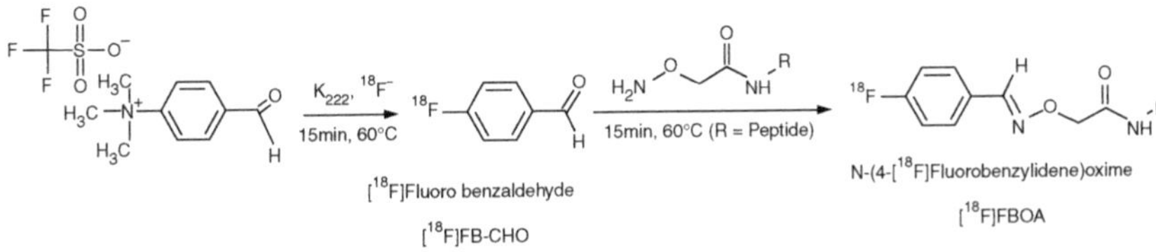

Figure 6   Formation of a N-fluorobenzylidene-oxime conjugate with peptides.

chloroacetylated model peptide, although the overall yield was not very high. A major improvement in the synthesis of fluorinated peptides was given by the group of Wester and presented in 2004 (45). They used a fast 2 step methodology for high yield radiofluorination (and radiohalogenation in general) of peptides, with a special emphasis on Octreotide. Their goal was based on the fact that appropriate radiofluorination methods for large scale production of [^{18}F]-peptides were lacking; they introduced a chemoselective synthesis of an oxime between a [^{18}F]-labeled aldehyde ([^{18}F]fluorobenzaldehyde) or ketone and an unprotected aminooxy-functionalized peptide, resulting in a N-fluorobenzylidene-oxime conjugate. They prepared a [^{18}F]fluorobenzilidene-oxime carbohydrated ana-logue of TOCA, studying parameters affecting the reaction, along with kinetics and biodistribution data. The conclusion was that this method combines rapid 2-step radiofluorination synthesis, stability against defluorination, favourable tumor uptake, and biodistribution. In Fig. 6 is a summary of these lately developed [^{18}F]fluorinated peptides.

The same group in 2004 expanded their work (63), detailing the synthesis of ^{18}F labeled glucose and cellobiose derivatives of TOCA via oxime formation with fluorobenzaldehyde. They compared the in-vitro internalization and mouse biodistribution with fluoropropionylated analogs and they found that, together with reduced synthesis time (50 minutes instead of 3 hours), the two carbohydrate-oxime analogs can be obtained in high yields (65–85%) and present high internalization rate (139 and 163% of the reference [^{125}I]TOC), high tumor accumulation (around 20–25%) in vivo, and high tumor:organ ratios. The carbohydration of SS analogs, along with oxime formation, showed to be very promising in these preclinical studies, opening wide perspectives for clinical applications of ^{18}F-Tyr^3-Octreotide derivatives. A recent publication showed (64) an automated module for the synthesis of N-succinimidyl-4-[^{18}F]fluoro-benzoate ([^{18}F]SFB), using a modified commercial [^{18}F]FDG synthesis module. In this way, large amounts of fluorinated peptides would be probably available in the future, thanks to the reduced operator exposure. A different approach to label peptides and proteins has been recently investigated by the group of Dollé; they synthesized a new [^{18}F]Fluoropyridine-based maleimide reagent to bind thiol groups with high chemoselectivity (65). In this precursor the [^{18}F]fluorine can be efficiently incorporated in a pyridine moiety via a nucleophilic heteroaromatic substitution and the maleimide function bring the chemoselectivity towards thiol groups, offering a valid alternative to the use of non selective carboxilate and amine reactive [^{18}F]-reagents.

Labeling with ^{68}Ga/^{66}Ga

The metallic behaviour of Ga^{3+} radioisotopes led them to replace diagnostic/therapeutic radiometals with the same or similar coordination chemistry (^{111}In, ^{90}Y). In particular the bifunctional chelator (BFC) approach, already developed for ^{111}In and ^{90}Y, has proven to be successful with $^{66/68}$Ga-radiopharmaceuticals.

As underlined by Heppeler, Maecke, and coworkers (66), ^{68}Ga was historically inserted in peptides (back to 1994), such as Octreotide, using the bifunctional chelator Desferrioxamine-B (DFO), which forms stable complexes with Fe(III) and Ga(III) through three hydroxamate groups. Although stable, this derivative presented low tumor:organ ratio and slow blood clearance, due to high binding to plasma proteins. Another way of labeling was a preformed chelate approach, via the 1,4,7-triazacyclononane-1-succinic acid-4,7-diacetic acid (NODASA). In this BFC, three carboxil groups together with three nitrogen atoms bind Ga, whereas another carboxilate is free for coupling to biomolecules (Fig. 7). This, according to the authors, may be crucial to achieve high specific activity radiopharmaceuticals.

Nevertheless, although a pre-labeling approach may be convenient, research is focusing on rapid, simple, and straightforward labeling reactions, thus to obtain the most pure radiopharmaceutical in the highest yield. In few words, the authors conclude that DOTA is a universal macrocyclic chelator for labeling peptides with different radioisotopes; in particular, being ^{68}Ga, a trivalent metal cation with similar chemical properties to ^{90}Y and ^{111}In, DOTA could be safely used with such a radioisotope. Many groups studied DOTA-conjugated

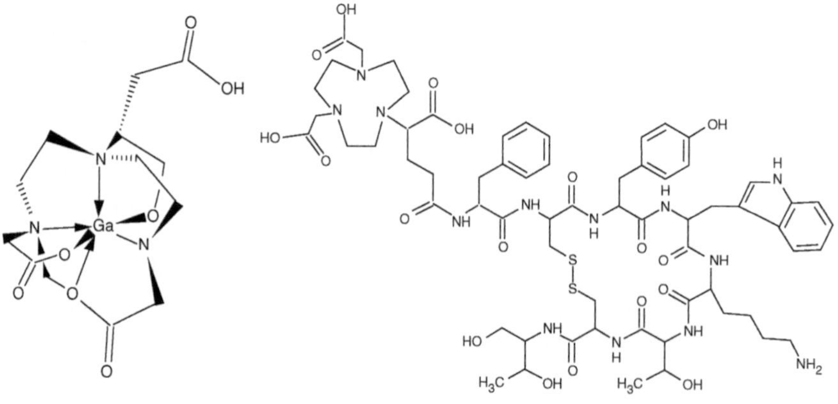

Figure 7 The complex ^{68}Ga-NODASA and the conjugate NODAGATOC.

peptides labeled with ^{68}Ga, investigating their pharmacokinetics and potential improvement of their biodistribution. Eisenwiener et al. published the synthesis of NODAGATOC, another chelator coupled SS analogue based on the NOTA core (a triaza-macrocyclic chelator), which can potentially be labeled with ^{68}Ga. They pointed out the structural x-ray differences between Y^{3+} and Ga^{3+} macrocyclic complexes, underlining the importance that steric hindrance and distance from the pharmacophoric side of the molecule may have on receptor binding and affinity (67). The rationale of this study was to investigate another chelator group which should allow to carry a spacer function between the chelator and the peptide (Fig. 7). Ugur studied the labeling of DOTATOC with ^{66}Ga and compared it with $^{67/68}$Ga. He successfully obtained labeling yields in the range 85–95% and radiochemical purities greater than 95%. The authors suggest that, thanks to the high positron energy (4.2 MeV), ^{66}Ga-DOTATOC can be used also for therapy treatments, provided that critical organs such as kidneys be protected (20).

From the radiopharmacist standpoint, special emphasis is paid to the work of Meyer et al, published in EJNM in 2004 (68). They studied and optimized a semi-automated ^{68}Ga-handling system for the labeling of DOTA-derivatised peptides such as DOTATOC. They implemented all the phases of the labeling, from the elution of the ^{68}Ga generator, the purification/concentration of the ^{68}Ga solution, the peptide labeling, and the final purification/sterilization. The system is remotely controlled and records all the key parameters of the procedure, in order to have a real-time idea of what is happening without any manipulation by the operator. They achieved very good results, with a labeling yield of 58% in only 20 minutes. Although it is a prototype, further efforts have been devoted to improve such a kind of automated module and it is hopeful that in the future it may be widely available (Fig. 8).

Velikyan, Beyer, and Långström published an interesting method to label ^{68}Ga-DOTA-peptides using microwave heating instead of conventional heating blocks (69). They showed that reaction kinetic was faster with microwave, allowing to obtain 100% of incorporation in only 5 minutes. Moreover, as the major fraction of the eluate contained about 60% of total activity in 1 mL, they used the fractionated elution to reduce reaction volume and they achieved 100% labeling in only 1 minute. With this method, together with eluate purification in the anionic form, they prepared ^{68}Ga-DOTATOC with final specific activity above 3GBq/nmol.

Maecke and colleagues recently reviewed the current status of ^{68}Ga-labeled peptides in tumor imaging (11). They stressed the attention on the different ^{68}Ge/^{68}Ga generators available (commercial and home-made) and the purification of the eluate that is needed to avoid metal contamination. This, as already known by the previous authors, can be made by forming the anionic complex $[^{68}GaCl_4]^-$ in concentrated HCl, which is retained on an anion exchange resin. It can then be recovered in a small volume using a concentration step, critical for labeling. The authors deal also with the aqueous coordination chemistry and

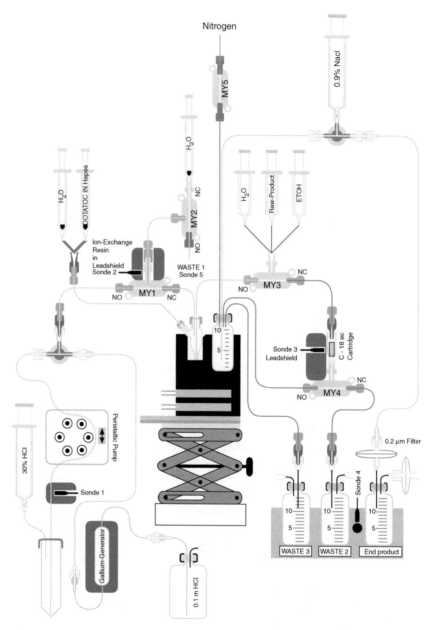

Figure 8 Semi-automated synthesis module for the radiolabeling of ^{68}Ga-DOTATOC.

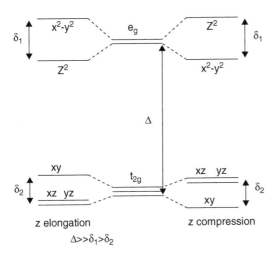

Figure 9 The Jahn-Teller distortion in the Cu(II) d^9-ion.

different chelators proposed for ^{68}Ga, showing that several peptides have been studied coupled to DOTA or analogue moyeties (DTPA, NOTA). To date, it appears that merging new labeling techniques (such as microwave heating) and optimized automated systems may lead to improving the quality standards of ^{68}Ga-labeled radiopharmaceuticals.

Labeling with ^{64}Cu

^{64}Cu has been considered as an alternative PET radiometal for labeling proteins, due to the double β^+/β^- emission that can be useful for both imaging and therapy of tumors. Although similar to other metal ions used in nuclear medicine, its chemistry is slightly different, and formation of chelates with poliazamacrocyclic ligands is not so simple. Cu(II) electron configuration, $[Ar]3d^9$, affect the stability of its complexes; in the ligand field theory, Cu(II) shows a degenerate electron state of the d orbitals, falling into the so called "Jahn-Teller effect." From the author's words; *"for a non linear molecule in an electronically degenerate state, distortion must occurr to lower the simmetry, remove the degeneracy, and lower the energy"*(70). Graphically this effect may be depicted with splitting of the t_{2g} and e_g orbitals, thus resulting in elongation/compression of the octahedral Cu(II) complexes (Fig. 9).

For this reason, Cu^{2+} azamacrocyclic complexes have been extensively studied. Kaden illustrated in 1993 (71) their structural complexity, showing that Cu may assume several conformations and coordination geometries depending on the structure and degree/type of derivatization of the azamacrocyclic rings. Anderson et al. in 1995 synthesized two new conjugates, TETA-D-Phe^1-octreotide (TETA = 1,4,8,11-tetraazacyclotetradecane-N,N',N'',N'''-tetraacetic acid), and

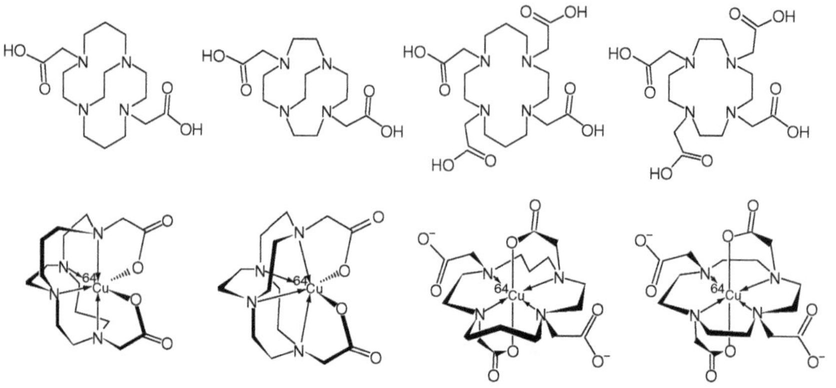

Figure 10 Different conventional and cross-bridged tetraazamacrocyclic Cu-complexes.

CPTA-D-Phe[1]-octreotide (CPTA = 4-[1,4,8,11-tetraazacyclotetradec-1-methyl]-benzoic acid) (72). They labeled both with ^{64}Cu and compared them to ^{111}In-DTPA-D-Phe[1]-octreotide. They prepared TETA and CPTA analogs with specific activity in the range 56-111GBq/mmol; the complexation kinetic of ^{64}Cu with TETA was more favourable than with CPTA, where only 85% was radiolabeled up to 18 hours, requiring thus a reversed phase purification. Their preparations were stable when gentisic acid was added, otherwise were subject to radiolysis. One point open to further investigation is the dissociation of the metal complex and relative metabolites analysis. Sun, Anderson, and colleagues published in 2004 (33) an in vivo evaluation of three different ^{64}Cu-monooxo-tetraazamacrocyclic ligands with different ring size and oxo-position. They found that, beside the good stability in rat serum, a costant high uptake was common in blood, liver, and kidneys, indicating a dissociation of ^{64}Cu from the complexes. The three oxo-complexes are +1 charged and the authors suggested that shifting the complex charge to neutral or negative may improve biodistribution. Anderson, Boswell et al. published the same year a comparative evaluation of ^{64}Cu conventional and cross-bridged tetrazamacrocyclic complexes useful for derivatization of peptide for tumor imaging. Previous works indeed demonstrated how ^{64}Cu is partially dissociated from conventional macrocyclics and subsequently bound to superoxide dismutase (SOD). This paper found out that the structurally enforcing cross-bridge enhances the in vivo stability by reducing metal losses (Fig. 10).

In another work, the authors then analyzed the labeling of ^{64}Cu-CB-TETA-Tyr^3-OctreoTATE and ^{64}Cu-CB-TE2A-Tyr^3-OctreoTATE, which was achieved at 95 °C at pH 7.0–8.0 in 1 hour, without the need for further purification, at maximal specific activity of 5.1mCi/µg (34). In 2005 Boswell, Anderson et al. studied the labeling and metabolites of ^{64}Cu-DOTA, ^{64}Cu-TETA, and their corresponding cross bridged analogs ^{64}Cu-CB-TE2A and ^{64}Cu-CB-DO2A by radio-LC-MS. The authors underline that for synthetic ligand, such as CB-TE2A, the presence of trace impurities is unavoidable. Moreover, the possible incorporation of ^{64}Cu into a trace chelator impurity may be favored under certain reaction conditions; great importance is thus given to the extensive characterization of radiolabeled complexes species, carried out with reliable hyphenate-chromatographic techniques, in order to develop these radiolabeled compounds as radiopharmaceuticals (73).

Labeling with ^{86}Y/^{110m}In

The two radiometals ^{86}Y/^{110m}In are chemically identical to their counterparts ^{90}Y/^{111}In. To successfully obtain ^{86}Y/^{110m}In-radiopharmaceuticals with high stability it is therefore possible to adopt the BFC approach, mainly with open chain (DTPA), and azamacrocyclic (DOTA) chelators. These types of binding moieties have already proven to be the gold standard for the cited ^{90}Y/^{111}In. Moreover, it is generally accepted that for In^{3+} DTPA should be preferred, but it is even more important to use cyclic chelators (such as DOTA and smaller modifications) for Y^{3+} because of the stability of the final complex. Care should be taken to the pH of the reaction (in the range 4.5–5.0), in order to obtain the highest RCY and purity. Many works described ^{86}Y/^{110m}In-labeled octreotide derivatives, concluding that the foreseen stability was confirmed by experimental data. Some clinical applications of these compounds will be discussed later.

Labeling with ^{124}I

Iodine (especially ^{123,125,131}I and recently ^{124}I) has historically played a major role in the labeling of proteins for medical purposes. As in the case of the pair ^{90}Y/^{86}Y, here the therapeutic potential of ^{131}I-radiopharmaceuticals can be better evaluated with PET imaging using ^{124}I analogs rather than with SPECT scintigraphy of a ^{123}I surrogate. Hence the importance of developing stable [^{124}I]-radiopharmaceuticals. Numerous iodinated molecules have been developed in the past for scintigraphic studies and the conventional labeling reaction proceeds via a direct electrophilic substitution on an activated aromatic ring. The two widely diffuse reagents to produce the electrophilic I$^+$ are Chloramine-T (CAT) and Iodogen. In the case of antibodies, this is rather easy because of the number of Tyr residues present; for peptides the challenge may be harder, in case of low molecular weight chains and Tyr-poor sequences. Therefore, prelabeling approaches have been developed, as in the case of ^{18}F, preparing [^{124}I]iodinated precursors ready to link the carrier molecule, for example via an amide bond formation. Precursors of such a type may be the classical Bolton-Hunter reagent or activated esters of m-[^{124}I]iodobenzoic acid. In 2003 Glaser and co-workers studied a ^{124}I derivative of annexin V obtained both with the direct CAT method and the indirect N-succinimidyl 3-[^{124}I]iodobenzoate ([^{124}I]m-SIB) method. With CAT they achieved 22% RCY, whereas with SIB they obtained 14–25% depending on the technique used. Both methods gave radiochemical purities

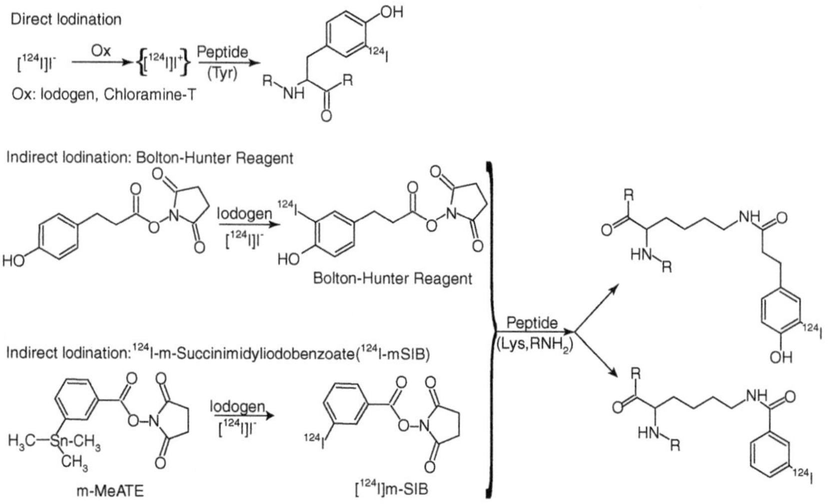

Figure 11 Synthetic strategies for [^{124}I]Iodination of peptides.

around 98% and the radiotracer could be stored for up to four days without significant radiodeiodination. In vitro binding studies with human leukaemic HL60 cells revealed the superiority of indirectly labeled annexin V compared to the direct labeling method (Fig. 11) (74).

OVERVIEW OF POSITRON-LABELED PEPTIDE FAMILIES USEFUL IN CANCER DIAGNOSIS AND THERAPY: CURRENT STATUS AND FUTURE PERSPECTIVES

Somatostatin/Somatostatin Receptor

SS receptor are widely expressed on neuroendocrine tumors and for many years the clinical use of radiolabeled octreotide derivatives has encountered favorable results. Several PET analogs have been developed in the last 10 years, especially with ^{18}F, ^{68}Ga and ^{64}Cu, and we present here a concise resume.

One of the first attempts to label octreotide with ^{18}F was made by Vaidyanathan and Zalutsky[55] using the N-Succinimidil-FluoroBenzoate (SFB) approach and by Guhlke in 1994, who succeeded using activated ^{18}F-fluoropropionic acid (56). Biodistribution studies of 2-[^{18}F]fluoropropionyl-D-Phe^1-octreotide (56,58) and 4-[^{18}F]fluorobenzoyl-D-Phe^1-octreotide (75) in rodents revealed low tumor uptake, poor tumor retention and unfavourable biokinetics. Later on, Wester (58) compared the pharmacokinetics of [^{18}F]-FluoropropionilOctreotide, ^{86}Y-DTPA-OC, and ^{67}Ga-DFO-OC. Although the uptake of ^{18}F analogue was rapid, the short tumor residence time and its hepatobiliary excretion imposed further developments, to obtain a more hydrophilic derivative. In 2002 Schottelius showed that the pharmacokinetic of radioiodinated TOC can be improved when conjugated to carbohydrates (61). This gave the biomolecule a more hydrophilic behaviour and partially overcame the drawback of ^{18}F liver uptake previously encountered. The idea then was to synthetize a carbohydrated analogue of ^{18}F-Octreotide, as the same group published in 2003 ([^{18}F]-FP-Gluc-TOCA) (5), this derivative showed receptor binding specificity and the affinity for sstr subtype 2 was very high (2.8nM), while LogP was rather low (-1.7). Subsequently, a novel fluorobenzilidene-oxime carbohydrated analogue of TOCA proved to be stable against defluorination and with favourable tumor uptake and biodistribution (63). If compared to the fluoropropionylated analog, the carbohydrate-oxime derivative present high in-vitro internalization rate (139 and 163% of the reference [^{125}I]TOC), high mouse tumor accumulation (around 20–25%) and high tumor:organ ratios, The carbohydration of SS analogs, along with oxime formation, showed to be very promising in these preclinical studies; glycosilated ^{18}F-Tyr^3-Octreotide showed encouraging biodistribution also in a pilot patient study[5].

Clinical developments of ^{68}Ga SS analogs are today focusing mainly on the gold standard DOTATOC, because of the high versatility of DOTA macrocyclic chelator to bind trivalent ions such as Y^{3+} and Ga^{3+}. In fact, Hoffman published recently some preliminary data on biokinetics and imaging with ^{68}Ga-DOTATOC. On the basis of eight patients, they found a fast, bi-exponential clearance from blood and no radioactive metabolites in serum. Moreover, tumor maximum accumulation was after 70 minutes and tumor:organ ratio ranged from 3:1 (for liver) to 100:1 (for CNS). They compared ^{68}Ga-DOTATOC with ^{111}In-Octreotide in detecting documented lesions and, while the first showed 100% of them, with ^{111}In planar or SPECT scintigraphy they revealed only 85%, thus demonstrating the superiority of ^{68}Ga-DOTATOC. In 2001 Henze published the first results with ^{68}Ga-DOTATOC in patients with meningiomas[2]; they found that, once injected, the radiotracer is rapidly cleared from the blood, with a bi-exponential kinetic (half lives of 3.5 and 63 minutes, respectively). They achieved high accumulation in even small meningiomas, which were clearly differentiated from healty brain tissue. Eisenwiener et al. (67) published in 2002 the synthesis of NODAGATOC, another chelator-coupled SS analogue based on the NOTA core (a triaza-macrocyclic chelator), which can potentially be labeled with ^{68}Ga. They studied the labeling with ^{111}In, ^{67}Ga, and ^{nat}Ga, obtaining high internalization rates, good specific activity, good in-vitro affinity to sstr2 and 5 receptor subtypes, as well as favorable biodistribution. In 2003 Kowalski published the first ^{68}Ga-DOTATOC results in patients with neuroendocrine tumors (14), comparing it to Octreoscan and evidencing a superior performance, especially with small lesions, due to the increased spatial resolution of the PET radioligand. These promising results were supported in 2004 by Henze and colleagues, when they showed, in the EJNM Image of the Month (12), an exceptional increase of ^{68}Ga-DOTATOC uptake in a pancreatic neuroendocrine tumor.

Very recently, Henze et al. published in JNM an extensive study on the pharmacokinetic of ^{68}Ga-DOTATOC in 21 patients with meningiomas. They assumed a two compartmental model (blood, receptors and meningioma cells) and compared the uptake and internalization in meningioma and nasal mucosa (reference tissue). They showed that the rate of uptake/release by the receptor and internalization/externalization from the cell were significantly and statistically different for the two groups, being 6- to 8-fold greater for the tumor compared to reference tissue.

Anderson and other colleagues published large amounts of data on ^{64}Cu-labeled octreotide (72). The derivatives of octreotide with two azamacrocyclic chelators, ^{64}Cu-TETA-D-Phe^1-octreotide and ^{64}Cu-CPTA-D-Phe^1-octreotide, were superior if compared to ^{111}In-DTPA-D-Phe^1-octreotide. In vitro binding studies indicated a 40- and 10- times greater receptor affinity. Animal biodistribution studies showed that the major drawback of CPTA-octreotide was its relevant liver uptake, which did not clear after 24 hours, while only TETA-OC seems to clear appreciably from the kidneys in 24 hours. The main point, as already underlined, was the stability of the conjugate; in fact 24 hours post injection, both tumor uptake, and tumor-to-non target organ ratios were greater for ^{111}In-DTPA-D-Phe^1-octreotide than each of the ^{64}Cu-analogs. Later on (75), they found that the radiotherapeutic efficacy of ^{64}Cu-TETA-D-Phe^1-Octreotide, in rat pancreatic tumors, can be improved using the analogue ^{64}Cu-TETA-D-Phe^1-OctreoTATE, and even more using ^{64}Cu-TETA-D-Phe^1-Tyr^3-OctreoTATE; substitution of Phe^3 for Tyr^3 and replacement of alcoholic function for a carboxilic one in the C-terminal amino acid led to improved pharmacokinetic and biodistribution. In 2001 the first results of ^{64}Cu-TETA-D-Phe^1-Octreotide in patients with neuroendocrine tumors were published in JNM (4). They showed that the PET radioligand was comparable to ^{111}In-DTPA-Octreotide, but was able to detect more lesions. Moreover pharmacokinetic studies showed that ^{64}Cu-TETA-D-Phe^1-Octreotide is rapidly cleared from the blood and about 60% of injected dose is excreted in the urine. One point open to further investigation is the dissociation of the metal complex and relative metabolites analysis; it was noticed that liver uptake increased with time and some dissociation of ^{64}Cu likely occurred, with subsequent binding to plasma protein, as already evidenced in rat liver by the same authors in a previous work. In 2004 (34) another paper dealt with ^{64}Cu and Tyr^3-OctreoTATE. They introduced a modified, cross-bridged macrocyclic chelator named CB-TE2A (formerly 4,11-bis-(carboxymethyl)-1,4,8,11-tetraazabicyclo(6.6.2)hexadecane) which was shown to confer ^{64}Cu improved in vivo clearance properties and compared to TETA chelator for the same peptide Tyr^3-OctreoTATE. Results were encouraging: in vitro affinities for pancreatic tumor SS receptors was comparable (TETA$=0.7$nM, CB-TE2A$=1.7$nM), while in biodistribution studies non-specific uptake in blood and liver was lower for CB-TE2A. The differences increased with time and at 4 hours blood and liver uptake were 4.3-fold and 2.4-fold lower respectively for ^{64}Cu-CB-TE2A-Tyr^3-OctreoTATE than for ^{64}Cu-TETA-Tyr^3-OctreoTATE. Interestingly, at the same time point, tumor uptake was more than 4 times greater for CB-TE2A analogue. Nevertheless, the cross-bridged analogue showed much slower kidney clearance than TETA-conjugate. The authors speculate that this may be due to different net charge (TETA = -1, CB-TE2A = + 1) of the molecule and suggest that a carboxil modification of CB-TE2A may additionally improve the biodistribution. However, a deep characterization of radiolabeled metabolites is mandatory in the development process of these compounds as radiopharmaceuticals.

In 1999 Rösch published a study on the uptake kinetic of ^{86}Y-DOTATOC in non-human primates (46), thus to allow the dosimetric calculations for the therapeutic ^{90}Y-analogue. They found that ^{86}Y-DOTATOC is highly stable in vivo both in serum and urine, whereas binding to blood cells and serum proteins is negligible and the compound is rapidly cleared from the blood pool. Kidneys were found to be the critical organs in a therapy regimen with ^{90}Y-DOTATOC and a concomitant amino acid coninfusion may reduce their uptake. An update on the dosimetry for therapy planning using ^{86}Y-DOTATOC was presented in 2001 by Förster, Rösch, and colleagues (47). They compared dosimetry obtained with the PET analogue and conventional dosimetry by ^{111}In-DTPA-OC; although doses to critical organs were quite similar, they found discrepancies for the doses delivered to the tumor, suggesting ^{86}Y-DOTATOC dosimetry to be preferred when possible to ^{111}In-DTPA-OC, since it has been found to underestimate the tumor dose. In 2002 a paper by Lubberink et al. appeared in JNM (52); they studied the PET analogue ^{110m}In-DTPA-OC for imaging of neuroendocrine tumors and compared it to the imaging performances of ^{111}In-DTPA-OC. The spatial resolution was demonstrated to be superior for the PET isotope; nevertherless, the short half life, and the need for a nearby cyclotron, are limiting factors for its clinical use. Jamar et al. in 2003 published (3) a phase I clinical study on ^{86}Y-DOTATOC. They investigated the pharmacokinetic and biodistribution with different amino acid coinfusion, finding that kidney protective agents significantly lowered critical organ uptake more than 20%, without affecting tumor uptake. They moreover found that prolongation of the infusion from 4 to 10 hours further enhances the protective effect on the kidneys.

Integrins/Angiogenesis/RGD

Integrins are transmembrane glycoproteins consisting of two subunits, α and β, and to date, 25 different integrin $\alpha\beta$ heterodimers have been reported. Integrins mediate cell adhesion to the extracellular matrix proteins or to the surfaces of other cells. Among the integrins, the $\alpha_V\beta_3$ receptor, also known as the vitronectin receptor, has been reported to be involved in tumor cell migration. The $\alpha_V\beta_3$ receptors are expressed on metastatic tumor cells and are involved in angiogenesis. Thus, the $\alpha_V\beta_3$ integrin participates in tumor metastasis and tumor-related angiogenesis. Angiogenesis, or formation of new blood vessels, is crucial for the growth of tumors from a few millimeters spots to bulky masses. In this highly regulated process, over the surface of endothelial cells is associated an overexpression of the integrin $\alpha_V\beta_3$. Characteristic of integrins is the recognition of the arginine-glicine-aspartic acid (RGD) motif. Therefore, another field in tumor imaging has been and currently is the labeling of RGD-type molecules to study the extention of angiogenesis.

Sutcliffe-Goulden et al. succeded in 2002 in radiolabeling linear RGD peptides using ^{18}F-fluorobenzoic acid (60), in fact in vitro studies demonstrated how the fluorobenzoyl prosthetic group had no effect on the binding on integrins. Unfortunately these compounds showed to be very unstable in vivo and the accumulation on the tumor is not RGD dependent. Another attempt was done by Ogawa et al. in 2003, who labeled cyclic RGD peptides by direct electrophilic fluorination with ^{18}F]acetyl-hypofluorite (76). The cyclic peptide had the highest affinity for $\alpha_V\beta_3$ receptor and the method used did not alter significantly the biochemical nature of the peptide. The affinity of the fluorinated RGD for $\alpha_V\beta_3$ receptor was similar to that of unlabeled peptide and was shown to be specific. Their biodistribution only in minor part was at the tumor site, whereas great uptake was found in the liver, kidneys, and intestine. This suggested a liver metabolic pathway leading to biliary excretion of radioactive metabolites. The major problem to face in this case is the carrier-added preparation, giving a low specific activity compound. In 2004 Chen et al. evaluated cyclic RGD labeled via ^{18}F]SFB. The compound showed a rapid blood clearance and tumor uptake was high and specific by blocking studies; the excretion proceeded both by liver and kidneys in glioblastoma mice (8). The same author in 2004 compared the detection of α_V integrins by [18]F- and ^{64}Cu-labeled RGD by microPET and autoradiography in breast cancer animal models (41). FB-RGD and ^{64}Cu-DOTA-RGD, despite the fast blood clearance, and high tumor/blood ratio, showed lower tumor uptake than ^{125}I-RGD. Especially FB-RGD showed fast tumor washout and accumulation in the hepatobiliary system. The authors conclude that the overall molecular charge and conjugate design have profound impact on the biodistribution of the radiotracer, claiming further developments, and optimization for prolonged tumor uptake and favourable biokinetics. The formation of a *N*-(4-^{18}F]fluorobenzylidene)oxime derivative of RGD, suggested in 2004 by Poethko, Wester et al. led to a conjugate which is predominantly excreted by kidneys (45). During the same year, Haubner, Schwaiger, and colleagues published a full paper on a glycosylated RGD peptide (^{18}F]Galacto-RGD) (77). This reaction involved the use of ^{18}F]-fluoropropionate as prosthetic group and the previous formation of Galacto-RGD conjugate. This radiotracer showed some degree of metabolic degradation in liver, blood, and kidneys, whereas in tumor was found intact for 87%. Nevertheless, this approach represents a second generation in the development of a more suitable candidate for imaging $\alpha_V\beta_3$ receptor; similar to the case of SS, glycosilation has proven to increase the hydrophilic behaviour of the molecule, confering it an improved biodistribution pattern. ^{18}F-RGD peptides have successfully been used to image the expression of the $\alpha_v\beta_3$ integrin in inflammatory diseases since integrin also plays an important role in angiogenesis induced by chronic inflammatory processes.

One of the few examples of ^{64}Cu-RGD conjugate was presented in 2004 by Chen (41), using DOTA as macrocyclic chelator. In breast cancer, mice tumor uptake was intermediate between ^{125}I-RGD and ^{18}F-RGD. Liver, kidneys, and intestine uptake were similar to the tumor and probably the insertion of the bulky DOTA moiety close to the pharmacophoric (RGD) site justifies the lowered tumor uptake compared to ^{125}I-RGD. As already noted for other molecules, improvements of the chelator are needed to avoid transchelation of ^{64}Cu towards plasma proteins in liver and blood. The group of Chen in 2004 prepared a PEGylated RGD and coupled it to DOTA, labeling it with ^{64}Cu in order to improve the unfavorable pharmacokinetic (78). The polyethylene-glycol chain was inserted as spacer between DOTA and RGD moiety, then the complex was radiolabeled and evaluated in brain tumor models. The radiotracer's IC$_{50}$ towards $\alpha_v\beta_3$ integrins was intermediate (around 67.5 nM). The liver uptake was significantly reduced and renal excretion was higher and more rapid than its analogue ^{64}Cu-DOTA-cycloRGD. This study demonstrated the suitability of a PEG moiety to improve the in vivo kinetics of a ^{64}Cu-RGD peptide tracer without compromising the tumor-targeting ability and specificity of the peptide. The same author presented (79) an evaluation of two ^{64}Cu-labeled dimeric RGD peptides. Compared to the monomer ^{64}Cu-DOTA-cycloRGD, the dimers showed more favorable in vivo characteristics with significantly lowered liver uptake, presumably due to their increased hydrophilicity. Moreover, a multimeric RGD peptide is expected to enhance the affinity of the receptor ligand interactions even more significantly through the phenomenon of polyvalency.

GRP/Bombesin

Bombesin (BN) is a 14 amino acid amphibian neuropeptide which shows, just as its mammalian counterpart gastrin-releasing peptide (GRP), high affinity for the human gastrin-releasing peptide receptor (GRP-r), which is overexpressed on several types of cancer, including prostate, breast, gastrointestinal, and small cell lung cancer. Thus, radiolabeled BN or BN analogs may prove to be specific tracers for diagnostic and therapeutic targeting of GRP-r positive tumors in nuclear medicine

Since the native BN peptide has a pyroglutamic acid at the N-terminus and an amide bond at the C-terminus, further modification and radiolabeling of this peptide with metallic radionuclides is not possible. Efforts have been made to design derivatized BN analogs for binding and pharmacokinetic studies. Because BN agonists are generally preferable to BN antagonists for receptor-specific internalization, most BN analogs with an amidated C-terminus that have been developed are agonists. Because the C-terminus is directly involved in the specific binding interaction with the GRP-r, the truncated C-terminal heptapeptide sequence Trp-Ala-Val-Gly-His-Leu-Met (BN (8–13)) must be maintained or minimally substituted. Several strategies have been applied to develop radiometallated BN analogous conjugates.

The first and unique study to date on ^{68}Ga-labeled BN analogue is the one published in JNM by Schuhmacher et al. in 2005 (80). They synthesized the PEGylated derivative DOTA-PEG$_2$-[DTyr[6], βAla[11],Thi[13],Nle[14]]BN (6–13) amide (BZH3). The ligand was labeled with [67,68]Ga and tested on rat pancreatic tumor model in vitro and in vivo. The diagnostic potential of ^{68}Ga-BZH3 was demonstrated by PET images, the ^{67}Ga analogue dissociation constant ($K_d = 0.46$ nM), and rapid internalization of the radioligand in tumor cells and fast clearance from GRP-r negative tissues.

Roger, Welch, and co-workers published in 2003 a study on a ^{64}Cu-DOTA labeled BN analogue, where between DOTA and BN an 8-aminooctanoic acid (Aoc) spacer was inserted (25). The BN fraction considered was the 8 C-terminal amino acids BN (7–13). The resulting DOTA-Aoc-BN (7–13) was evaluated, labeled with ^{64}Cu, in vitro and in vivo towards prostate carcinoma cell lines and animal models. The dissociation constant for the radioligand was above 6 nM and internalization was up to 21% at 240 minutes. The uptake in tumor was good but localization in healty tissues was rather higher than in other BN analogs considered. Thus the authors conclude that further improvements, including charge modification of the chelator, are needed. In 2004 Chen suggested ^{64}Cu-DOTA-[Lys[3]]-BN as alternative radioligand for imaging GRP-r positive tissues (39). It showed high affinity and selective binding in vitro in prostate carcinoma cells. Tumor uptake was high (around 10% ID/g at 30 minutes) and radioligand was mainly cleared via renal pathway.

Melanoma/α-MSH

α-Melanocyte stimulating hormone (α-MSH) is a 13 amino acid peptide regulating melanoma cell proliferation and function. The presence of high affinity MSH receptor on melanoma cell lines drove researchers towards the development of radiolabeled MSH analogue, mainly DTPA or DOTA conjugates.

Because of the instability of α-MSH, the more stable [Nle[4],D-Phe[7]]-α-MSH was developed. It was labeled using the N-succinimidyl-4-[^{18}F]-fluorobenzoate by Vaidyanathan and Zalutsky (81). However it remains to be determined if this α-MSH analogue can be prepared with sufficient specific activity needed for PET imaging of melanoma receptors.

In 2004 Froidevaux developed an α-MSH analogue (DOTA-NAPamide) (17), suitable for labeling with the positron emitter [68]Ga. They improved a previously reported DOTA-α-MSH, DOTA-MSH$_{oct}$, where DOTA was linked to the N-terminus of the peptide, coupling the chelator to the ε-amino group of C-terminal Lys[11]. [67/68]Ga-DOTA-NAPamide showed to be superior to the analogue ^{111}In-DOTA-MSH$_{oct}$ by a 7-fold binding potency. The high tumor uptake was relevant especially when the amount of injected peptide was low, underlining the importance of high specific activity preparations. An extensive overview has been published very recently in JNM by the same author, dealing with DOTA-α-MSH congeners and studying the parameters affecting tumor and kidney uptake (82). Compared to the previous DOTA-NAPamide, which was found to selectively accumulate in melanoma in mouse model, structural modification, including shifting the DOTA chelator position and changing the hydrophobicity and charge of the whole molecule, were applied. The authors observed that kidney uptake of DOTA-α-MSH analogs may be reduced, without affecting the affinity for the receptor, by neutralizing the charge of Lys[11].

Apoptosis/Annexin V

Apoptosis, or programmed cell death, plays a crucial role in development of cancer. Cells that are deficient in their apoptotic response can potentially become tumorigenic. Annexin V is a 36-kDa protein that binds with high affinity (dissociation constant about 10 nM) to phosphatidylserine (PS), a phospholipid that is normally found only on the interior of the cell membrane but is redistributed to the exterior of the cell membrane in the early stages of apoptosis. The highly regulated apoptosis pathway can thus be imaged in its early phase by specific binding with radiolabeled annexin V.

Zijlstra et al. proposed in 2003 (83) a fluorinated annexin V derivative, obtained via [^{18}F]SFB. Biological binding properties were checked with PS liposomes and binding to Jurkat T-cell lymphoblast after induced apoptosis were promising. More recently, Yagle and colleagues published (84) an evaluation of ^{18}F-annexin V as imaging agent of apoptosis in animal models. They pre-induced liver apoptosis in rats which were injected and imaged, then sacrificed and dissected. Compared to control, the uptake of ^{18}F-annexin V in apoptotic liver cells was 3- to 9-fold increased, whereas biodistribution analysis of normal rats showed highest uptake of ^{18}F-annexin V in the kidneys and urinary bladder, indicating rapid renal clearance of ^{18}F-annexin V metabolites.

In 2003 Glaser and co-workers studied a ^{124}I derivative of annexin V obtained both with the direct CAT method and the indirect [^{124}I]m-SIB method. In vitro binding studies with human leukaemic HL60 cells revealed the superiority of indirectly labeled annexin V towards the direct method (74). In the last months, three papers appeared in Nuclear Medicine and Biology by Dekker, Zweit et al. In a first paper (85), they developed a maltose-binding protein/annexin V chimera (MBP-annexin V) in order to obtain a radiolabeled analogue useful for imaging apoptotic cells. They hypothesize that MBP fusion protein is advantageous for the ease of purification and in the improved specificity in immunological detection techniques. Radiolabeling of MBP-annexin V was carried out with Iodogen and CAT methods, retaining its PS binding properties, but when high amounts of oxidizing agents are used, specificity is compromised. Secondly (86), they published another work in which they report metabolite analysis of ^{124}I annexin V and correlation of its uptake to apoptotic density. The specificity of PS binding was confirmed by a radiolabeled [124]I-ovalbumin control which did not show increased uptake in apoptotic cells. In vivo uptake of [124]I annexin V well fitted with apoptotic cell density obtained from histology. Moreover, their last work (87) pointed out the differences of annexin V labeled directly (with CAT method) and indirectly (with [[124]I]m-SIB) with [124]I. The data suggest that [[124]I]4IB-annexin V, produced with the indirect method, had a higher rate of PS binding compared to [124]I annexin V, higher kidney and urine uptake, a lower thyroid and stomach uptake, greater plasma stability, and a lower rate of plasma clearance. Finally, binding ratio of apoptotic cell over normal cell was lower for [[124]I]4IB-annexin V than for [124]I annexin V, making the latter more promising for further investigations.

CONCLUSION

Over the last two decades the pre- and clinical scenario of positron radiolabeled molecules has shifted from few pioneering works to a wide range of applications with the goal of an accurate cancer diagnosis for a potential successful treatment. Radiolabeled peptides described herein represent a new important tool for therapy planning, still under development and expansion. Thanks to the efforts and the creativity of many scientists, now available are several radiolabeling strategies of peptides with PET radionuclides: currently under improvement are not only the radiochemical yields, but also the radiopharmaceutical safety, behaviour and biodistribution of these tracers. [18]F is the most common PET radionuclide and is extensively used for its favorable physical properties; nevertheless production and handling of ^{18}F requires a high technology facility, and fluorination of a molecule like a peptide is not a straighforward task, but fine tuning of the synthesis equipment, together with carefully trained personnel, are mandatory. On the other hand, ^{68}Ga is readily available as an in-house [68]Ge/^{68}Ga generator, the labeling of DOTA-conjugated peptides is rather well established, and some remote synthesis modules are going to become commercially available. Moreover, considering the role that positron-radiolabeled peptides assume in a well planned cancer treatment, it is required to mantain the highest similarity between the diagnostic and therapeutic radiopharmaceuticals. This is particularly important when working with fluorinated analogs, where in some cases the ^{18}F-prosthetic group gives the molecule a hydrophobic behavior, altering the in-vivo biodistribution. For this purpose several strategies were required to improve the biodistribution of the ^{18}F-labeled peptide, especially when planning treatment is based on dosimetric studies with peptide PET. On the contrary, when using a metallic positron emitting radioisotope of the same element or with similar labeling chemistry (^{68}Ga or [86]Y for ^{90}Y), there is no need of chemical modification that may alter the in vivo behaviour of the radiopharmaceutical and the same molecule can be directly used both for diagnosis or therapy.

At the time of writing other experimental data and in-vivo studies are adding more and more data to what is written in this chapter, and this is the proof that positron radiolabeled peptides are a fundamental tool for cancer therapy.

REFERENCES

1. Lundqvist H, Tolmachev V. Targeting peptides and positron emission tomography. Biopolymers (Pept Sci) 2002; 66:381–392.
2. Henze M, Schuhmacher J, Hipp P, Kowalski J, Becker DW, Doll J, Macke HR, Hoffmann M, Debus J, Haberkorn U. PET imaging of somatostatin receptors using [68Ga]DOTA-D-Phe[1]-Tyr[3]-octreotide: first results in patients with meningiomas. J Nucl Med 2001; 42:1053–1056.
3. Jamar F, Barone R, Mathieu I, Walrand S, Labar D, Carlier P, de Camps J, Schran H, Chen T, Smith MC, Bouterfa H, Valkema R, Krenning EP, Kvols LK, Paulwels S. 86Y-DOTA0-D-Phe[1]-Tyr[3]-octreotide (SMT487): a phase 1 clinical study—pharmacokinetics, biodistribution, and renal protective effect of different regimens of amino acid coinfusion. Eur J Nucl Med 2003; 30:510–518.
4. Anderson CJ, Dehdashti F, Cutler PD, Schwarz SW, Laforest R, Bass LA, Lewis JS, McCarthy DW. 64Cu-TETA-octreotide as a PET imaging agent for patients with neuroendocrine tumors. J Nucl Med 2001; 42:213–221.
5. Wester HJ, Schottelius M, Scheidhauer K, Meisetschlager G, Herz M, Rau FC, Reubi JC, Schwaiger M. PET imaging of somatostatin receptors: design, synthesis, and preclinical evaluation of a novel 18F-labelled, carbohydrated analogue of octreotide. Eur J Nucl Med 2003; 30:117–122.
6. Pichler BJ, Kneilling M, Haubner R, Braumuller H, Schwaiger M, Rocken M, Weber WA. Imaging of delayed-type hypersensitivity reaction by PET and 18F-Galacto-RGD. J Nucl Med 2005; 46:184–189.
7. Laking GR, Price PM. Positron emission tomographic imaging of angiogenesis and vascular function. Br J Radiol 2003; 76:S50–S59.
8. Chen X, Park R, Shahinian AH, Tohme M, Khankaldyyan V, Bozorgzadeh MH, Bading JR, Moats R, Laug WE, Conti PS. 18F-labeled RGD peptide: initial evaluation for imaging brain tumor angiogenesis. Nucl Med Biol 2004; 31:179–189.
9. Puduvalli VK, Sawaya R. Antiangiogenesis—therapeutic strategies and clinical implications for brain tumors. J Neurooncol 2000; 50:189–200.
10. Stöcklin GL. Is there a future for clinical fluorine-18 radiopharmaceuticals (excluding FDG)? Eur J Nucl Med 1998; 25:1612–1616.
11. Maecke HR, Hofmann M, Haberkorn U. 68Ga-labeled peptides in tumor imaging. J Nucl Med 2005; 46:172s–178s.
12. Henze M, Schuhmacher J, Dimitrakopoulou-Strauss A, Strauss LG, Macke ME, Haberkorn U. Exceptional increase in somatostatin receptor expression in pancreatic neuroendocrine tumor, visualised with 68Ga-DOTATOC PET. Eur J Nucl Med 2004; 31:466.
13. Kowalski J, Henze M, Schuhmacher J, Maecke HR, Hofmann M, Haberkorn U. Evaluation of positron emission tomography imaging using [68Ga]-DOTA-D-Phe[1]-Tyr[3]-octreotide in comparison to [111In]-DTPAOC SPECT. First results in patients with neuroendocrine tumors. Mol Imaging Biol 2003; 5:42–48.

14. Breeman WAP, De Jong M, De Blois E, Bernard BF, Konijnenberg M, Krenning EP. Radiolabeling DOTA-peptides with [68]Ga. Eur J Nucl Med 2005.

15. Hofmann M, Maecke H, Borner R, Weckesser E, Schoffski P, Oei L, Schumacher J, Henze M, Heppler A, Meyer J, Knapp H. Biokinetics and imaging with the somatostatin receptor PET radioligand ^{68}Ga-DOTATOC: preliminary data. Eur J Nucl Med 2001; 28:1751–1757.

16. Deutsch E. Clinical PET: its time has come? J Nucl Med 1993; 34:1132–1133.

17. Froidevaux S, Calame-Christe M, Schuhmacher J, Tanner H, Saffrich R, Henze M, Eberle AN. A gallium-labeled DOTA-alpha-melanocyte-stimulating hormone analog for PET imaging of melanoma metastases. J Nucl Med 2004; 45:116–123.

18. Hofmann M, Machtens S, Stief C, Maecke H, Boerner AR, Knapp WH. Feasibility of Ga-68-DOTABOM PET in prostate carcinoma patients. J Nucl Med 2004; 45:449P.

19. Schuhmacher J, Maecke H, Hauser H, et al. In vivo and in vitro characterization of a [67,68]Ga-labeled bombesin (6-14) analog for receptor scintigraphy with PET. Nuklearmedizin 2004; 43:A145.

20. Ugur O, Kothari PJ, Finn RD, Zanzonico P, Ruan S, Guenther I, Maecke HR, Larson SM. Ga-66 labeled somatostatin analogue DOTA-D-Phe[1]-Tyr[3]-octreotide as a potential agent for positron emission tomography imaging and receptor mediated internal radiotherapy of somatostatin receptor positive tumors. Nucl Med Biol 2002; 29:147–157.

21. Froidevaux S, Eberle AN, Christe M, Sumanovski L, Heppeler A, Schmitt JS, Eisenwiener K, Beglinger C, Macke HR. Neuroendocrine tumor targeting: study of novel gallium-labeled somatostatin radiopeptides in a rat pancreatic tumor model. Int J Cancer 2002; 98:930–937.

22. Graham MC, Pentlow KS, Mawlawi O, Finn RD, Daghighian F, Larson SM. An investigation of the physical characteristics of [66]Ga as an isotope for PET imaging and quantification. Med Phys 1997; 24:317–326.

23. Obata A, Kasamatsu S, McCarthy DW, Welch MJ, Saji H, Yonekura Y, Fujibayashi Y. Production of therapeutic quantities of ^{64}Cu using a 12 MeV cyclotron. Nucl Med Biol 2003; 30:535–539.

24. McCarthy DW, Shefer RE, Klinkowstein RE, Bass LA, Margeneau WH, Cutler CS, Anderson CJ, Welch MJ. The efficient production of high specific activity Cu-64 using a biomedical cyclotron. Nucl Med Biol 1997; 24:35–43.

25. Li WP, Lewis JS, Kim J, Bugaj JE, Johnson MA, Erion JL, Anderson CJ. DOTA-D-Tyr1-octreotate: a somatostatin analogue for labeling with metal and halogen radionuclides for cancer imaging and therapy. Bioconj Chem 2002; 13:721–728.

26. Rogers BE, Bigott HM, McCarthy DW, Della Manna D, Kim J, Sharp TL, Welch MJ. MicroPET imaging of a gastrin-releasing peptide receptorpositive tumor in a mouse model of human prostate cancer using a ^{64}Cu-labeled bombesin analogue. Bioconj Chem 2003; 14:756–763.

27. Lewis MR, Wang M, Axworthy DB, Theodore LJ, Mallet RW, Fritzberg AR, Welch MJ, Anderson CJ. In vivo evaluation of pretargeted 64Cu for tumor imaging and therapy. J Nucl Med 2003; 44:1284–1292.

28. Lewis JS, Laforest R, Lewis MR, Anderson CJ. Comparative dosimetry of copper-64 and yttrium-90-labeled somatostatin analogs in a tumor-bearing rat model. Cancer Biother Radiopharm 2000; 15:593–604.

29. Anderson CJ, Jones LA, Bass LA, Sherman EL, McCarthy DW, Cutler PD, Lanahan MV, Cristel ME, Lewis JS, Schwarz SW. Radiotherapy, toxicity, and dosimetry of copper-64-TETA-yoctreotide in tumor-bearing rats. J Nucl Med 1998; 39:1944–1951.

30. Lewis JS, Lewis MR, Cutler PD, Srinivasan A, Schmidt MA, Schwarz SW, Morris MM, Miller JP, Anderson CJ. Radiotherapy and dosimetry of ^{64}Cu-TETA-Tyr^3-octreotate in a somatostatin receptor-positive, tumor-bearing rat model. Clin Cancer Res 1999; 5:3608–3616.

31. Lewis J, Laforest R, Buettner T, Song S, Fujibayashi Y, Connett J, Welch M. Copper-64-diacetyl-bis(N 4-methylthiosemicarbazone): an agent for radiotherapy. Proc Natl Acad Sci USA 2001; 98:1206–1211.

32. Apelgot S, Coppey J, Gaudemer A, Grisvard J, Guille E, Sasaki I, Sissoeff I. Similar lethal effect in mammalian cells for two radioisotopes of copper with different decay schemes, ^{64}Cu, and ^{67}Cu. Int J Radiat Biol 1989; 55:365–384.

33. Sun X, Kim J, Martell AE, Welch MJ, Anderson CJ. In vivo evaluation of copper-64-labeled monoxo-tetraazamacrocyclic ligands. Nucl Med Biol 2004; 31:1051–1059.

34. Sprague JF, Peng Y, Sun X, Weisman GR, Wong EH, Achilefu S, Anderson CJ. Preparation and biological evaluation of copper-64-labeled Tyr^3-octreotate using a cross-bridged macrocyclic chelator. Clin Cancer Res 2004; 10:8674–8682.

35. Weisman GR, Wong EH, Hill DC, Rogers ME, Reed DP, Calabrese JC. Synthesis and transition-metal complexes of new cross-bridged tetraamine ligands. J Chem Soc Chem Commun 1996;947–948.

36. Wong EH, Weisman GR, Hill DC, Hill DC, Reed DP, Rogers ME, Condon JS, Fagan MA, Calabrese JC, Lam KC, Guzei IA, Rheingold AL. Synthesis and characterization of cross-bridged cyclams and pendant-armed derivatives and structural studies of their copper (II) complexes. J Am Chem Soc 2000; 122:10561–10572.

37. Boswell CA, Sun X, Niu W, Weisman GR, Wong EH, Rheingold AL, Anderson CJ. Comparative in vivo stability of copper-64-labeled cross-bridged and conventional tetraazamacrocyclic chelators. J Med Chem 2004; 47:1465–1474.

38. Sun X, Wuest M, Weisman GR, Wong EH, Reed DP, Boswell CA, Motekaitis R, Martell AE, Welch MJ, Anderson CJ. Radiolabeling and in vivo behaviour of copper-64-labeled cross-bridged cyclam ligands. J Med Chem 2002; 45:469–477.

39. Chen X, Park R, Hou Y, Tohme M, Shahinian AH, Bading JR, Conti PS. MicroPET and autoradiographic imaging of GRP receptor expression with ^{64}Cu-DOTA-[Lys^3] bombesin in human prostate adenocarcinoma xenografts. J Nucl Med 2004; 45:1390–1397.

40. Thakur ML, Aruva MR, Gariepy J, Acton P, Rattan S, Prasad S, Wickjstrom E, Alavi A. PET imaging of oncogene overexpression using ^{64}Cu-vasoactive intestinal peptide (VIP) analog: comparison with 99mTc-VIP analog. J Nucl Med 2004; 45:1381–1389.

41. Chen X, Park R, Tohme M, Shahinian AH, Bading JR, Conti PS. MicroPET and autoradiographic imaging of breast cancer (α-integrin expression using ^{18}F- and ^{64}Cu-labeled RGD peptide. Bioconj Chem 2004; 15:41–49.

42. Rösch F, Qaim SM, Stöcklin G. Production of the positron emitting radioisotope ^{86}Y for nuclear medical application. Appl Radiat Isot 1993; 44:677–681.

43. Herzog H, Rösch F, Stöcklin G, Lueders C, Qaim SM, Feinendegen LE. Measurement of pharmacokinetics of yttrium-86 radiopharmaceuticals with PET and radiation dose calculation of analogous yttrium-90 radiotherapeutics. J Nucl Med 1993; 34:2222–2226.

44. Rösch F, Herzog H, Plag C, Neumaier B, Braun U, Muller-Gratner HW, Stocklin G. Radiation doses of yttrium-90-citrate and yttrium-90-EDTMP. Eur J Nucl Med 1996; 23:958–966.

45. Poethko T, Schottelius M, Thumshirn G, Thumshirn G, Hersel U, Herz M, Henriksen G, Kessler H, Schwaiger M, Wester HJ. Two-step methodology for high-yield routine radiohalogenation of peptides: ^{18}F-labeled RGD and octreotide analogs. J Nucl Med 2004; 45:892–920.

46. Rösch F, Herzog H, Stolz B, Brockmann J, Kohle M, Muhlensiepen H, Marbach P, Muller-Gartner HW. Uptake kinetics of the somatostatin receptor ligand $[^{86}Y]$DOTA-DPhe^1-Tyr^3-octreotide ($[^{86}Y]$SMT487) using positron emission tomography in non-human primates and calculation of radiation doses of the ^{90}Y-labelled analogue. Eur J Nucl Med 1999; 26:358–366.

47. Förster GJ, Engelbach MJ, Brockmann JJ, Reber HJ, Buchholz HG, Macke HR, Rosch FR, Herzog HR, Bartenstein PR. Preliminary data on biodistribution and dosimetry for therapy planning of somatostatin receptor positive tumors: comparison of ^{86}Y-DOTATOC and ^{111}In-DTPA-octreotide. Eur J Nucl Med 2001; 28:1743–1750.

48. Pentlow KS, Graham MC, Lambrecht RM, Daghighian F, Bacharach SL, Bendriem B, Finn RD, Jordan K, Kalaigian H, Karp JS, Robeson WR, Larson SM. Quantitative imaging of iodine-124 with PET. J Nucl Med 1996; 37:1557–1562.

49. Herzog H, Tellmann L, Qaim SM, Spellerberg S, Schmid A, Coenen HH. PET quantization and imaging of the non-pure positron-emitting iodine isotope ^{124}I. Appl Radiat Isot 2002; 56:673–679.

50. Lubberink M, Tolmachev V, Widström C, Bruskin A, Lundqvist H, Westlin J. 110mIn-DTPA-D-Phe1-octrotide for imaging of neuroendocrine tumors with PET. J Nucl Med 2002; 43:1391–1397.

51. Adams S, Baum R, Rink T, Schumm-Drager PM, Usadel KH, Hor G. Limited value of fluorine-18 fluorodeoxyglucose positron emission tomography for the imaging of neuroendocrine tumors. Eur J Nucl Med 1998; 25:79–83.

52. Kilbourn MR, Dence CS, Welch MJ, Mathias CJ. Fluorine-18 labeling of proteins. J Nucl Med 1987; 28:462–470.

53. Vaidyanathan G, Zalutsky MR. Labeling proteins with fluorine-18 using N-succinimidyl 4- $[^{18}F]$fluorobenzoate. Nucl Med Biol 1992; 19:275–281.

54. Vaidyanathan G, Zalutsky MR. Improved synthesis of N-succinimidyl-4-$[^{18}F]$fluoro-benzoate and its application to the labeling of a monoclonal antibody fragment. Bioconj Chem 1994; 5:352–356.

55. Wester HJ, Hamacher K, Stöcklin G. A comparative study of N.C.A. fluorine-18 labeling of proteins via acylation and photochemical conjugation. Nucl Med Biol 1996; 23:365–372.

56. Guhlke S, Wester HJ, Bruns C, Stocklin G. (2-$[^{18}F]$fluoropropionyl-(D)Phe^1)-octreotide, a potential radiopharmaceutical for quantitative somatostatin receptor imaging with PET: synthesis, radiolabeling, in vitro validation and biodistribution in mice. Nucl Med Biol 1994; 21:819–825.

57. Downer JB, McCarthy TJ, Edwards WB, Anderson CJ, Welch MJ. Reactivity of p-[^{18}F]fluorophenacylbromide for radiolabeling of proteins and peptides. Appl Radiat Isot 1997; 48:907–916.

58. Wester HJ, Brockmann J, Rösch F, Wutz W, Herzog H, Smith-Jones P, Stolz B, Bruns C, Stocklin G. PET-pharmacokinetics of ^{18}F-octreotide: a comparison with ^{67}Ga-DFO-octreotide and ^{86}Y-DTPA-octreotide. Nucl Med Biol 1997; 24:275–286.

59. Okarvi SM. Recent progress in fluorine-18 labelled peptide radiopharmaceuticals. Eur J Nucl Med 2001; 28:929–938.

60. Sutcliffe-Goulden JL, O'Doherty MJ, Marsden PK, Hart IR, Marshall JF, Bansal SS. Rapid solid phase synthesis and biodistribution of ^{18}F-labelled linear peptides. Eur J Nucl Med 2002; 29:754–759.

61. Schottelius M, Wester HJ, Reubi JC, Senekowitsch-Schmidtke R, Schwaiger M. Improvement of pharmacokinetics of radioiodinated Tyr^3-octreotide by conjugation with carbohydrates. Bioconj Chem 2002; 13:1021–1030.

62. Glaser M, Karlsen H, Solbakken M, Arukwe J, Brady F, Luthra SK, Cuthbertson A. ^{18}F-Fluorothiols: a new approach to label peptides chemoselectively as potential tracers for positron emission tomography. Bioconj Chem 2004; 15:1447–1453.

63. Schottelius M, Poethko T, Herz M, Reubi JC, Kessler H, Schwaiger M, Wester HJ. First ^{18}F-labeled tracer suitable for routine clinical imaging of sst receptor-expressing tumors using positron emission tomography. Clin Cancer Res 2004; 10:3593–3606.

64. Mäding P, Füchtner F, Wüst F. Module-assisted synthesis of the bifunctional labelling agent N-succinimidyl 4-[^{18}F]fluorobenzoate ([^{18}F]SFB). Appl Rad Isot 2005; 63:329–332.

65. De Bruin B, Kuhnast B, Hinnen F, Yaouancq L, Amessou M, Johannes L, Samson A, Boisgard R, Tavitian B, Dolle F. 1-[3-(2-[^{18}F]fluoropyridin-yloxy)propyl]pyrrole-2,5-dione: design, synthesis, and radiosynthesis of a new [^{18}F]fluoropyridine-based maleimide reagent for the labeling of peptides and proteins. Bioconj Chem 2005; 16:406–420.

66. Heppeler A, Froidevaux S, Eberle AN, Maecke HR. Receptor targeting for tumor localization and therapy with radiopeptides. Curr Med Chem 2000; 7:971–994.

67. Eisenwiener KP, Prata MI, Buschmann I, Zhang HW, Santos AC, Wenger S, Reubi JC, Macke HR. NODAGATOC, a new chelator-coupled somatostatin analogue labeled with [$^{67/68}$Ga] and [^{111}In] for SPECT, PET, and targeted therapeutic applications of somatostatin receptor (hsst2) expressing tumors. Tumors Bioconj Chem 2002; 13:530–541.

68. Meyer GJ, Mäcke HR, Schuhmacher J, Knapp WH, Hofmann M. ^{68}Ga-labelled DOTA-derivatised peptide ligands. Eur J Nucl Med Mol Imaging 2004; 31:1097–1104.

69. Velikyan I, Beyer GJ, Långström B. Microwave-supported preparation of ^{68}Ga bioconjugates with high specific radioactivity. Bioconj Chem 2004; 15:554–560.

70. Jahn HA, Teller E. Stability of polyatomic molecules in degenerate electronic states I—orbital degeneracy. Proc Roy Soc London Series A 1937; 161:220–235.

71. Kaden TA. Structural aspects of metal complexes with functionalized azamacro-cyclic ligands. Pure Appl Chem 1993; 65:1477–1483.

72. Anderson CJ, Pajeau TS, Edwards WB, Sherman ELC, Rogers BE, Welch MJ. In vitro and in vivo evaluation of copper-64-octreotide conjugates. J Nucl Med 1995; 36:2315–2325.

73. Boswell CA, McQuade P, Weisman GR, Wong EH, Anderson CJ. Optimization of labeling and metabolite analysis of copper-64-labeled azamacrocyclic chelators by radio-LC-MS. Nucl Med Biol 2005; 32:29–38.

74. Glaser M, Collingridge DR, Aboagye EO, Bouchier-Hayes L, Hutchinson OC, Martin SJ, Price P, Brady F, Luthra SK. Iodine-124 labelled annexin-V as a potential radiotracer to study apoptosis using positron emission tomography. Appl Rad Isot 2003; 58:55–62.

75. Hostetler ED, Edwards WB, Anderson CJ, Welch MJ. Synthesis of 4-[^{18}F]fluoro-obenzoyl octreotide and biodistribution in tumor-bearing lewis rats. J Labelled Cpd Radiopharm 1999; 42:S720–S721.

76. Ogawa M, Hatano K, Oishi S, Kawasumi Y, Fujii N, Kawaguchi M, Doi R, Imamura M, Yamamoto M, Ajito K, Mukai T, Saji H, Ito K. Direct electrophilic radiofluorination of a cyclic RGD peptide for in vivo $\alpha_v\beta_3$ integrin related tumor imaging. Nucl Med Biol 2003; 30:1–9.

77. Haubner R, Kuhnast B, Mang C, Weber WA, Kessler H, Wester HJ, Schwaiger M. [^{18}F]Galacto-RGD: synthesis, radiolabeling, metabolic stability, and radiation dose estimates. Bioconj Chem 2004; 15:61–69.

78. Chen X, Hou Y, Tohme M, Park R, Khankaldyyan V, Gonzales-Gomez I, Bading JR, Laug WE, Conti PS. Pegylated Arg-Gly-Asp peptide: ^{64}Cu labeling and PET imaging of brain tumor $\alpha_v\beta_3$-integrin expression. J Nucl Med 2004; 45:1776–1783.

79. Chen X, Liu S, Hou Y, Tohme M, Park R, Bading JR, Conti PS. MicroPET imaging of breast cancer (α-integrin expression with ^{64}Cu-labeled dimeric RGD peptides. Mol Imaging Biol 2004; 6:350–359.

80. Schuhmacher J, Zhang H, Doll J, Macke HR, Matys R, Hauser H, Henze M, Haberkorn U, Eisenhut M. GRP receptor-targeted PET of a rat pancreas carcinoma xenograft in nude mice with a ^{68}Ga-labeled bombesin(6-14) analog. J Nucl Med 2005; 46:691–699.

81. Vaidyanathan G, Zalutsky MR. Fluorine-18-lebeled [Nle^4,D-Phe^7]-α-MSH, an α-melanocyte stimulating hormone analogue. Nucl Med Biol 1997; 24:171–178.

82. Froidevaux S, Calame-Christe M, Tanner H, Eberle AN. Melanoma targeting with DOTA-α-melanocyte-stimulating hormone analogs: structural parameters affecting tumor uptake and kidney uptake. J Nucl Med 2005; 46:887–895.

83. Zijlstra S, Gunawan J, Burchert W. Synthesis and evaluation of a ^{18}F-labelled recombinant annexin-V derivative, for identification and quantification of apoptotic cells with PET. Appl Rad Isot 2003; 58:201–207.

84. Yagle KJ, Eary JF, Tait JF, Grierson JR, Link JM, Lewellen B, Gibson DF, Krohn KA. Evaluation of ^{18}F-annexin V as a PET imaging agent in an animal model of apoptosis. J Nucl Med 2005; 46:658–666.

85. Dekker B, Keen H, Lyons S, Disley L, Hastings D, Reader A, Ottewell P, Watson A, Zweit J. MBP-annexin V radiolabeled directly with iodine-124 can be used to image apoptosis in vivo using PET. Nucl Med Biol 2005; 32:241–252.

86. Keen HG, Dekker BA, Disley L, Hastings D, Lyons S, Reader AJ, Ottewell P, Watson A, Zweit J. Imaging apoptosis in vivo using ^{124}I-annexin V and PET. Nucl Med Biol 2005; 32:395–402.

87. Dekker B, Keen H, Shaw D, Disley L, Hastings D, Hadfield J, Reader A, Allan D, Julyan P, Watson A, Zweit J. Functional comparison of annexin V analogues labeled indirectly and directly with iodine-124. Nucl Med Biol 2005; 32:403–413.

5

Radiolabeling DOTA-Peptides with ^{90}Y and ^{177}Lu to a High Specific Activity

Wouter A. P. Breeman, Erik de Blois, and Willem H. Bakker

Department of Nuclear Medicine, Erasmus MC Rotterdam, Rotterdam, The Netherlands

Eric P. Krenning

Department of Nuclear Medicine, and Department of Internal Medicine, Erasmus MC Rotterdam, Rotterdam, The Netherlands

RADIOLABELING DOTA-PEPTIDES WITH ^{90}Y AND ^{177}LU TO A HIGH SPECIFIC ACTIVITY

DOTA-conjugated peptides, such as the stable somatostatin analogs [DOTA^0,Tyr^3]octreotate (DOTA-tate) and [DOTA^0,Tyr^3]octreotide (DOTATOC), can be readily labeled with radionuclides such as ^{90}Y and ^{177}Lu. In order for these radiolabeled peptides to be successfully used in peptide receptor radionuclide therapy (PRRT) (1–6), high specific activities (SA) are required (7). There are a number of biological factors that dictate the need for high SA. First, for in vivo use the amount of (radio)ligand that can be administered is limited by affinity and amount of receptors. Above the optimal dose a further increase in ligand will increase the competition between unlabeled and labeled ligand for the same receptor and consequently lower the uptake of radiolabel into receptor-positive tissue (4). Second, for peptides that display pharmacological effects, such as substance P or bombesin, including their DOTA-analogs, even less quantities of peptide are tolerated. The amount that can be administered intravenously is for some peptides limited to 0.2–0.5 nmol per minute (8,9). The higher the SA, the lower the amount of peptide is needed for the administration for imaging and/or therapy. Third, endocytotic mechanisms that affect the cellular internalization of peptides may become desensitised at high peptide concentration (10), also resulting in lower uptake of radionuclide into target tissue. Moreover, in vitro investigations aimed at measuring receptor-binding affinities require low concentrations of these radioligands (e.g., 10^{-10} M) in order to measure accurately. Unfortunately, the need for high SA is often compromised by conflicting radiochemical parameters that determine reaction rates and yields, i.e., the rate of formation of the metal-DOTA complexes increases with pH (11), but the solubility of Y^{3+} and Lu^{3+} decreases with pH due to formation of colloids or hydroxides (12).

Reaction Conditions: The Effects of pH and Temperature

Studies are performed to determine the optimal conditions for radiolabeling DOTA-peptides, using the radionuclide ^{90}Y and ^{177}Lu, and DOTATOC and DOTA-tate as model reactants. The effects of ever-present contaminants such as nuclides formed by decay of the radionuclides are summarised (13). Successful labeling of DOTA-analogs with ^{90}Y and ^{177}Lu in the presence of sodium acetate is also reported at pH 7–8 (14,15). However, solubility problems may occur at high concentrations of these radionuclides (37 GBq per mL ^{90}Y represents 2.10^{-5} M solution of Y) at pH 7–8 (13). Reaction kinetics with ^{90}Y and ^{177}Lu were found to be optimal at pH 4–4.5, with a steep decrease at lower pH [13]. In addition, the % incorporation at pH $\geq$ 5 became non-reproducable; after centrifugation in these reaction vials precipitation is found (13). The binding kinetics are time- and temperature-dependent. With ^{90}Y and ^{177}Lu the reaction is complete after 20 minutes at 80 °C (Fig. 1). In Table 1 the highest SA of ^{90}Y and ^{177}Lu achieved are presented, implying a mol/mol ratio of DOTA over nuclide of 3½ and 6, respectively (see also Legend Table 1). The rate of incorporation is > 99%, even at a mol/mol ratio (DOTA-peptide over $^{176+177}Lu$) of 1.2 (13). Radiochemical purity (RCP) of the radiolabeled DOTATOC and DOTA-tate are studied at room temperature in the presence of 4 mM DTPA pH 5 and virtually no transchelation is measured (13). If samples are taken in the absence of a chelator (as DTPA), non-incorporated $^{90}Y^{3+}$ and $^{177}Lu^{3+}$ will stick to the carrier of ITLC and/or HPLC, and will result in a false-positive good incorporation (ITLC) and poor recoveries (HPLC), and thus an unreliable RCP (15,16). See also *DTPA-addition reroutes free radionuclide.*

Maximal Achievable SA, and Effects of Contaminants

Ions of Hf^{4+} and Zr^{4+}, decay products of ^{177}Lu and ^{90}Y, respectively, and Sr^{2+} (parent of ^{90}Y) have no effect on the % incorporation of both radionuclides in the DOTA-peptide, indicating that these nuclides are no competitor under the

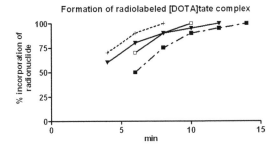

Figure 1 Formation of radiolabeled DOTA-tate at pH 4 as function of time of incubation, as measured by the % incorporation of the radionuclide. Similar results are reported with DOTATOC as ligand (13). ^{177}Lu at 80° (+) and 100° C (▼), ^{90}Y at 80° (■) and 100° C (□).

reaction conditions (13). In contrast, the addition of ions of nuclides, such as Fe and Cd, clearly showed that these metals are strong competitors for the incorporation of radionuclide in the DOTA-peptide, as shown in Table 2. The ingrowth of Hf did not affect the maximal achievable SA; high SA are measured even two weeks after production of ^{177}Lu (13).

Table 1 Production Methods, Target Materials, Decay Products, Physical Constants and Maximal SA of ^{90}Y and ^{177}Lu

	^{90}Y	^{177}Lu
Production method	Generator	Reactor (n)
Target	^{90}Sr	^{176}Lu
Decay product	^{90}Zr	^{177}Hf
Physical constants		
T1/2 [in days]	2.67	6.71
Pmoles per MBq	0.55	1.4
Maximal SA [MBq per pmol]		
Theory[a]	1.8	0.7
In practice[b]	0.5	0.1[b] and 0.4[c]

Note: The highest SA of ^{90}Y and ^{177}Lu achieved are presented, this implies a mol/mol ratio of DOTA over nuclide of $3\frac{1}{2}$ and 6 respectively. The latter needs extra explanation, since, due to the production process, the current achievable SA (and only in high flux reactors) is 0.7–0.9 MBq per mg Lu (specifications Missouri University Reactor Research and NRG), while the maximal achievable SA in theory is 4 GBq per mg Lu.

[a] Since 1 nmol DOTA can incorporate 1 nmol (radio)nuclide, this number indicates the maximal theoretical SA of the radiolabeled DOTA-peptides.

[b] Highest value achieved, this implies a ratio of DOTA over radionuclide practice (b).

[c] 0.1 GBq per nmol with (n, γ) produced ^{177}Lu via ^{176}Lu, and 0.4 GBq per nmol from ^{176}Yb target.

Abbreviation: SA, specific activity, expressed as MBq per pmol.

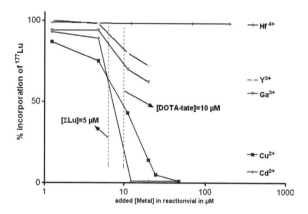

Figure 2 Effects of contaminants on the incorporation of ^{177}Lu in DOTA-tate by the controlled addition of nuclides (13), and the results of the additions are summarized in Table 2. The concentration of $^{176/177}$Lu and DOTA-tate in the reaction vial were approximately 5 and 10 μM, resp. Similar results are reported with ^{90}Y and with DOTA-tate as ligand (13).

Ligands and Radionuclides

In general the DOTA-peptides are dissolved in 0.01–0.05 M acetic acid in Milli-Q water. Sodium ascorbate (25 mM final, as buffer and quencher) and gentisic acid (50 mM final as quencher) (15,16) are dissolved in 50 mM sodium acetate (13). Currently good quality ^{90}Y, enabling radiolabeling DOTA-peptides at high specific activities, is available (1,13,15,16). Highly enriched ^{176}Lu is irradiated in high flux reactors. Missouri University Reactor Research (MURR), St Louis, MO, U.S.A., and NRG, Petten, the Netherlands (distributed by IDB Holland, Baarle Nassau, The Netherlands) are producing high quality ^{177}Lu and in high quantities (>200 GBq per week). The radionuclides are delivered in 0.01–0.1 N HCl. A typical standardized mixture for four patients contains 40 GBq of ^{177}LuCl$_3$ in 1 mL, mixed with 1 mg of DOTA-tate, 105 mg ascorbic acid, and 525 mg gentisic

Table 2 Effects of Metal Ions as Contaminants in Reaction Vial on Incorporation of Radionuclides in DOTA-Ligand

0	Ag^+	Hf^{4+}	Hg^{2+}	Sr^{2+}	Zr^{4+}			
+	Ga^{3+}	Y^{3+}						
+ +	Cd^{2+}	Co^{2+}	Cu^{2+}	In^{3+}	Fe^{2+}	Lu^{3+}	Ni^{2+}	Zn^{2+}

Classification of effects: the concentration of the metal ions and corresponding effects on the incorporation of radionuclides in DOTA-ligand 0: ≤10% at 10 μM; +: ≥10% at 1-10 μM; + +: ≥10% at 1 μM. From Table 2 can be seen that Hf^{4+} is no competitor for Lu in the incorporation in DOTA. This implies that the ingrowth of Hf has no consequences for the maximal achievable SA. In addition, high SA can still be achieved even 2 weeks after production of ^{177}Lu.
Abbreviation: SA, specific activities.

acid in 2.5 mL. Recently ^{177}Lu produced via ^{176}Yb (17) is commercially available (www.mds.nordion.com), the quality hereof was investigated, and the maximal achievable SA increased from 0.1 to 0.4 GBq per nmol DOTA-peptides (unpublished results from the author, see also Table 1). The amount of ligand can thus be lowered, or the amount of radioactivity can be concordantly be increased.

DTPA-Addition Reroutes Free Radionuclide

The incorporation of ^{90}Y and ^{177}Lu in DOTA-peptides is typically $\geq 99.5\%$, however, there is always a free fraction ($=$ non-incorporated ^{90}Y^{3+} or ^{177}Lu^{3+}), and since therapeutically doses are involved, the absolute amount of free ^{90}Y^{3+} and ^{177}Lu^{3+} can be significant. Moreover, free ^{90}Y^{3+} and ^{177}Lu^{3+} acts as Ca^{2+} mimic, and will by consequence accumulate in bone with unwanted bone marrow irradiation. Based on the knowledge that DTPA-ligands are rapidly excreted via the kidneys, studies were performed in rats. After radiolabeling DOTA-peptides, an excess of DTPA is added and complexes the fraction of free ^{90}Y^{3+} or ^{177}Lu^{3+} into ^{90}Y-DTPA or ^{177}Lu-DTPA, and these are cleared via the kidneys (18,19). As an example for the above-mentioned reaction mixture, post radiolabeling 1 mL 10 mM DTPA is added prior to patient administration. This resulted in lowered specifications of incorporation for the radiolabeled DOTA-peptides to 97%.

CONCLUSIONS

1. DOTA-peptides can be radiolabeled at high SA
2. Reactions can be influenced by contaminants, hereby reducing the maximal achievable specific activity of the radiolabeled DOTA-peptide
3. Reaction kinetics differ per radionuclide; conditions were optimal with ^{90}Y and ^{177}Lu at pH 4–4.5 and the reactions were complete after 20 minutes at 80 °C
4. After labeling DOTA-peptides with ^{90}Y or ^{177}Lu, the addition of DTPA prior to intravenous administration is recommended.

ACKNOWLEDGMENTS

Stimulation discussions within COST B12 working group three is greatly acknowledged.

REFERENCES

1. Otte A, Jermann E, Behe M, et al. DOTATOC: a powerful new tool for receptor-mediated radionuclide therapy. Eur J Nucl Med 1997; 24:792–795.
2. Erion JL, Bugaj JE, Schmidt MA, Wilhelm RR, Srinivasan A. High radiotherapeutic efficacy of [Lu-177]-DOTA-Y3-octreotate in a rat tumor model. J Nucl Med 1999; 40:223.
3. Krenning EP, Valkema R, Kooij PP, et al. The role of radioactive somatostatin and its analogues in the control of tumor growth. Recent Results Cancer Res 2000; 153:1–13.
4. Breeman WA, de Jong M, Kwekkeboom DJ, et al. Somatostatin receptor-mediated imaging and therapy: basic science, current knowledge, limitations and future perspectives. Eur J Nucl Med 2001; 28:1421–1429.
5. Kwekkeboom D, Krenning EP, de Jong M. Peptide receptor imaging and therapy. J Nucl Med 2000; 41:1704–1713.
6. Kwekkeboom DJ, Bakker WH, van der Pluijm ME, et al. Lu-177-DOTA-Tyr3-Octreotate: comparison with In-111-DTPA-octreotide in patients. Eur J Nucl Med 2000; 27:273.
7. Bernhardt P, Kolby L, Johanson V, Nilsson O, Ahlman H, Forssell-Aronsson E. Biodistribution of 111in-DTPA-D-Phe1-octreotide in tumor-bearing nude mice: influence of amount injected and route of administration. Nucl Med Biol 2003; 30:253–260.
8. Basso N, Lezoche E, Speranza V. Studies with bombesin in man. World J Surg 1979; 3:579–585.
9. van Hagen PM, Breeman WA, Reubi JC, et al. Visualization of the thymus by substance P receptor scintigraphy in man. Eur J Nucl Med 1996; 23:1508–1513.
10. Bunemann M, Hosey MM. G-protein coupled receptor kinases as modulators of G-protein signalling. J Physiol 1999; 517:5–23.
11. Szilagyi ETE, Kovacs Z, Platzek J, Radüchel B, Brücher E. Equilibria and formation kinetics of some cyclen derivative complexes of lanthanides. Inorganica Chemica Acta 2000; 298:226–234.
12. Moerlein SM, Welch MJ. The chemistry of gallium and indium as related to radiopharmaceutical production. Int J Nucl Med Biol 1981; 8:277–287.
13. Breeman WA, De Jong M, Visser TJ, Erion JL, Krenning EP. Optimizing conditions for radiolabelling of DOTA-peptides with 90Y, 111In and 177Lu at high specific activities. Eur J Nucl Med Mol Imaging 2003; 30:917–920.
14. Kukis DL, DeNardo SJ, DeNardo GL, O'Donnell RT, Meares CF. Optimized conditions for chelation of yttrium-90-DOTA immunoconjugates. J Nucl Med 1998; 39:2105–2110.
15. Liu S, Edwards DS. Stabilization of (90)y-labeled DOTA-biomolecule conjugates using gentisic acid and ascorbic acid. Bioconjug Chem 2001; 12:554–558.
16. Liu S, Ellars CE, Edwards DS. Ascorbic acid: useful as a buffer agent and radiolytic stabilizer for metalloradiopharmaceuticals. Bioconjug Chem 2003; 14:1052–1056.
17. Lebedev NA, Novgorodov AF, Misiak R, Brockmann J, Rosch F. Radiochemical separation of no-carrier-added 177Lu as produced via the 176Yb(n,gamma)177Yb—> 177Lu process. Appl Radiat Isot 2000; 53:421–425.

18. Breeman WA, van der Wansem K, Bernard BF, et al. The addition of DTPA to [177Lu-DOTA0,Tyr3]octreotate prior to administration reduces rat skeleton uptake of radioactivity. Eur J Nucl Med Mol Imaging 2003; 30:312–315.

19. Breeman WA, De Jong MT, De Blois E, Bernard BF, De Jong M, Krenning EP. Reduction of skeletal accumulation of radioactivity by co-injection of DTPA in [90Y-DOTA0,Tyr3]octreotide solutions containing free 90Y3+. Nucl Med Biol 2004; 31:821–824.

6

Peptide Receptor Radionuclide Therapy: Preclinical Findings

Astrid Capello, Wouter A. P. Breeman, Bert Bernard,
and Marion de Jong
Department of Nuclear Medicine, Erasmus MC Rotterdam, Rotterdam,
The Netherlands

Eric P. Krenning
Department of Nuclear Medicine, and Department of Internal Medicine,
Erasmus MC Rotterdam, Rotterdam, The Netherlands

INTRODUCTION

Somatostatin is a cyclopeptide that has a broad inhibitory effect on the secretion of hormones such as growth hormone, glucagon, and insulin. The finding that somatostatin inhibits hormone secretion of various glands led to the application of somatostatin in the treatment of diseases based on, for instance, overproduction of hormones by tumors. The native peptide somatostatin itself is unsuitable for routine treatment, as after intravenous administration it has a very short half-life due to rapid enzymatic degradation. Therefore, somatostatin analogs that are more resistant to enzymatic degradation were synthesized; the molecule was modified in various ways with preservation of the biological activity of the original molecule. Introduction of D-amino acids, an amino-alcohol Thr-ol at the C-terminus, and shortening of the molecule resulted e.g., in the 8 amino acids-containing somatostatin analog octreotide, having a long and therapeutically useful plasma half-life. The diagnostic radiolabeled peptide [^{111}In-DTPA]octreotide (OctreoScan, ^{111}In-pentetreotide) was approved by the FDA on June 2, 1994 for scintigraphy of

Table 1 Affinity Profiles (IC_{50}, nM) for Human sst_2, sst_3 and sst_5

Peptide	sst_2	sst_3	sst_5
SS-28	2.7	7.7	4.0
[In-DTPA]octreotide	22	182	237
[Y-DOTA,Tyr^3]octreotide (DOTATOC)	11	389	114
[Y-DOTA]lanreotide (DOTALAN)	23	290	16
[DOTA,Tyr^3]octreotate (DOTATATE)	1.5	>1,000	547
[Y-DOTA, 1-Nal^3]octreotide	3.3	26	10

Source: From Refs. 8, 9.

patients with neuroendocrine tumors. Nowadays somatostatin analogs are widely used in the treatment of symptoms due to neuroendocrine-active tumors, such as growth hormone-producing pituitary adenomas and gastroenteropancreatic tumors (1–4). Recently, improvement of quality of life has been demonstrated with long-acting depot formulations.

Somatostatin effects are mediated by high-affinity G-protein coupled membrane receptors, integral membrane glycoproteins. Five different human somatostatin receptor subtypes have been cloned (5–7). Somatostatin binds to all subtypes with high affinity, while the affinity of the different somatostatin analogs for these subtypes differ considerably. Octreotide e.g. binds with high affinity to the somatostatin receptor subtype 2 (sst_2), and with lower affinities to sst_5 and sst_3. It shows no binding to sst_1 and sst_4 (Table 1) (6).

Peptide receptor scintigraphy with radioactive octreotide, first [^{123}I-Tyr^3] octreotide and nowadays mostly [^{111}In-DTPA]octreotide (OctreoScan$^®$), appeared to be sensitive and specific for in vivo visualization of the presence and abundance of somatostatin receptors on the primary as well as metastatic tumor sites of a variety of neuroendocrine tumors, like carcinoids, islet cell tumors, and paragangliomas (10–15).

As soon as the success of peptide receptor scintigraphy for tumor visualization became clear, the next logical step was to try to label these peptides with therapeutic radionuclides, emitting α- or β-particles, or Auger or conversion electrons, and to perform peptide receptor radionuclide therapy (PRRT) with these radiolabeled peptides, as no effective general anti-tumor treatment is available for metastasized neuroendocrine tumors and only symptomatic relief can be achieved using somatostatin analogs and interferon.

OCTREOTIDE

The molecular basis of the use of radiolabeled octreotide in scintigraphy and radionuclide therapy is receptor-mediated internalization and cellular retention of the radionuclide. Internalization of radiolabeled [DTPA]octreotide in somatostatin receptor-positive tumors and tumor cell lines has been investigated (16–18) and it appeared that this process is receptor-specific and temperature dependent. Receptor-mediated internalization of [^{111}In-DTPA]octreotide results in degradation to the final radiolabeled metabolite ^{111}In-DTPA-D-Phe in the lysosomes (19). This metabolite is not capable passing the lysosomal and/or other cell membrane(s), and will therefore stay in the lysosomes, causing the long retention time of ^{111}In in sst$_2$-positive (tumor) cells.

Internalization of [^{111}In-DTPA]octreotide is especially important for radionuclide therapy of tumors when radionuclides emitting therapeutical particles with very short path lengths are used, like those emitting Auger electrons (e.g., ^{111}In). These electrons are only effective in a short distance of a few nm up to μm from their target, the nuclear DNA.

Recently, Hornick et al. (20) and Wang et al. (21) described in vitro cellular internalization, nuclear translocation, and DNA binding of radiolabeled somatostatin analogs, which significantly increased after prolonged exposure.

In a clonogenic assay in vitro the therapeutic potential of [^{111}In-DTPA]-octreotide was investigated (22). In this study 200 CA20948 tumor cells per well were plated in six-well plates; in this way the distance between the cells was long enough to rule out the option of crossfire between the cells when distributed equally in the well. In this in vitro system, [^{111}In-DTPA]octreotide could completely control the tumor growth; the effects (Table 2) were dependent on incubation time, radiation dose, and specific activity used. The longer the incubation period, the higher a tumoricidal effect was reached. When a higher specific activity was used (B vs. A&C) with the same amount of radioactivity (A vs. B), a higher tumor kill was reached. Similar concentrations of ^{111}In-DTPA, which is not internalized into sst$_2$-positive tumor cells like [^{111}In-DTPA]octreotide, did not influence tumor survival. So, ^{111}In-labeled peptides are therefore suitable for both scintigraphy and radionuclide therapy, all the more so as the decay of Auger electron emitter has recently been shown to lead to a "bystander effect," an in vivo, dose-independent inhibition or retardation of tumor growth in nonradiotargeted cells by a signal produced in Auger electron-labeled cells (23).

Table 2 Effects of Incubation Time, Concentration and Specific Activity of [^{111}In-DTPA]octreotide on the Cell Survival of CA20948 Cells After PRRT. Cells Were Incubated for 1, 3 and 5 Hours with 0.37 or 3.7 MBq [^{111}In-DTPA]octreotide at 37 °C Using Two Different Specific Activities [B vs. (A&C)].

	Incubation period		
Concentration/specific activity	1 hour	3 hours	5 hours
3.7 MBq (10^{-8} mol/L) (A)	28.48 ± 7.10	11.13 ± 6.90	11.18 ± 3.23
3.7 MBq (10^{-7} mol/L) (B)	47.04 ± 8.67	21.09 ± 7.38	20.31 ± 4.82
37 MBq (10^{-7} mol/L) (C)	18.68 ± 3.46	3.93 ± 3.12	0.54 ± 0.55

In our preclinical radionuclide therapy studies in vivo, we also used the rat pancreatic CA20948 tumor as a model for receptor-targeted scintigraphy and radionuclide therapy using radiolabeled somatostatin analogs. This tumor is transplantable in Lewis rats, not only subcutaneously in the flank, but also metastasized to the liver. The latter is achieved by inoculation of tumor cells in the portal vein of the liver. The CA20948 tumor has been shown to be somatostatin receptor-positive, being an excellent model to study receptor-targeted scintigraphy and radionuclide therapy in rats using radiolabeled somatostatin analogs (24).

We performed radionuclide therapy using [^{111}In-DTPA]octreotide in the CA20948 liver metastases model (25). Radionuclide therapy with administrations of 370 MBq (coupled to 0.5 µg octreotide) [^{111}In-DTPA]octreotide after intraportal CA20948 tumor cell inoculation induced a significant decrease in the number of hepatic metastases at day 21. Co-injection with 1 mg unlabeled octreotide resulted in inhibition of the tumor response to radionuclide therapy, pointing to a receptor-dependent therapeutic effect. Also, dose-dependent effects of radionuclide therapy by injection of 370, 37 or 3.7 MBq [^{111}In-DTPA]octreotide one day after tumor inoculation were investigated (26). The 370 MBq dosage had significantly more therapeutic effects and inhibited the increase of liver weight due to tumor growth more than the 37 or 3.7 MBq doses. The findings hold promise for application of radionuclide therapy with ^{111}In-labeled octreotide in an adjuvant, micrometastatic setting, e.g., after surgery to eradicate occult metastases.

As ^{111}In emits therapeutic Auger electrons with mean particle ranges of less than one cell diameter, radiation emitted from a receptor-positive tumor cell cannot kill neighboring receptor-negative cells in tumors with receptor heterogeneity. In clinical studies an anti-tumor response of high doses of [In-111-DTPA]octreotide was found; however, the radiopeptide was not very effective in end-stage patients and in patients with large tumors (27–32). Consequently, various research groups aimed to develop somatostatin analogs that can be linked via a chelator to a therapeutic radionuclide, which emits β-particles with longer particle ranges, such as ^{90}Y and ^{177}Lu. In addition, new somatostatin analogs were synthesized to improve receptor affinity.

OCTREOTIDE ANALOGS

Various chelator-peptide constructs have been synthesized and evaluated concerning their receptor affinity, internalization capacities, and biodistribution in vivo (Table 1) (33). The analogs tested included [DTPA,Tyr^3]octreotide and [DTPA,Tyr^3]octreotate (in octreotate the C-terminal threoninol has been replaced with the native amino acid threonine) in comparison to [DTPA]octreotide. Phe^3-residues were replaced with Tyr to increase the hydrophylicity of the peptides. Octreotate was synthesized to investigate the effects of an additional negative charge on clearance and cellular uptake. We concluded that radiolabeled

[DTPA,Tyr^3]octreotate and second best [DTPA,Tyr^3]octreotide, and also their DOTA-coupled counterparts, were most promising for scintigraphy and radionuclide therapy of octreotide receptor-positive tumors in humans (33).

DOTA is a universal chelator capable of formation of stable complexes with metals like ^{111}In, ^{67}Ga, ^{68}Ga, ^{86}Y, and ^{64}Cu for imaging as well as with ^{90}Y (high energy β-particle emitter) and with radiolanthanides like ^{177}Lu (low energy β-particle and gamma emitter) for receptor-mediated radionuclide therapy. Reubi et al. (8) evaluated the in vitro binding characteristics of labeled (indium, yttrium, gallium) and unlabeled [DOTA,Tyr^3]octreotide, [DOTA]octreotide, [DOTA]-lanreotide, [DOTA]vapreotide (RC-160), [DTPA,Tyr^3]octreotate, and [DOTA,-Tyr^3]octreotate using cell lines transfected with the human somatostatin receptor subtypes sst$_1$, sst$_2$, sst$_3$, sst$_4$, and sst$_5$ (Table 1). They found that small structural modifications, chelator substitution, or metal replacement considerably affected the receptor binding affinity. A marked improvement of sst$_2$ affinity was found for [Ga-DOTA,Tyr^3]octreotide (IC$_{50}$ 2.5 nM) compared with the Y-labeled compound and [In-DTPA]octreotide. An excellent binding affinity for sst$_2$ in the same range was also found for [In-DTPA,Tyr^3]octreotate (IC$_{50}$ 1.3 nM) and for [Y-DOTA,Tyr^3]octreotate (IC$_{50}$ 1.6 nM). Of ^{111}In-, ^{88}Y- and ^{177}Lu-labeled [DOTA,Tyr^3]octreotate, biodistribution and tumor uptake were compared in CA20948 tumor-bearing rats (34). In vivo, for all three radiolabeled analogs a rapid clearance from the blood and very high, specific uptake in sst$_2$-positive organs and tumor was found. For tumor and sst$_2$-positive organs it was found that uptake of ^{111}In- ≈ ^{88}Y- < [^{177}Lu-DOTA,Tyr^3]octreotate uptake, making the latter analog most promising for radionuclide therapy. Schmitt et al. (35) investigated [^{177}Lu-DOTA,Tyr^3]octreotate in nude mice with human small cell lung cancer and concluded that the tumor had a higher activity concentration compared to all measured normal tissues at all time points tested, pointing to the therapeutic potential of [^{177}Lu-DOTA,Tyr^3]octreotate for small cell lung cancer.

A therapeutic comparison between radiolabeled octreotide and octreotate was performed in vitro, after labeling with ^{177}Lu or ^{90}Y in a colony-forming assay using the rat pancreatic tumor cell line CA20948 (36). Both Tyr^3-octreotide and Tyr^3-octreotate labeled with either ^{177}Lu or ^{90}Y were able to control tumor growth in a dose-dependent manner. In all concentrations used, radiolabeled Tyr^3-octreotate had a higher tumor kill capacity compared to radiolabeled Tyr^3-octreotide, labeled with ^{177}Lu (Fig. 1) or ^{90}Y.

A comparison between radiolabeled octreotide and octreotate analogs was also performed in rats using ^{64}Cu-labeled analogs, reaching the same conclusion, that because of its high tumor uptake in comparison to that of the other analogs tested, [Tyr^3]octreotate was selected for future PET imaging and targeted radiotherapy studies. New stable analogs of somatostatin with high affinity for different somatostatin receptors are currently being developed. An interesting example is [DOTA, 1-Nal^3]octreotide, which has high affinity for sst$_2$, sst$_3$, and sst$_5$ (9,37). This compound may allow PRRT of tumors which do not bind octreotide and octreotate with high affinity, i.e., sst$_3$- and sst$_5$-positive tumors.

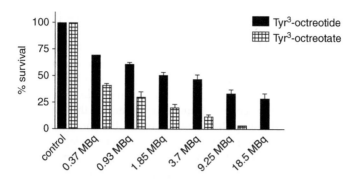

Figure 1 Inhibitory effect of ^{177}Lu coupled to either octreotide or octreotate on the tumor cell survival of the CA20948 cell line. Cells were incubated for 1 hour at 37 °C with increasing amounts of ^{177}Lu-octreotate or ^{177}Lu-octreotide. Data are expressed as mean ± SEM.

A problem during radionuclide therapy may be caused by the high uptake of radioactivity in the kidneys; small peptides in the blood plasma are filtered through the glomerular capillaries in the kidneys and subsequently reabsorbed by and retained in the proximal tubular cells, thereby reducing the scintigraphic sensitivity for detection of small tumors in the perirenal region and the possibilities for radionuclide therapy. The renal uptake of radiolabeled octreotide in rats could be reduced by positively charged amino acids, e.g., with about 50% by single intravenous administration of 400 mg/kg L- or D-lysine (38,39). Therefore, during PRRT an infusion containing the positively charged amino acids L-lysine and L-arginine (in patients e.g., 25 g lysine and 25 g arginine infused in 4 hours) can be given during and after the infusion of the radiopharmaceutical, in order to reduce the kidney uptake (40,41).

After ^{111}In, the next radionuclide investigated was ^{90}Y, emitting β-particles with a high maximum energy (2.27 MeV) and a long maximum particle range (> 10 mm). The first somatostatin analog radiolabeled with ^{90}Y and applied for PRRT in animals and patients was [^{90}Y-DOTA,Tyr[3]]octreotide, in which, in comparison with octreotide, the phenylalanine residue at position 3 has been replaced with tyrosine; this makes the compound more hydrophilic and increases the affinity for sst_2, leading to higher uptake in sst_2-positive tumors both in preclinical studies and in patients (33,42).

We compared the radiotherapeutic effect of different doses [^{90}Y-DOTA,-Tyr[3]]octreotide in rats bearing pancreatic CA20948 tumors of different size in the flank (43). After the highest dose, i.e., 370 MBq [^{90}Y-DOTA,Tyr[3]]octreotide, 50% complete response was reached for the small tumors (< 1 cm^2), whereas only growth delay was found in the very large tumors (> 12 cm^2). Medium-sized tumors (about 8 cm^2), however, showed 100% cure after this same dose of [^{90}Y-DOTA,Tyr[3]]octreotide. So, in this study a difference is found in the radio-therapeutic effects in CA20948 tumors of different size. In larger tumors more clonogenic, presumably hypoxic, cells will be present, thereby limiting radiocurability. The small tumors on the other hand, will not absorb all energy emitted by ^{90}Y, thereby decreasing tumor curability.

Significant tumor growth delay was also found in rats bearing small CA20948 tumors after radionuclide therapy with up to 3×740 MBq [^{64}Cu-TETA,Tyr^3]octreotide or [^{64}Cu-TETA,Tyr^3]octreotate (44,45), the first compound given either fractionated or as a single dose. Dose fractionation in two doses induced significantly increased tumor growth inhibition compared with rats given a single dose. However, in this study the single 555 MBq dose was bound to twice the amount of peptide compared to the two 278 MBq doses. So, partial saturation of the receptors using the single high dose and therefore relatively lower uptake of radioactivity in the tumor may have contributed to these findings.

Tumor growth inhibition in the same model was also found after treatment of CA20948 tumor-bearing rats with [^{90}Y-DTPA-benzyl-acetamido-Tyr^3]octreotide (46). Using 370 MBq/kg of [^{90}Y-DOTA,Tyr^3]octreotide, the same group observed even complete tumor reduction in five out of seven rats (47).

Clinical studies to determine the therapeutic efficacy of [^{90}Y-DOTA-Tyr^3]octreotide in cancer patients are ongoing at various institutions in Basel, Milano, Brussels, and Rotterdam (41,48–56). The most promising rate of complete plus partial responses seen in the various [^{90}Y-DOTA-Tyr^3]octreotide studies consistently surpasses that obtained with [In-111-DTPA]octreotide.

The next analog investigated in preclinical radionuclide therapy studies was [^{177}Lu-DOTA,Tyr^3]octreotate. ^{177}Lu emits gamma radiation with a suitable energy for imaging and therapeutic β-particles with low to medium energy (maximum 0.50 MeV), so the same complex can be used for both imaging and dosimetry and radionuclide therapy, thus obviating the need for a pretherapeutic diagnostic study. The approximate range of the β-particles is 20 cell diameters, whereas the range of those emitted by ^{90}Y is 150 cell diameters. Less "cross-fire" induced radiation damage in the renal glomeruli can therefore be expected with ^{177}Lu. Also, in comparison with ^{90}Y, a higher percentage of the ^{177}Lu radiation energy will be absorbed in very small tumors and (micro)metastases.

We investigated the anti-tumor effects of [^{177}Lu-DOTA,Tyr^3]octreotate in various models, including a rat liver micrometastatic model, mimicking disseminated disease, and a solid tumor model. [^{177}Lu-DOTA,Tyr^3]octreotate showed anti-tumoral effects in the rat liver tumor metastases model leading to significant better survival in the treated rats (57).

In the radionuclide therapy studies using ^{177}Lu-labeled octreotate for therapy in solid tumors, 100% cure was found in the groups of rats bearing small (≤ 1 cm^2) CA20948 tumors after two repeated doses of 277.5 MBq or after a single dose of 555 MBq [^{177}Lu-DOTA,Tyr^3]octreotate (estimated tumor dose 60 Gy) (34). After therapy with the same doses of [^{177}Lu-DOTA,Tyr^3]octreo*tide*, that has a lower tumor uptake than the octreotate analog, these data were 50% and 60% cure in rats bearing small tumors. In rats bearing larger (≥ 1 cm^2, range 1.4–10 cm^2) tumors, 40% and 50% cure were found in the groups that received one or two 277.5 MBq injections of [^{177}Lu-DOTA,Tyr^3]octreotate, respectively (34). However, in another study in a different rat pancreatic tumor model (AR42J), in which a more favorable tumor dose was reached after 555 MBq [^{177}Lu-DOTA,Tyr^3]octreotate (140 Gy), all rats but one were cured irrespective of the size of their tumor (unpublished result). So, [^{177}Lu-DOTA,Tyr^3]octreotate showed excellent therapeutic results in the rats bearing small to big tumors, and the findings for the small tumors were in accordance with those of an earlier study (58).

Patients treated with [^{177}Lu-DOTA,Tyr3]octreotate showed complete or partial remissions in an impressive 30% of the patients, and a minor response in 12% (59).

In a different set of preclinical experiments the combination of [^{177}Lu-DOTA,Tyr^3]octreotate and [^{90}Y-DOTA,Tyr^3]octreotide (at a constant total dose) was studied in rats that each bore both a small (0.1 cm^2) and a large tumor (8 cm^2), to mimic the clinical situation, in which large tumors and small metastases are usually present in the same patient. The rats treated with the combination of 50% [^{177}Lu-DOTA,Tyr^3]octreotate plus 50% [^{90}Y-DOTA,Tyr^3]-octreotide/or octreotate showed a longer survival than those treated with 100% [^{90}Y-DOTA,Tyr^3]octreotide/octreotate or [^{177}Lu-DOTA,Tyr^3]octreotate (60). This underscores the great promise of ^{177}Lu- and ^{90}Y-labeled somatostatin analogs for radionuclide therapy and the potential of the combination of these radionuclides with different β-energies and particle ranges to achieve higher cure rates in the presence of tumors of different size.

We conclude that [^{177}Lu-DOTA,Tyr^3]octreotate is a very promising somatostatin analog for radionuclide therapy in patients suffering from sst$_2$-expressing tumors. In patients with tumors of different size, including small metastases, combinations of radionuclides are also interesting, e.g., ^{90}Y and ^{177}Lu, to obtain the widest range of tumor curability.

Because in animal experiments ^{90}Y-labeled somatostatin analogs are more effective for larger tumors, and ^{177}Lu-labeled somatostatin analogs are more effective for smaller tumors, whereas their combination was found to be most effective (see above), a very interesting treatment will be [^{90}Y-DOTA,Tyr^3]octreotide and [^{177}Lu-DOTA,Tyr^3]octreotate. Apart from the combination of analogs labeled with different radionuclides, future directions to improve this therapy may also include efforts to upregulate the somatostatin receptor expression on the tumors, as well as studies to the effects of the use of radiosensitizers.

LANREOTIDE

Virgolini et al. developed an ^{111}In-/^{90}Y- labeled somatostatin analog, [DOTA]-lanreotide, for tumor diagnosis and therapy (61–64). They described that ^{111}In-/^{90}Y-labeled [DOTA]lanreotide bound with high affinity to a number of primary human tumors. [^{111}In-DOTA]lanreotide bound with high affinity to

$hsst_2$, $hsst_3$, $hsst_4$, and $hsst_5$ and with lower affinity to $hsst_1$ expressed on COS7 cells, making it a universal receptor binder (65). In Sprague Dawley rats, [^{90}Y-DOTA]lanreotide was rapidly cleared from the circulation and concentrated in somatostatin receptor-positive tissues, such as pancreas or pituitary. It was concluded that this radiolabeled peptide can be used for somatostatin receptor-mediated diagnosis as well as systemic radiotherapy of human tumors. However, Reubi et al. found in vitro in cell lines transfected with the different somatostatin receptor subtypes that whereas [Y-DOTA]lanreotide had a good affinity for the sst_5, it had a low affinity for sst_3 (IC_{50} 290 nM) and sst_4 (IC_{50} > 10,000 nM) (8). Thereby, they challenged the concept that lanreotide is a universal binder to the different somatostatin receptors. Froidevaux et al. (66) concluded from their comparison study of among other things [DOTA,Tyr^3]octreotide and [DOTA]-lanreotide in rats that radiolabeled [DOTA,Tyr^3]octreotide has more potential for clinical application than [DOTA]lanreotide.

Lanreotide was the second analog labeled with ^{90}Y and used for clinical PRRT studies. Virgolini et al. (62) reported on the biodistribution, safety, and radiation-absorbed dose of [^{111}In-DOTA]lanreotide. [^{90}Y-DOTA]lanreotide treatment was further studied at different centers in the MAURITIUS (Multicenter Analysis of a Universal Receptor Imaging and Treatment Initiative, a European Study) trial (63). Overall treatment results in 70 patients indicated stable tumor disease in 35% of patients and regressive tumor disease in 10% of tumor patients with different tumor entities expressing hSSTR. In two-thirds of patients with neuroendocrine tumor lesions, [^{90}Y-DOTA,Tyr^3]octreotide showed a higher tumor uptake than [^{90}Y-DOTA]lanreotide, which can be explained by the lower affinity of [^{90}Y-DOTA]lanreotide for sst_2.

RC-160

Several reports have been published on the in vitro receptor binding to somatostatin receptors of another somatostatin analog, the octapeptide RC-160 (vapreotide). It has been reported that RC-160 has a higher affinity than octreotide for the somatostatin receptors in human breast, ovarian, exocrine pancreatic, prostatic, and colonic cancer, explained by the much higher affinity of RC-160 for sst_4 (67,68). Therefore, the possible binding of RC-160 to a somatostatin receptor subtype that does not bind octreotide (sst_4), should offer a potential advantage for RC-160 over octreotide. However, different experiments showed that [^{111}In-DTPA]RC-160 does not seem to have advantages over [^{111}In-DTPA]oc-treotide as a radiopharmaceutical for somatostatin receptor scintigraphy, despite the fact that [^{111}In-DTPA]RC-160 shows specific high-affinity binding to somatostatin receptor-positive organs (69–71). This is in accordance with the findings of Reubi et al. (8), who showed that the affinities of [DOTA]RC-160 and [^{90}Y-DOTA]RC-160 for the human sst_2 and sst_3 are in the same range as that of [^{111}In-DTPA]octreotide. The affinities (IC_{50}) of the RC-160 analogs for the sst_4, however, were found to be low, around 700 nM (for [^{111}In-DTPA]octreotide the IC_{50} for the sst_4 was > 1000 nM), in contrast to the above mentioned findings. Furthermore, unlike (radioiodinated) RC-160 that passes the blood-brain barrier, it was also shown that [^{111}In-DTPA]RC-160 and [^{111}In-DTPA]octreotide do not pass the blood-brain barrier organs (69–71). Also Froidevaux et al. (66) concluded from biodistribution studies in experimental animals comparing [DOTA]RC-160 and other DOTA-coupled somatostatin analogs (lanreotide, octreotide, [Tyr^3] octreotide) and from clinical data that [DOTA-Tyr^3]octreotide has a better potential in the clinic than RC-160.

Rhenium-188 coupled to the analog RC-160 has also been used to establish the feasibility of treating tumors with radiolabeled peptides (72–74). In different experimental tumor models in nude mice, treatment resulted in significant reduction or elimination of tumor burden. Long-term studies with ^{188}Re-RC-160 demonstrated a protracted reduction of tumor volume and a positive effect on animal survival. Neither RC-160 by itself nor an ^{188}Re-labeled peptide unrelated to somatostatin demonstrated the reduction in tumor mass observed with ^{188}Re-RC-160.

RGD-OCTREOTATE

As described above, a large variety of radiolabeled somatostatin derivatives have been prepared for radionuclide therapy purposes and are in various stages of investigation. Furthermore, cell matrix interactions are fundamental to tumor invasion and formation of metastases as well as to tumor-induced angiogenesis. Integrins, heterodimeric transmembrane glycoproteins, composed of an alpha- and beta-subunit, play a key role in these interactions. One of these integrins, the $\alpha_v\beta_3$ receptor, is able to bind a number of extracellular matrix proteins via an Arg-Gly-Asp (RGD) sequence (75). This receptor is expressed on various malignant human tumors and upregulated in proliferating endothelial cells. Based on the RGD sequence, several compounds have been designed as $\alpha_v\beta_3$ antagonists. In tumor models using the $\alpha_v\beta_3$, antagonists not only blocked tumor-angiogenesis but in some cases also resulted in tumor regression (76,77).

In addition, several procaspases also contain potential RGD-binding motifs near the site necessary for activation to the mature caspase. Caspases are proteases that are critical in programmed cell death (78). Buckley and coworkers (79) demonstrated that RGD peptides are able to directly activate caspase-3 and thereby induce apoptosis. Other work has shown that molecules specific for GPIIb/IIIa integrins can also stimulate caspase-3 activity (80). Since caspase-3 is one of the key executioner proteases (81) in the apoptosis pathway, it seems likely that this enzyme will be an important site of action for targeted therapeutics that are designed to selectively induce cell death.

To further enhance the therapeutic potential of the somatostatin analogs, we hypothesize that the synergistic effects of an apoptosis-inducing factor, such as an Arg-Gly-Asp (RGD) motif, can increase the radiotherapeutic efficacy of these peptides. We combined the characteristics of the somatostatin analog

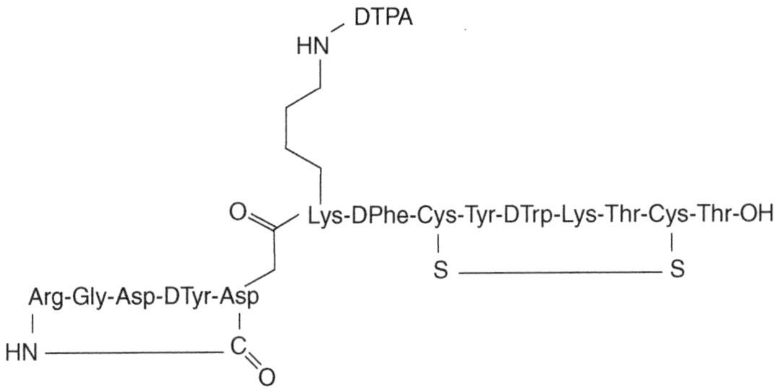

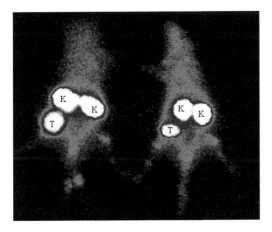

Figure 2 Structure of RGD-octreotate [c(Arg-Gly-Asp-D-Tyr-Asp)-Lys(DTPA)-Phe-c(Cys-Tyr-D-Trp-Lys-Thr-Cys)-Thr].

Tyr^3-octreotate and RGD in one compound by synthesizing the hybrid peptide RGD-DTPA-octreotate [c(Arg-Gly-Asp-D-Tyr-Asp)-Lys(DTPA)-Phe-c(Cys-Tyr-D-Trp-Lys-Thr-Cys)-Thr] (Fig. 2) (82).

In biodistribution studies in rats we showed that there is a high receptor-specific uptake in sst$_2$-positive tissues and tumors of RGD[^{111}In-DTPA]-octreotate (Fig. 3) and comparable to the uptake of [^{111}In-DOTA,Tyr^3]octreotate in sst$_2$-positive tissues and tumors. A decreased uptake in sst$_2$-positive tissues and tumors was found after co-injection of RGD[^{111}In-DTPA]octreotate with 500 μg unlabeled octreotide. A drawback of the new hybrid compound is the high renal uptake and retention of radioactivity, limiting the therapeutic dose that can be administered, as the kidneys are the first dose-limiting organs in radionuclide

Figure 3 Scan of two rats bearing a CA20948 tumor on their right hind leg, 24 hours post injection of RGD[^{111}In-DTPA,Tyr^3]octreotate. *Abbreviations*: K, kidney; T, Tumor.

therapy using somatostatin analogs. D-lysine injection resulted in 40% reduction of the renal uptake.

In an in vitro study the tumoricidal effects of the ^{111}In-labeled peptide RGD-DTPA-octreotate in comparison with ^{111}In-labeled RGD and Tyr[3]-octreotate were evaluated using a colony-forming assay (83). Tumor cell survival after incubation with 9.25 MBq for 1 hour with ^{111}In-labeled RGD, octreotate, and RGD-DTPA-octreotate were 81%, 68% and 43%, respectively, in the CA20948 cell line, showing that the radiolabeled RGD-DTPA-octreotate has a more pronounced tumoricidal effect than [^{111}In-DTPA]RGD and [^{111}In-DTPA]octreotate. The superior tumoricidal effect is probably the result of increased apoptosis, as is shown by an increased caspase-3 activity after incubation with ^{111}In-labeled RGD-DTPA-octreotate.

These results show that the ^{111}In-labeled peptide RGD-DTPA-octreotate promotes apoptosis in comparison with the two monopeptides RGD and Tyr[3]-octreotate, via an increase in caspase-3 levels. The ^{111}In-labeled hybrid peptide can therefore significantly enhance the therapeutic efficacy of somatostatin-based agents. Because of the high kidney uptake of this hybrid peptide it is also very interesting to use the unlabeled peptide RGD(DTPA)octreotate for a adjuvant therapy.

CONCLUSION

This chapter shows that radionuclide therapy with radiolabeled somatostatin analogs is a most promising new treatment modality for patients bearing sst_2-positive tumors.

A variety of other peptide-based radioligands, like bombesin, gastrin/cholecystokinin, and neurotensin analogs, which receptors are expressed on different major cancers, and RGD peptides, which can be targeted to many major tumors because of their binding to receptors expressed on newly formed blood vessels and which can induce apoptosis, is currently under development.

In conclusion, radiolabeled peptides have opened a new era in nuclear oncology, not only for diagnosis but also for radionuclide therapy.

REFERENCES

1. Kvols LK, Moertel CG, O'Connell MJ, Schutt AJ, Rubin J, Hahn RG. Treatment of the malignant carcinoid syndrome. Evaluation of a long-acting somatostatin analogue. N Engl J Med 1986; 315:663–666.
2. Eriksson B, Oberg K. Summing up 15 years of somatostatin analog therapy in neuroendocrine tumors: future outlook. Ann Oncol 1999; 10:S31–S38.
3. Lamberts SW, Krenning EP, Reubi JC. The role of somatostatin and its analogs in the diagnosis and treatment of tumors. Endocr Rev 1991; 12:450–482.
4. Lamberts SW, Reubi JC, Krenning EP. Somatostatin analogs in the treatment of acromegaly. Endocrinol Metab Clin North Am 1992; 21:737–752.

5. Patel YC, Greenwood MT, Panetta R, Demchyshyn L, Niznik H, Srikant CB. The somatostatin receptor family. Life Sci 1995; 57:1249–1265.

6. Patel YC. Somatostatin and its receptor family. Front Neuroendocrinol 1999; 20:157–198.

7. Schonbrunn A. Somatostatin receptors present knowledge and future directions. Ann Oncol 1999; 10:S17–S21.

8. Reubi JC, Schar JC, Waser B, et al. Affinity profiles for human somatostatin receptor subtypes SST1-SST5 of somatostatin radiotracers selected for scintigraphic and radiotherapeutic use. Eur J Nucl Med 2000; 27:273–282.

9. Wild D, Schmitt JS, Ginj M, et al. DOTA-NOC, a high-affinity ligand of somatostatin receptor subtypes 2, 3 and 5 for labelling with various radiometals. Eur J Nucl Med Mol Imaging 2003; 30:1338–1347.

10. Krenning EP, Kwekkeboom DJ, Oei HY, et al. Somatostatin receptor scintigraphy in carcinoids, gastrinomas and Cushing's syndrome. Digestion 1994; 55:54–59.

11. Krenning EP, Kwekkeboom DJ, Oei HY, et al. Somatostatin-receptor scintigraphy in gastroenteropancreatic tumors. An overview of European results. Ann NY Acad Sci 1994; 733:416–424.

12. Krenning EP, Kwekkeboom DJ, Bakker WH, et al. Somatostatin receptor scintigraphy with [111In-DTPA-D-Phe1]- and [123I- Tyr3]-octeotide: the Rotterdam experience with more than 1000 patients. Eur J Nucl Med 1993; 20:716–731.

13. Krenning EP, Bakker WH, Breeman WA, et al. Localisation of endocrine-related tumors with radioiodinated analogue of somatostatin. Lancet 1989; 1:242–244.

14. Krenning EP, Bakker WH, Kooij PP, et al. Somatostatin receptor scintigraphy with indium-111-DTPA-D-Phe-1- octreotide in man: metabolism, dosimetry and comparison with iodine-123- Tyr-3-octreotide. J Nucl Med 1992; 33:652–658.

15. Bakker WH, Albert R, Bruns C, et al. [111In-DTPA-D-Phe1]-octreotide, a potential radiopharmaceutical for imaging of somatostatin receptor-positive tumors: synthesis, radiolabeling and in vitro validation. Life Sci 1991; 49:1583–1591.

16. Andersson P, Forssell-Aronsson E, Johanson V, et al. Internalization of indium-111 into human neuroendocrine tumor cells after incubation with indium-111-DTPA-D-Phe1-octreotide. J Nucl Med 1996; 37:2002–2006.

17. De Jong M, Bernard BF, De Bruin E, et al. Internalization of radiolabelled [DTPA0]octreotide and [DOTA0,Tyr3]octreotide: peptides for somatostatin receptor-targeted scintigraphy and radionuclide therapy. Nucl Med Commun 1998; 19:283–288.

18. Hofland LJ, van Koetsveld PM, Waaijers M, Lamberts SW. Internalization of isotope-coupled somatostatin analogues. Digestion 1996; 57:2–6.

19. Duncan JR, Stephenson MT, Wu HP, Anderson CJ. Indium-111-diethylenetriamine-pentaacetic acid-octreotide is delivered in vivo to pancreatic, tumor cell, renal, and hepatocyte lysosomes. Cancer Res 1997; 57:659–671.

20. Hornick CA, Anthony CT, Hughey S, Gebhardt BM, Espenan GD, Woltering EA. Progressive nuclear translocation of somatostatin analogs. J Nucl Med 2000; 41:1256–1263.

21. Wang M, Caruano AL, Lewis MR, Meyer LA, VanderWaal RP, Anderson CJ. Subcellular localization of radiolabeled somatostatin analogues: implications for targeted radiotherapy of cancer. Cancer Res 2003; 63:6864–6869.

22. Capello A, Krenning EP, Breeman WA, Bernard BF, de Jong M. Peptide receptor radionuclide therapy in vitro using [111In-DTPA0]octreotide. J Nucl Med 2003; 44:98–104.

23. Xue LY, Butler NJ, Makrigiorgos GM, Adelstein SJ, Kassis AI. Bystander effect produced by radiolabeled tumor cells in vivo. Proc Natl Acad Sci USA 2002; 99:13765–13770.

24. Bernard BF, Krenning E, Breeman WA, et al. Use of the rat pancreatic CA20948 cell line for the comparison of radiolabelled peptides for receptor-targeted scintigraphy and radionuclide therapy. Nucl Med Commun 2000; 21:1079–1085.

25. Slooter GD, Breeman WA, Marquet RL, Krenning EP, van Eijck CH. Antiproliferative effect of radiolabelled octreotide in a metastases model in rat liver. Int J Cancer 1999; 81:767–771.

26. De Jong M, Breeman WA, Bernard HF, et al. Therapy of neuroendocrine tumors with radiolabeled somatostatin- analogues. Q J Nucl Med 1999; 43:356–366.

27. Valkema R, De Jong M, Bakker WH, et al. Phase I study of peptide receptor radionuclide therapy with [In- DTPA]octreotide: the Rotterdam experience. Semin Nucl Med 2002; 32:110–122.

28. Krenning EP, de Jong M, Kooij PP, et al. Radiolabelled somatostatin analogue(s) for peptide receptor scintigraphy and radionuclide therapy. Ann Oncol 1999; 10:S23–S29.

29. Fjalling M, Andersson P, Forssell-Aronsson E, et al. Systemic radionuclide therapy using indium-111-DTPA-D-Phe1-octreotide in midgut carcinoid syndrome. J Nucl Med 1996; 37:1519–1521.

30. Anthony LB, Woltering EA, Espenan GD, Cronin MD, Maloney TJ, McCarthy KE. Indium-111-pentetreotide prolongs survival in gastroenteropancreatic malignancies. Semin Nucl Med 2002; 32:123–132.

31. McCarthy KE, Woltering EA, Anthony LB. In situ radiotherapy with 111In-pentetreotide. State of the art and perspectives. Q J Nucl Med 2000; 44:88–95.

32. McCarthy KE, Woltering EA, Espenan GD, Cronin M, Maloney TJ, Anthony LB. In situ radiotherapy with 111In-pentetreotide: initial observations and future directions. Cancer J Sci Am 1998; 4:94–102.

33. de Jong M, Breeman WA, Bakker WH, et al. Comparison of (111)In-labeled somatostatin analogues for tumor scintigraphy and radionuclide therapy. Cancer Res 1998; 58:437–441.

34. de Jong M, Breeman WA, Bernard BF, et al. [177Lu-DOTA(0),Tyr3] octreotate for somatostatin receptor-targeted radionuclide therapy. Int J Cancer 2001; 92:628–633.

35. Schmitt A, Bernhardt P, Nilsson O, et al. Biodistribution and dosimetry of 177Lu-labeled [DOTA0,Tyr3]octreotate in male nude mice with human small cell lung cancer. Cancer Biother Radiopharm 2003; 18:593–599.

36. Capello A, Krenning EP, Breeman WA, Bernard BF, Konijnenberg MW, de Jong M. Tyr3-octreotide and Tyr3-octreotate radiolabeled with 177Lu or 90Y: peptide receptor radionuclide therapy results in vitro. Cancer Biother Radiopharm 2003; 18:761–768.

37. Schmitt JS, Wild D, Ginj M, et al. DOTA-NOC, a high affinity ligand of the somatostatin receptor subtypes 2, 3 and 5 for radiotherapy. J Labelled Cpd Radiopharm 2001; 44:s697–s699.

38. de Jong M, Rolleman EJ, Bernard BF, et al. Inhibition of renal uptake of indium-111-DTPA-octreotide in vivo. J Nucl Med 1996; 37:1388–1392.

39. Bernard BF, Krenning EP, Breeman WA, et al. D-lysine reduction of indium-111 octreotide and yttrium-90 octreotide renal uptake. J Nucl Med 1997; 38:1929–1933.

40. Rolleman EJ, Valkema R, de Jong M, Kooij PP, Krenning EP. Safe and effective inhibition of renal uptake of radiolabelled octreotide by a combination of lysine and arginine. Eur J Nucl Med Mol Imaging 2003; 30:9–15.

41. Bodei L, Cremonesi M, Zoboli S, et al. Receptor-mediated radionuclide therapy with 90Y-DOTATOC in association with amino acid infusion: a phase I study. Eur J Nucl Med Mol Imaging 2003; 30:207–216.

42. Kwekkeboom DJ, Kooij PP, Bakker WH, Macke HR, Krenning EP. Comparison of 111In-DOTA-Tyr3-octreotide and 111In-DTPA-octreotide in the same patients: biodistribution, kinetics, organ and tumor uptake. J Nucl Med 1999; 40:762–767.

43. de Jong M, Breeman WA, Bernard BF, et al. Tumor response after [(90)Y-DOTA(0),Tyr(3)]octreotide radionuclide therapy in a transplantable rat tumor model is dependent on tumor size. J Nucl Med 2001; 42:1841–1846.

44. Anderson CJ, Jones LA, Bass LA, et al. Radiotherapy, toxicity and dosimetry of copper-64-TETA-octreotide in tumor-bearing rats. J Nucl Med 1998; 39:1944–1951.

45. Lewis JS, Lewis MR, Cutler PD, et al. Radiotherapy and dosimetry of 64Cu-TETA-Tyr3-octreotate in a somatostatin receptor-positive, tumor-bearing rat model. Clin Cancer Res 1999; 5:3608–3616.

46. Stolz B, Smith-Jones P, Albert R, et al. Somatostatin analogues for somatostatin-receptor-mediated radiotherapy of cancer. Digestion 1996; 57:17–21.

47. Stolz B, Weckbecker G, Smith-Jones PM, Albert R, Raulf F, Bruns C. The somatostatin receptor-targeted radiotherapeutic [90Y-DOTA-DPhe1,Tyr3]octreotide (90Y-SMT 487) eradicates experimental rat pancreatic CA 20948 tumors. Eur J Nucl Med 1998; 25:668–674.

48. de Jong M, Krenning E. New advances in peptide receptor radionuclide therapy. J Nucl Med 2002; 43:617–620.

49. De Jong M, Kwekkeboom D, Valkema R, Krenning EP. Radiolabelled peptides for tumor therapy: current status and future directions. Plenary lecture at the EANM 2002. Eur J Nucl Med Mol Imaging 2003; 30:463–469.

50. De Jong M, Valkema R, Jamar F, et al. Somatostatin receptor-targeted radionuclide therapy of tumors: preclinical and clinical findings. Semin Nucl Med 2002; 32:133–140.

51. Otte A, Herrmann R, Heppeler A, et al. Yttrium-90 DOTATOC: first clinical results. Eur J Nucl Med 1999; 26:1439–1447.

52. Otte A, Mueller-Brand J, Dellas S, Nitzsche EU, Herrmann R, Maecke HR. Yttrium-90-labelled somatostatin-analogue for cancer treatment [letter]. Lancet 1998; 351:417–418.

53. Paganelli G, Bodei L, Chinol M, et al. Receptor mediated radiotherapy with 90Y-DOTATOC: results of a phase I study. J Nucl Med 2001; 42:36.

54. Waldherr C, Pless M, Maecke HR, Haldemann A, Mueller-Brand J. The clinical value of [90Y-DOTA]-D-Phe1-Tyr3-octreotide (90Y-DOTATOC) in the treatment of neuroendocrine tumors: a clinical phase II study. Ann Oncol 2001; 12:941–945.

55. Waldherr C, Pless M, Maecke HR. Tumor response and clinical benefit in neuro-endocrine tumors after 7.4 GBq ^{90}Y-DOTATOC. J Nucl Med 2002; 43:610–616.

56. Bushnell D, O'Dorisio T, Menda Y, et al. Evaluating the clinical effectiveness of 90Y-SMT 487 in patients with neuroendocrine tumors. J Nucl Med 2003; 44:1556–1560.

57. Breeman WA, Mearadji A, Capello A, et al. Anti-tumor effect and increased survival after treatment with [177Lu-DOTA0,Tyr3]octreotate in a rat liver micrometastases model. Int J Cancer 2003; 104:376–379.

58. Erion JL, Bugaj JE, Schmidt MA, Wilhelm RR, Srinivasan A. High radiotherapeutic efficacy of [Lu-177]-DOTA-Y3-octreotate in a rat tumor model. J Nucl Med 1999; 40:223.

59. Kwekkeboom DJ, Bakker WH, Kam BL, et al. Treatment of patients with gastro-entero-pancreatic (GEP) tumors with the novel radiolabelled somatostatin analogue [177Lu-DOTA(0),Tyr3]octreotate. Eur J Nucl Med Mol Imaging 2003; 30:417–422.

60. De Jong M, Bernard HF, Breeman WAP, van Gameren A, Krenning EP. Combination of ^{90}Y- and ^{177}Lu-labeled somatostatin analogs is superior for radionuclide therapy compared to ^{90}Y- or ^{177}Lu-labeled analogs only. J Nucl Med 2002; 43:P123–P124.

61. Virgolini I, Traub T, Novotny C, et al. Experience with indium-111 and yttrium-90-labeled somatostatin analogs. Curr Pharm Des 2002; 8:1781–1807.

62. Virgolini I, Szilvasi I, Kurtaran A, et al. Indium-111-DOTA-lanreotide: biodistri-bution, safety and radiation absorbed dose in tumor patients. J Nucl Med 1998; 39:1928–1936.

63. Virgolini I, Britton K, Buscombe J, Moncayo R, Paganelli G, Riva P. In- and Y-DOTA-lanreotide: results and implications of the MAURITIUS trial. Semin Nucl Med 2002; 32:148–155.

64. Virgolini I, Kurtaran A, Angelberger P, Raderer M, Havlik E, Smith-Jones P. "MAURITIUS": tumor dose in patients with advanced carcinoma. Ital J Gastroenterol Hepatol 1999; 31:S227–S230.

65. Smith-Jones PM, Bischof C, Leimer M, et al. DOTA-lanreotide: a novel somatostatin analog for tumor diagnosis and therapy. Endocrinology 1999; 140:5136–5148.

66. Froidevaux S, Heppeler A, Eberle AN, et al. Preclinical comparison in AR4-2J tumor-bearing mice of four radiolabeled 1,4,7,10-tetraazacyclododecane-1,4,7,10-tetraacetic acid- somatostatin analogs for tumor diagnosis and internal radiotherapy. Endocrinology 2000; 141:3304–3312.

67. Srkalovic G, Cai RZ, Schally AV. Evaluation of receptors for somatostatin in various tumors using different analogs. J Clin Endocrinol Metab 1990; 70:661–669.

68. Liebow C, Reilly C, Serrano M, Schally AV. Somatostatin analogues inhibit growth of pancreatic cancer by stimulating tyrosine phosphatase. Proc Natl Acad Sci USA 1989; 86:2003–2007.

69. Breeman WA, Hofland LJ, Bakker WH, et al. Radioiodinated somatostatin analogue RC-160: preparation, biological activity, in vivo application in rats and comparison with [123I- Tyr3]octreotide. Eur J Nucl Med 1993; 20:1089–1094.

70. Breeman WA, Hofland LJ, van der Pluijm M, et al. A new radiolabelled somatostatin analogue [111In-DTPA-D-Phe1]RC-160: preparation, biological activity, receptor scintigraphy in rats and comparison with [111In-DTPA-D-Phe1]octreotide. Eur J Nucl Med 1994; 21:328–335.

71. Breeman WAP, van Hagen PM, Kwekkeboom DJ, Visser TJ, Krenning EP. Somatostatin receptor scintigraphy using [111In-DTPA0]RC-160 in humans: a comparison with [111In-DTPA0]octreotide. Eur J Nucl Med 1998; 25:182–186.

72. Zamora PO, Bender H, Knapp FF, Jr., Rhodes BA, Biersack HJ. Targeting peptides for pleural cavity tumor radiotherapy: specificity and dosimetry of Re-188-RC-160. Hybridoma 1997; 16:85–91.

73. Zamora PO, Gulhke S, Bender H, et al. Experimental radiotherapy of receptor-positive human prostate adenocarcinoma with 188Re-RC-160, a directly-radio-labeled somatostatin analogue. Int J Cancer 1996; 65:214–220.

74. Zamora PO, Bender H, Gulhke S, et al. Pre-clinical experience with Re-188-RC-160, a radiolabeled somatostatin analog for use in peptide-targeted radiotherapy. Anticancer Res 1997; 17:1803–1808.

75. Varner JA. The role of vascular cell integrins alpha v beta 3 and alpha v beta 5 in angiogenesis. EXS 1997; 79:361–390.

76. Brooks PC, Montgomery AM, Rosenfeld M, et al. Integrin alpha v beta 3 antagonists promote tumor regression by inducing apoptosis of angiogenic blood vessels. Cell 1994; 79:1157–1164.

77. Brooks PC, Stromblad S, Klemke R, Visscher D, Sarkar FH, Cheresh DA. Antiintegrin alpha v beta 3 blocks human breast cancer growth and angiogenesis in human skin. J Clin Invest 1995; 96:1815–1822.

78. Salvesen GS, Dixit VM. Caspases: intracellular signaling by proteolysis. Cell 1997; 91:443–446.

79. Buckley CD, Pilling D, Henriquez NV, et al. RGD peptides induce apoptosis by direct caspase-3 activation. Nature 1999; 397:534–539.

80. Adderley SR, Fitzgerald DJ. Glycoprotein IIb/IIIa antagonists induce apoptosis in rat cardiomyocytes by caspase-3 activation. J Biol Chem 2000; 275:5760–5766.

81. Wolf BB, Green DR. Suicidal tendencies: apoptotic cell death by caspase family proteinases. J Biol Chem 1999; 274:20049–20052.

82. Bernard BF, Capello, A, van Hagen PM. Radiolabeled RGD-DTPA-Tyr[3]-octreotate for receptor-targeted radionuclide therapy. Cancer Biother Radiopharm 2004; 19:273–280.

83. Capello A, Krenning EP, Bernard BF, Breeman WA, van hagen M, de Jong M. Increased cell death after therapy with an Arg-Gly-Asp linked somatostatin analog. J Nucl Med 2004; 45:1716–1720.

7

Pathological Evaluation and Biochemical Characterization of Peptide Receptors Other Than Somatostatin Receptors as Potential Tumor Targets for Radionuclide Diagnosis and Therapy

Giuseppe Pelosi, Michele Masullo, and Giuseppe Viale

Division of Pathology and Laboratory Medicine, European Institute of Oncology and University of Milan School of Medicine, Milan, Italy

INTRODUCTION

Recent in vitro studies have shown that several peptide receptors can be overexpressed in a variety of neoplasms, including neuroendocrine tumors, meningiomas, mesenchymal tumors, lymphomas, gliomas, blastomas, and several types of carcinomas from kidney, lung, liver, prostate, stomach, nasopharynx, and ovary (reviewed in Reubi, 2003) (1). Most of these studies have dealt with the characterization and distribution of somatostatin receptors on tumor cells, whereas less is known on the occurrence in different tumors of other receptors, including those binding vasoactive intestinal peptide (VIP), cholecystokinin (CCK), bombesin/gastrin-releasing peptide, neurotensin, α-melanocyte-stimulating hormone (MSH), neuropeptide Y, luteinizing hormone-releasing hormone (LHRH), calcitonin, atrial natriuretic peptide (ANP), glucagon-like peptide-1, oxytocin, endothelin and substance P. This review focuses on the distribution and the biochemical characterization of several peptide receptors other than somatostatin in different tumor types, and on the clinical relevance of their pathological assessment on tissue samples as an important tool for the proper diagnosis and therapy of different malignancies.

In the recent past, it has been demonstrated that several peptide receptors could be used as targets for in vivo detection of human cancers using low molecular weight-radiolabelled peptides (2) much more effectively than radiolabeled antibodies, because the excessive molecular mass of the latter could affect their in vivo distribution or target binding (3). This has prompted a great deal of in vitro and immunohistochemical investigations to unveil the molecular basis for targeting, showing that peptide receptors can be expressed at high levels by several tumor types (4,5). In particular, it has been documented that co-expression of several peptide receptors may occur in tumor cells, especially of neuroendocrine lineage. This is a further aspect of the inherent vast biological diversity of these neoplasms, but may also be used as a molecular background for the choice of the most suitable radiopeptides to be used—either singly or in association—for in vivo tumor diagnosis, metastasis localization, and therapy (5). The clinical advantage of this multireceptorial tumor targeting with radiolabeled molecular cocktails is that it makes it possible to target different tumors at the same time, or several co-expressed peptide receptors in a single tumor. The rationale of using several receptor-selective radiopeptides simultaneously is to facilitate tumor detection by increasing the scintigraphic signal or to improve the efficacy of targeted radiotherapy by taking into account tumor heterogeneity in the expression of peptide receptors. A further advantage of the combined use of different radiopeptides is that different isotopes with different radiation-emitting properties may be used simultaneously. All these approaches reduce the risk of a loss of efficacy during peptide radiotherapy or in vivo diagnostic tumor localization because of nonhomogeneous distribution of receptors within individual tumors (1,5,6). Moreover, different β-emitters with different ranges can be simultaneously used for obtaining the optimal radiotherapy of large and small neoplastic lesions (7).

To select the most suitable radiopeptides to be used in an individual patient for the best diagnostic or therapeutic results, the peptide receptors and their affinity profile may be preliminarily assayed on the tumor cells using a biopsy sample as an ex vivo model. Indeed, the direct assessment of the patients by scintigraphy is much more time-consuming, cumbersome, expensive, and may be hampered by high background signal due to radiopeptide binding to normal tissues. The precise knowledge of the distribution of peptide receptors at the cellular level in different tumor types, as well as of the prevalence of co-expressed receptors within individual tumors, are prerequisites for a successful clinical application of radiopeptides (8). Radiolocalization is an in vivo, indirect demonstration of functional receptor status, but does not dissect the different subtypes of individual peptide receptor, nor does it assess whether receptors are expressed by the neoplastic or non-neoplastic cell populations or both (4). As a matter of fact, it has been demonstrated that somatostatin receptor expression is not restricted to neoplastic cells of neuroendocrine or, to a lesser extent, non-neuroendocrine tumors, but may be also a feature of intratumoral lymphocytes, endothelia, and necrotic areas. This has to be taken into account in the evaluation of octreoscan findings, because the in vivo procedures do not allow to assess the cellular localization of the receptors. Moreover, most peptide receptors exist as multiple subtypes, which should be individually assessed not only for the best chances of optimal targeting for diagnosis and therapy, but also for ascertaining the pathobiological characteristics of the different tumors being labelled (1,5). Accordingly, the choice of the best in vitro methodology and molecular parameters to provide the required information is of primary relevance to the proper management of patients with peptide receptor-expressing tumors. The following section will discuss the methodological aspects of this assessment, paying special attention to the assays for peptide receptors other than somatostatin that have clinical relevance or are instrumental for translational research.

METHODOLOGICAL ASPECTS

Tumor peptide receptors have been extensively mapped by several techniques, which offer different results according to the specific questions to be addressed. Given that the receptor protein itself is the ultimate target of either the natural or the synthetic ligand, it is conceivable that protein-detecting methods are more useful than those highlighting the occurrence of specific mRNAs. In general, the first choice method should enable the assessment of the number of receptors harbored by tumor cells, be sensitive enough to detect even small amounts of molecules, and be characterized by a resolution high enough to localize the receptor binding sites at the subcellular levels, at the cell membrane, or in the cytoplasm or in the nuclei. Last but not least, the receptor assay should be easy to perform in most laboratories, with high intra- and inter-laboratory reproducibility, inexpensive, and not time-consuming, and possibly suitable for *routine* formalin-fixed and paraffin-embedded tissues to allow investigations of large retrospective or prospective series of tumors, especially when dealing with rare neoplasms like neuroendocrine tumors. Unfortunately, an assay with all the above characteristics has not been developed thus far, because all the currently available assays are affected by their own inherent limitations and drawbacks, either related to the type of material needed or the peculiar characteristics of the assay itself. For example, autoradiography is a highly sensitive method but it requires fresh frozen tissue, it cannot be applied to large retrospective series, and its signals are not permanent; immunohistochemistry, in turn, provides subcellular resolution, but essentially is a semiquantitative technique that does not allow a precise assessment of the amount of receptors expressed by tumor cells. The most commonly used assays will be dealt with in this section, paying particular attention to their methodological aspects, indications, and limitations or drawbacks.

Autoradiography

In vitro receptor autoradiography likely is the assay of first choice for its high diagnostic accuracy, because it allows simultaneously a highly sensitive localization of the receptors, together with the assessment of their functional activity (9). Moreover, it identifies the precise binding site of the receptor proteins, which will be targeted by radioligands, and used in vivo for diagnostic and therapeutic purposes. A subtype-specific autoradiography may be also used to detect the co-expression of multiple peptide receptor subtypes within individual tumors (10,11). The main drawbacks of this technique are that it requires fresh frozen tissue, thus making very difficult the analysis of large retrospective series of uncommon tumors unless an expensive and time-consuming tissue banking strategy is in place; furthermore, the final histological preparations are not permanent, and the results must be documented and stored as sets of photomicrographs. Briefly, the tissue frozen sections are reacted at room temperature with the radioligand (most often using ^{125}I radiolabeling) in a solution containing bovine serum albumine, bacitracin, and $MgCl_2$ to inhibit endogenous protease, and including some unlabelled ligand to reduce non-specific binding (5). Incubated sections are repeatedly washed first in the incubation buffer containing bovine serum albumine and then in buffer alone, to eliminate the excess of unlabelled radioligand and to ensure binding specificity. After quickly drying, the sections are apposed to film and exposed for an appropriate time in x-ray cassettes. To identify specific protein receptor subtypes in a given tumor, displacement experiments can be carried out using adjacent tissue sections and increasing concentrations of various unlabeled ligands under evaluation (5). Finally, autoradiograms are quantified by means of computer-assisted image processing system, and the assay is scored positive whenever the total binding absorbance is at least twice that of non-specific binding in the control section (12). When assessing multiple receptor subtypes belonging to the same receptor family in the same tumor, only receptors with a density equal to or greater than a given threshold value (conventionally stated at 10%) of the density of the most abundantly expressed receptor subtype are recorded as positive. When different receptor subtypes are known to partially compete with each other for the binding to the same radioligand (for example sst_1 and sst_5), a correction must be introduced in assaying the receptor status of a given tumor by subtracting the density value corresponding to the cross-reaction from the value measured (13). Another important aspect to be accounted for whenever detecting multiple peptide receptors in the same tumor—especially when a subtype-selective autoradiography is used with universal radioligands—is that the signal of a given receptor expressed at very low level on tumor cells could be partially or completely masked by another receptor subtype expressed at higher levels (8).

Immunohistochemistry

Immuno(cyto)histochemistry is becoming an emerging new diagnostic technique for peptide receptor assessment, especially in the study of large, either prospective or retrospective tumor series, in virtue of its diagnostic accuracy, low cost, and high reproducibility, and high cellular resolution when applied to paraffin-embedded tumor tissues (1,4). This assay precisely localizes the binding site of receptor proteins at the subcellular level, either cell membrane, cytoplasm, or nucleus, and detects co-expression of different peptide receptor subtypes by using antibodies with different specificities on adjacent tumor sections (4,14). Most of the receptor proteins detected by immuno(cyto)histochemical methods appear as a linear signal highlighting the entire cell membrane (4,14–16), whereas the detection of an intracellular immunostaining is currently an intriguing and not fully understood occurrence (17).

Briefly, immuno(cyto)histochemistry relies on the detection of a specific receptor protein in tumor sections by means of specific primary antibodies, either monoclonal or polyclonal; the resulting immune complex is subsequently revealed by directly labelled secondary antibodies or more sensitive, multi-layered "sandwich" systems, the latter allowing a higher number of enzyme or fluorochrome molecules to bind to the sites of primary reaction (18). For enzyme-based methods, appropriate chromogenic solutions are eventually applied to tumor sections to obtain a final colored immunoreaction product confined to the site of the immune complex and its immediate neighborhood. The results of the immunohistochemical assays depend on the quality, sensitivity, and specificity of the antibodies used, which are currently available for a large range of peptide receptors (1).

The major advantages of immuno(cyto)histochemistry, besides its higher cellular resolution than autoradiography, is that it provides permanent preparations and can be easily applied to *routine* histological or cytological samples. The main drawback is that it allows only a semiquantitative evaluation of the results, which can be scored as percentage of labelled cells, but not as the amount of peptide receptor proteins per individual tumor cells. This is because there is no direct relationship between staining intensity of tumor cells and the number of receptor molecules in the cell membrane. Additionally, immunohis-tochemical assays may identify an epitope different from the actual binding site, and therefore these assays do not provide information on the functional capability of tumor receptors. The comparative evaluation of the results stemming from immunohistochemical and reverse transcriptase-polymerase chain reaction (RT-PCR) assays or in vivo octreoscan tests demonstrated a high grade of correlation among the different assays in the detection of peptide receptor in tumor samples (14). Moreover, it has been clearly shown that an occasional immunoreactivity for peptide receptors can also be found in lymphocytes, stromal cells, endothelia, and necrotic tumor areas, which represent possible causes of false-positive results to be considered for a proper evaluation of in vivo octreoscans, when it is not possible to ascertain the precise tissue distribution of the signal (4,14). Therefore, immunohistochemistry may powerfully complement radionuclear investigations, either in vivo or in vitro, to better characterize the cellular content, and distribution of peptide receptors and their subtypes in a wide range of human tumors (1).

Molecular Assays for Detecting mRNA

Northern blot, RT-PCR, real-time RT-PCR, and in situ hybridization (ISH) may detect mRNA transcripts with high diagnostic accuracy, but without any morphological correlates (with the exception of ISH) as compared with autoradiography and immuno(cyto)histochemistry (4). RT-PCR and ISH have been used in several studies dealing with the detection of specific peptide receptor mRNAs in a variety of human cancers.

1. RT-PCR may identify very low levels of mRNAs, occurring either singly or concomitantly (reviewed in Reubi 2003) (1). The amount of mRNAs in tumors, however, appears generally higher than expected based on the findings of receptor binding or immunohistochemical assays (19–21). It is unclear whether the conflicting data are due to the outstanding sensitivity of the PCR technique or to the amplification of mRNA molecules from nontumoral adjacent tissues. Moreover, the occurrence of alternative splicing variants not consistently translated into significant amounts of the respective receptor subtype proteins or responsible for truncated and functionally inactive proteins may partially account for these discrepancies. Therefore, care should be taken to avoid an over-estimation of the expression of peptide receptors as documented by ultrasensitive methods such as RT-PCR, especially because it should be considered that the ultimate target of the ligands used in the current clinical applications is the receptor protein located on the cell membrane and not its mRNA (1). Another drawback of the RT-PCR assays on tissue homogenates is that it makes it impossible to assess the precise site of expression of the receptor, thus distinguishing between the specific signals from tumor cells and the nonspecific signals from the surrounding or intermingled normal cells. The use of highly purified cell preparations with laser-assisted microdissection procedures or tumor tissue sections with high tumor cellularity and low contamination by stromal cells and leukocytes may greatly increase the specificity of RT-PCR assays (22).

2. Recent studies dealing with real-time RT-PCR indicate that mRNA transcripts can be quantified precisely in tumor cells (23), though the exquisite sensitivity of this technique allows detection of extremely low levels of target mRNA that may not be translated into a functional amount of the corresponding peptide receptors (1).

3. ISH using specific probes labeled with either radioactive or non-radioactive has been widely applied to tumor samples for detecting peptide receptor mRNAs, especially because it can be reliably used on paraffin-embedded tissue sections (4,24,25). Compared with RT-PCR, ISH is less sensitive but enables a precise anatomical localization of the target, with good resolution to a subcellular level and good sensitivity, even when the target sequence is expressed only by a minor fraction of the tumor cell population (25). Remarkably concordant data have been derived from ISH, RT-PCR, and immunoistochemical assays in assessing receptor expression in tumor cells (4), and the combined application of ISH and immunohistochemistry, either on adjacent tumor sections or by double staining of the very same section, has resulted in more complete information on the highly dynamic process of gene transcription and translation, thus unveiling the pathways of peptide receptor synthesis and storage by specific tumors (25,26).

Choosing the Best Means to Detect Peptide Receptors

Because extensive in vitro information about the occurrence and density of receptors in a given tumor is an essential prerequisite to perform in vivo investigations in humans, it is mandatory to select the best approaches to peptide receptor assessment for successful clinical applications (1). To predict the in vivo peptide receptor status of a tumor as accurately as possible, the in vitro methods should evaluate the peptide receptors in both primary tumors and their metastases, defining at the same time the threshold value of peptide receptors in normal tissue representing the background signal. This is why morphological methods represent the first choice assays to precisely identify receptor expression at the cellular level, which is not possible with extractive assays on tissue homogenates. It remains difficult, however, to standardize all the variables related to tissue sampling and processing, because the sample size (biopsy, surgical resection) may not be adequate and representative enough of the whole tumor; the delay after sampling (surgery, autopsy) may be prolonged, thus hampering the preservation of antigens and mRNA molecules in the tumor tissue, and the sample processing (fresh, frozen, fixed; diverse method of fixation) may differ among laboratories or require specific reagents. Moreover, even peritumoral tissues may be affected by pathological changes able to induce receptor (over)expression, that can only be identified by an accurate morphological evaluation of receptor distribution using autoradiography or immuno(cyto)histochemistry. As discussed previously, the former assay allows reliable protein quantification at the cost of lesser morphological details, whereas the latter has better cellular resolution but provides only a semiquantitative evaluation. Whenever the methods assessing receptor contents at the protein level fail to provide the necessary data (e.g., the characterization of receptor subtypes), these can be sought for by looking at mRNA expression by means of RT-PCR, real-time RT-PCR, or ISH (1,8).

BIOCHEMICAL AND FUNCTIONAL CHARACTERIZATION OF PEPTIDE RECEPTORS AND THEIR NORMAL DISTRIBUTION

In this section, the main biochemical and functional characteristics of peptide receptors other than somatostatin will be briefly summarized, that currently have clinical applications in the oncological diagnosis and therapy. These include receptors for VIP/pituitary adenylate cyclase activating peptide (PACAP), cholecystokinin/gastrin, bombesin/gastrin releasing peptide (GRP), neurotensin, substance P, neuroepeptide Y, α-MSH, LHRH, calcitonin, ANP, glucagon-like-peptide-1 (GLP-1), oxytocin, and endothelin.

Vasoactive Intestinal Peptide/Pituitary Adenylate Cyclase Activating Peptide and Their Receptor Subtypes

VIP is a 28-amino acid-long neuroepeptide belonging to the family of secretin-like, G protein-coupled receptors (27). PACAP, in turn, is a structurally homologous, 27 to 38-amino acid-long peptide, and both molecules act as either neurotransmitters in the gut and central nervous system or general modulators of the immune response (28,29). Upon binding to ligands, the corresponding G-coupled receptors are activated and internalized, inducing specific adenylate cyclase activity, which eventually exerts the peptide-mediated biochemical effects in target organs (30). Several receptor subtypes have been described within the VIP/PACAP family, including two VIP receptors, namely $VPAC_1$ and $VPAC_2$, both recognizing VIP, and PACAP with high affinity, and distinguishable pharmacologically by two different $VPAC_1$- and $VPAC_2$-selective ligands, and at least one PACAP (PAC_1) receptor, with higher affinity for PACAP than VIP (1). Recently, several alternative splicing variants of PAC_1 receptor, derived from a complex post-transcriptional regulation of the receptor, have been described with distinct pharmacological behavior (31). In normal tissues, VIP/PACAP receptors, especially $VPAC_1$ receptor, are found in the brain, lymphoid tissue, and in the majority of epithelial cells of the gastrointestinal, respiratory, and urothelial tract (32,33), and in myoenteric neurons as well (34). Other tissues, such as adrenal medulla, pituitary gland, and myoenteric plexus of the gut wall, express preferably PAC_1 receptor (11,34). $VPAC_2$ receptors are distributed in smooth muscle cells at different anatomical sites, including the gastrointestinal tract, uterus, prostate, and blood vessels, in neuroendocrine cells (34), and in Cajal's pacemaker cells of the intestinal wall (11,35).

Cholecystokinin/Gastrin Receptors

CCK and gastrin exist in different molecular forms, all deriving from pro-hormones processed to peptides of variable length, but characterized by the same five terminal amino acid sequences at the C-terminus extremity. They function as neurotransmitters in the central nervous system and as regulatory/growth factors in the gastroenteropancreatic tract and in the derived tumors (36). The best characterized CCK and gastrin receptors are CCK_1 and CCK_2 receptors (37–39), the former with low and the latter with high affinity for gastrin, but additional CCK receptors have been described (40). The binding of gastrin or CCK to their common cognate receptor triggers the activation of multiple signal transduction pathways that relay the mitogenic signal to the nucleus and promote cell proliferation. A rapid increase in the synthesis of lipid-derived second messengers with subsequent activation of protein phosphorylation cascades, including mitogen-activated protein kinase, is an important early response to these signaling peptides. Gastrin and CCK also induce rapid Rho-dependent actin remodeling and coordinate tyrosine phosphorylation of cellular proteins including the non-receptor tyrosine kinases p125fak and Src and the adaptor proteins p130cas and paxillin (reviewed by Rozengurt & Walsh, 2001) (41). CCK_1 receptors are detectable in gallbladder and gastric smooth muscle and in the peripheral nervous system, especially in afferent vagal neurons and in the myoenteric plexus (35,42,43), whereas CCK_2 receptors are distributed into the brain and epithelial cells of the gut and endocrine pancreas (42,44) and in normal C-cells of the thyroid (45).

Bombesin/Gastrin-Releasing Peptide Receptors

Bombesin is a 14-amino-acid peptide of amphibians, whereas its human counterpart, GRP, consists of 27 amino acids., The two molecules differ by only one of the 10 C-terminus residues. GRP acts at the level of either brain or intestine, regulating diverse physiological activities such as satiety, thermo-regulation, circadian rhythm, smooth muscle contraction, immune function, and the release of other peptide hormones. At least four G protein-coupled receptors on cell membranes have been described (46), namely the neuromedin B receptor subtype (BB_1), the GRP receptor subtype (BB_2), and the BB_3 and BB_4 subtypes. Their distribution and function in human tissues are poorly known, with the remarkable exception of the GRP receptors that have been fully described in the gastrointestinal epithelial cells (35,47,48).

Neurotensin Receptors

Neurotensin is a tridecapeptide detectable in the central nervous system and the gastrointestinal tract (49). In the former, it acts as neurotransmitter or neuromodulator of dopamine transmission and anterior pituitary gland hormone secretion, showing also striking hypothermic and analgesic effects (50); in the gastrointestinal tract, it functions as an endocrine/paracrine, and growth regulator of the digestive tract (50,51) and of the gut- and lung-associated lymphoid tissue immune response (52,53). The physiological effects of neurotensin are mediated by the interaction of the peptide with at least three different high-affinity cell membrane receptors, namely NTR1 (54), NTR2 (55), and NTR3 (56), that are internalized after interaction with the ligand according to a temperature-dependent process (57,58). The downstream signaling pathways of the NTR1 receptor-neurotensin complex at the cell membrane include mitogen-activated protein kinase activation eventually leading to stimulated cell proliferation (59), whereas the effects of the activation of the other two receptors are less known.

Substance P Receptors

Substance P, an 11-amino acid-long peptide widely distributed into the central and peripheral nervous system and vessels independent of their anatomical localization, acts through the binding to three highly specific receptors at the cell membrane, namely NK_1, NK_2 and NK_3, and plays a role in pain perception and vasodilatation (60,61). Substance P is also able to trigger the growth of malignant tumor cells, such as human pancreatic cancer (62).

Neuropeptide Y (NPY) Receptors

NPY is a member of a 36-amino acid-long peptide family including also peptide YY and pancreatic polypeptide, and acts mainly as a neurotransmitter at both the central and the peripheral nervous system, where it regulates a wide variety of complex physiological functions, such as feeding behavior, inhibition of anxiety, vasoconstriction, regulation of gastrointestinal motility, and secretion, insulin release, and renal function (63–68). The functions of this peptide are mediated by several receptor subtypes (Y_1-Y_6), of which Y_1, Y_2, Y_4, and Y_5 have been better characterized in their distribution (69).

Miscellany of Other Peptide Receptors

1. *α-MSH* is a tridecapeptide produced by pituitary gland cells from pro-opiomelanocortin and stimulates melanin production by melanocytes. It is unclear whether it is also able to stimulate cell growth. After binding with its high-affinity but low-density cognate receptor (α-MSH-R), the complex is rapidly internalized (70). 2. *LHRH* is a hypothalamic decapeptide controlling the release of LH by adenohypophysis acting via negative feedback mechanisms. Specific receptors, namely LHRH-R and low-affinity GnRH-II subtype (71), have been described in pituitary gland cells, and in cancers of breast, prostate, endometrium, and ovary (72–74). LHRH analogs suppress the function of the pituitary-gonadal axis, decreasing the levels of circulating LH, FSH, estrogen, and prolactin (75). These molecules are also likely to directly inhibit the growth and proliferation of tumor cells (71). 3. *Calcitonin* is a 32-amino acid-long peptide produced by neurally derived C cells of the thyroid and involved primarily in calcium homeostasis through its effects on osteosclasts and the kidney (76). Furthermore, it plays a role also in cell growth regulation, differentiation, and tissue development (77). The human calcitonin receptor (H-CTR), belonging to a

subclass of seven transmembrane G protein-coupled receptors, has been found in many different normal and malignant tissues and cell lines (78). Six H-CTR isoforms generated by alternatively spliced mRNA have been described with different distribution, indicating the existence of a complex post-transcriptional gene regulation (78). 4. *ANP*, a 28-amino acid-long peptide produced in the cardiac atrium and playing a role in fluid-electrolyte homeostasis, acts through at least three differentially distributed receptors, namely the ANP_A and ANP_B types supplied with guanylate cyclase-dependent activity, and the ANP_C type lacking this activity (79). These receptors have been found in high density in the kidney, lung, and adrenal gland (1,80). 5. *Glucagon-like peptide-1-(7-36)-amide (GLP-1)* is a potent blood glucose-lowering hormone, produced by entero-endocrine L-cells of the distal intestine after ingestion of a meal. GLP-1 binds with high affinity to G protein-coupled receptor (GLP-1-R) located on pancreatic β-cells, thereby stimulating insulin gene transcription, insulin biosynthesis, and insulin secretion. Moreover, it acts as a growth factor, triggering formation of new pancreatic islets (neogenesis) while slowing beta-cell death (apoptosis) (81,82). GLP-1-R mRNA and protein have also been found in several areas of the human brain, including hypothalamus and brainstem, where the receptor is likely involved in feeding behavior (83), learning, and neuroprotection (84). The proliferative effects of GLP-1 are mediated by multiple intracellular pathways, including stimulation of Akt, activation of protein kinase Czeta, and transactivation of the epidermal growth factor receptor (EGFR) through c-src kinase. GLP-1 receptor activation also promotes cell survival in β-cells and neurons via increased levels of cAMP leading to cAMP response element binding protein activation, enhanced insulin receptor substrate-2 activity and, ultimately, activation of Akt. The effects of GLP-1 are responsible for the expansion of β-cell mass and the enhanced resistance to beta-cell injury in experimental models of diabetes in vivo (85). 6. *Oxytocin* is a 9-amino acid peptide with central and peripheral activities, whose specific receptor (OT-R) and corresponding mRNA have consistently been found in mammary gland, myometrium, and chorion/decidua during parturition (86–88). The OT receptor, mapping to the gene locus 3p25–3p26.2 and spanning 17kb with 3 introns and 4 exons, is a typical class IG protein-coupled receptor that is primarily coupled via G(q) proteins to phospholipase C-beta; moreover, the high-affinity receptor state requires both $Mg(2+)$ and cholesterol, which probably function as allosteric modulators (89). 7. *Endothelin* is a 21-amino acid-long potent vasoconstrictor peptide whose functions are mediated by two receptors, ET_A and ET_B, expressed by a variety of normal cells, including hepatocytes, biliary epithelium, vascular endothelium and smooth muscle cells (90), anterior segment of human eye (91), prostate (92), and colon (93). Endothelin can act by itself as a mitogen, but its effects are enhanced when it acts as a co-mitogen in association with a variety of other growth factors, such as basic fibroblast growth factor, insulin-like growth factor, and platelet derived growth factor. When acting in conjunction with vascular endothelial growth factor, it plays a major role in tumor angiogenesis (92).

ASSESSING PEPTIDE RECEPTOR EXPRESSION IN HUMAN TUMORS

The clinical implications of an accurate assessment of the expression of diverse peptide receptors in human tumors affect both diagnostic (allowing the selection of the most valuable tracers for tumor localization and assessing the degree of biological activity of the tumors) and therapeutic (choice of radioligands or nonradioactive, noncytotoxic peptide analogs) issues (1). In this respect pathologists play a pivotal role, not only for their histological expertise needed to ascertain the precise subcellular localization of the receptors, but also for their capability to select the most suitable technique for investigating the different tissue samples according to the specific clinical questions. In the next paragraphs, the expression of peptides other than somatostatin receptors in different tumor types will be summarized.

Vasoactive Intestinal Peptide/Pituitary Adenylate Cyclase Activating Peptide Receptors

Despite the considerable knowledge on VIP/PACAP receptors and mRNA expression in neoplasms gathered from the evaluation of tumor cell lines (94–96), relatively few studies are available thus far concerning human tumors (34). $VPAC_1$ receptor has been found in a variety of carcinomas of the lung, stomach, colon-rectum, breast, prostate, pancreas, liver, and urinary bladder (34), as well as in most ileal and bronchial carcinoids, insulinomas, gastrinomas, glucagonomas, and VIPomas (5), whereas $VPAC_2$ receptors are distributed in mesenchymal neoplasms, such as leiomyomas (11), and gastrointestinal stromal tumors (97), in meningiomas, and less frequently in carcinoids, insulinomas, gastric and breast cancer, and pheochromocytoma (34). PAC_1 receptor expression is more ubiquitous, being especially encountered in neoplasms of neuroendocrine lineage, such as gliomas, neuroblastomas, pituitary adenomas (98,99), and paragangliomas (11), but also in non-neuroendocrine tumors, such as endometrial carcinoma (11), meningioma, and breast cancer, and rarely in cancers of the stomach, liver, colon-rectum, thyroid, and prostate (34). A uniformly abundant expression of all the VIP/PACP receptor subtypes is an exclusive feature of glioblastomas (34), whereas medullary carcinomas of the thyroid are among the rare tumors not expressing any type of VIP/PACAP receptors (100).

Cholecystokinin/Gastrin Receptors

CCK_1 receptors have been detected in less that 50% of ileal carcinoids and functioning pancreatic gastrinomas, in meningiomas, in few pancreatic VIPomas and bronchial carcinoids, and in some neuroblastomas, but in none of 26 insulinomas, and 3 glucagonomas (5,10,101). CCK_2 receptors, in turn, are much more commonly expressed in human tumors, with a higher prevalence in most medullary thyroid carcinomas (45), small cell lung cancers (1), astrocytomas, medulloblastomas, sex-cord stromal ovarian tumors (10), functioning pancreatic insulinomas, glucagonomas, VIPomas, and in bronchial carcinoids (1), but also in a minority of breast and endometrial carcinomas, and of leiomyosarcomas (102). Differentiated thyroid, gastrointestinal, renal, prostate, and non-small cell lung carcinomas notably fail to express any type of CCK receptors (1,103). CCK mRNA has been identified in Ewing's sarcoma, and increasing levels of circulating pro-CCK have been found in the plasma of these patients according to the tumor size, and it has been suggested that it could serve as a novel tumor marker (104).

Bombesin/Gastrin-Releasing Peptide Receptors

In general, human tumors express preferentially individual bombesin/GRP receptor subtypes, especially high affinity-GRP-R, and less frequently low affinity-NMB-R (neuromemdin receptor) or the ligand-orphan BB_3-receptor (bombesin subtype 3 receptors) (46,48). Potent bombesin-like peptides have recently been developed for GRP receptor targeting of tumors, that distinguish the various receptor subtypes on the basis of the rank order of their affinity for GRP (48,105). GRP receptor mRNA or protein has been detected in various tumor cell lines and cancers of the gastrointestinal tract, lung, breast, and prostate (106–108), and immunohistochemically or by binding methods in neuroblastomas (109), carcinomas of the kidney (110), breast (111) and prostate (112), and neuroendocrine tumors (5). In particular, a subset of ileal carcinoids has been shown to express NMB-R but not GRP-R or BB_3-R, whereas the opposite was for functioning pancreatic insulinoma, gastrinoma, glucagonoma, and VIPoma, and pulmonary carcinoid, and small-cell lung cancer (5,113). The occurrence of aberrant and possibly mutated GRP receptors may account for the difficulty of highlighting these proteins in some tumors (107). The massive expression of GRP receptors in invasive adenocarcinoma and intraepithelial neoplasia of the prostate and in most bone metastases, but only rarely in prostate hyperplasia and not at all in the normal glands, emphasizes the possible role of these receptors in the development and progression of prostatic cancer, and indicates a possible use of this marker in differentiating benign from malignant prostate proliferation and in treating advanced stage tumors (1,112). Similar considerations hold true for breast carcinomas that show high GRP expression in both primary and metastatic settings, and could be treated with radionuclide therapy using GRP/bombesin analogs (111,114).

Neurotensin Receptors

Neurotensin receptor protein and mRNA have been reported in a variety of human tumors. NTR1 is particularly expressed by meningiomas, Ewing's sarcoma and pancreatic adenocarcinomas (115–117), and to a lower level also by astrocytomas, medulloblastomas, medullary thyroid carcinomas, and small-cell lung cancers (1). On the contrary, non-small cell lung cancers, neuroendocrine tumors of the gut, and pituitary gland, lymphomas, neurogenic soft tissue tumors, and carcinomas of the breast, colon-rectum, prostate, ovary, kidney, and liver rarely express NTR1 (1). Both NTR1 and NTR3 stimulate tumor growth in several in vitro studies dealing with tumor cell lines of various origin (118,119), thereby suggesting the existence of a stimulatory autocrine loop as shown for the GRP system (116).

Substance P

NK_1 subtype is the best characterized of the three substance P receptors, and it is expressed by medullary thyroid carcinoma, small-cell lung cancer, astrocytoma and glioblastoma, pancreatic, and mammary carcinoma, with a preferential localization in tumoral and peritumoral vessels, irrespective of the tumor type (1,61,62).

Neuropeptide Y Receptors

Contrary to many other peptide receptors, NPY-binding proteins (NYP-R) have not been often associated with human cancers. A recent in vitro study of breast carcinoma, however, indicated that these receptors, especially the Y_1 subtype, are demonstrable in most primary tumors, either invasive or intraductal, and their lymph node metastasis, but not in human non-small cell lung cancer, colorectal cancer, and prostate carcinoma (1,105). The high density of Y_1 in more than 85% of breast cancers opens the possibility of targeting this receptor for diagnosis and therapy with NYP analogs (1). Using in vitro autoradiography with ^{125}I-labeled peptide YY and receptor subtype selective analogs, Y_1 or Y_2 receptors or both have recently been found in all stromal tumors of the ovary, including granulosa-cell tumor, Leydig cell tumor, and Sertoli-Leydig cell tumors, fibroma, and fibrothecoma, but only in one third of common adenocarcinomas (120), suggesting a role of NYP receptors in the pathogenesis and also in the pathophysiology of ovarian malignancies. Moreover, receptors were observed in intra- and peritumoral blood vessel, independent of tumor types. The effects of NYP receptors on tumor growth regulation are conflicting, with either inhibition or stimulation of tumor growth being on record (12,121).

Miscellany of Other Peptide Receptors

1. *α-MSH receptors* are expressed at low density in melanoma cell membranes and have been proposed as potential targets for radionuclide therapy (122). 2. Specific *receptors for LHRH* have been described in cancers from breast, prostate, endometrium, and ovary (72–74), and the treatment with LHRH-R-blocking analogs (123,124)—able to either suppress the function of pituitary-gonadal axis (75) or directly inhibit the growth and proliferation of tumor cells (71)—has successfully been used for cancer care. 3. *Calcitonin* receptors have been variably found in giant-cell tumors of the bone (78), medullary carcinomas of the thyroid (125), breast cancer (77), and human myeloid leukemia cells (126), but

very limited information exists for other primary human tumors and the clinical applications of these receptors are still unsettled (1). 4. Likewise, little is known on the prevalence of *ANP receptors* in human tumors, apart from the occurrence of the subtype A in neuroblastomas (127). Aldosteronomas express mainly ANP type A receptor mRNA, whereas the corresponding binding sites for ANP are greatly reduced in most of these tumors, indicating the existence of somatic mutations or post-transcriptional tuning (80). 5. *Glucagon-like peptide-1-(7-36)-amide (GLP-1) receptors* have recently been found in a minority of ileal and bronchial carcinoids and of functioning pancreatic VIPomas, whereas most insulinomas, gastrinomas, and glucagonomas expressed these receptors at very high levels (5). Therefore, the use of GLP-1 receptor targeting in some neuroendocrine tumors, especially insulinomas and gastrinomas, could improve considerably not only the in vivo detection of these tumors in comparison with traditional octreoscan, but also their successful radiotherapy, thanks to the high receptor density on tumor cells. This receptor could also be used for a new stimulatory diagnostic test, by administering the ligand GLP-1 that is highly effective in stimulating insulin release from normal pancreatic β-cells- for the detection of early stage insulinomas (81). 6. *Oxytocin receptors* have been localized in glial tumors, neuroblastoma, osteosarcoma, Kaposi's sarcoma, choriocarcinoma, small-cell lung cancer, and breast, ovary, and endometrial carcinomas (128–135). Moreover, the recent development of a new potent radioligand, such as ^{111}In-labeled 1,4,7,10-tetraazacyclododecane-N,N′,N″,N″-tetraacetic acid-lys(8)-vasotocin (136)—which in turn can be linked to the DOTA chelant agent to form radiomolecules with high affinity for oxytocin receptors (137)—enables high efficacy radiotargeting of oxytocin receptor-overexpressing tumors for both diagnosis and therapy. 7. *Endothelin receptors* have been reported in gliomas and meningiomas (138), melanomas (139), and in cancers of the breast, ovary, thyroid, and lung (140–144), suggesting an autocrine role in promoting growth and progression, and neoangiogenesis of some of these tumors (145). For instance, the activation of endothelin receptors in medullary thyroid carcinoma has been proven to facilitate tumor cell proliferation, survival, neoangiogenesis, and bone metastases (146). Therefore, endothelin receptor antagonists are likely to become promising new options for targeted therapy of several human malignancies (147).

CO-EXPRESSION OF PEPTIDE RECEPTORS IN TUMORS: A NEW CHALLENGE FOR THE PATHOLOGIST

It is well known that many different peptide receptors are co-expressed by tumor cells (5), which show a complex phenotype characterized by a different spatial-temporal distribution of receptors depending on the tumor type and stage. Therefore, for the best selection of radiotracers or analogs to be used in diagnosis and therapy, and in general for a better knowledge of the tumor biology, it is most useful: (1) to investigate surgically resected specimens or tissue biopsies rather than tumor cell lines, because the latter cannot retain the same type and amount of receptor expression as in vivo; (2) to comparatively investigate both primary tumors and their metastases, because radiometabolic therapies are generally administered to patients with advanced-stage disease, and there may be changes in the peptide receptor status along with tumor progression; (3) to evaluate the possible occurrence of multiple receptor expression, assaying the most commonly expressed one(s) in a given malignancy, not only for academic purposes, but especially to increase the local damage on tumor cells of either radionuclides or non-radioactive analogs; and (5) to distinguish the tumor-specific expression from the background noise due to intermingled stromal or parenchymal nonneoplastic cells, because this distinction is not feasible using in vivo scintigraphy. Moreover, the accurate patholological evaluation of human tumors for peptide receptor content allows precise correlations between the receptor status and clinicopathological variables that can be useful for better predicting the patients' prognosis (1).

The simultaneous expression of distinct receptors by tumor cells is a common feature of several human malignancies, including neuroendocrine tumors (5) and breast cancer (8). Accordingly, the use of a cocktail of somatostatin receptor of type 2, GLP-1, CCK_2 and GRP radioligands would offer optimal targeting of gastrinomas for both diagnosis and therapy. This holds particularly true when considering that the receptors are not co-expressed at similar levels by the tumors, e.g. CCK_1 and CCK_2 in ileal carcinoids (5), and a combination of radiopeptides may be more effective in destroying more than one receptor-expressing tumor area. Furthermore, the risk of loss of efficacy of peptide radiotherapy or of an inaccurate diagnosis due to dedifferentiated tumor areas lacking some but not all peptide receptors is minimized by the use of ligand cocktails (5). β-emitters of different ranges may also be administered to the patients, achieving optimal radiotherapy for large and small tumoral lesions (7). The recent development of novel and more potent radioligands and analogs with high affinity for peptide receptors has paved the way for a more efficient and powerful in vivo multi-receptor targeting of tumors to be used both for diagnosis and therapy (1,5,136,137).

In this scenario, the pathologist has the great responsibility not only of assessing correctly the individual peptide receptor profile of the tumor(s) under evaluation by means of the assays described above (especially those highlighting the proteins that are the ultimate targets of radioligands and analogs), but also of emphasizing the possible heterogeneity in receptor expression by primary or metastatic tumors, or the changes in receptor status as a consequence of concomitant or previous therapies. Although most primary and metastatic gastrointestinal neuroendocrine tumors and breast cancers generally retain similar profiles and amounts of peptide receptor expression (1,8), there are other tumor types showing considerable differences of receptor status between primary lesions and derived metastases, such as the case of hormone-responsive prostate cancer primaries giving rise to hormone-resistant metastases (148).

This emphasizes the need of a double assessment of primary tumors and their metastases, either simultaneously or at the appearance of the metastases. Along this line, we have recently demonstrated, in patients with advanced-stage non-small cell carcinoma (NSCLC) treated with induction neoadjuvant chemotherapy, that chemotherapy may actually induce EGFR expression in originally EGFR-negative tumors (149). EGFR is expressed by 40% to 80% of NSCLC, where it is associated with increased tumor growth rate and proliferation, and poor prognosis. The current striking interest in EGFR as a potential target for therapy derives from the development of orally active drugs designed to specifically inhibit its kinase activity domain, such as gefitinib [Iressa (ZD18390); AstraZeneca, Wilmington, DE, USA]. The switch in peptide receptor status of NSCLC is consistent with the hypothesis that the EGFR ligand could be used as a survival factor to rescue tumor cells from chemotherapy-induced damage. Therefore, even the timing of in vivo sampling may be relevant for the clinical response, and it is recommended to re-evaluate for EGFR expression post-chemotherapy biopsies. This may prove useful for proper therapeutic interventions in patients with initially EGFR-negative lung cancer treated with neoadjuvant chemotherapy (149). Changes of peptide receptor expression may be induced by various substances, as already observed in several experimental conditions, showing that hormones can actually alter the profile and density of peptide receptors (150).

CONCLUSIVE REMARKS AND FUTURE PERSPECTIVES

The most promising developments of peptide receptor targeting are the diagnostic implications and the new therapeutic approaches with cyotoxic radiolabeled peptides (136,137), whereas targeting tumors with non-radio-labelled, noncytotoxic ligands supplied with long-term antiproliferative activity through their binding to cognate receptors has made slower progress in the past (1). In both situations, however, the pathologist plays a critical role, because a detailed knowledge of peptide receptor distribution in different human tumors is pivotal to subsequent decision making, by providing basic information on the receptor biology and pathobiology in normal and cancer cells and by unveiling the molecular mechanisms of the in vivo interaction between receptors and their cognate ligand(s). In this setting, the comparative analysis of normal and neoplastic tissues is of paramount relevance not only for assessing the actual expression of receptors by tumor cells over the background signal of the normal cell counterpart, but also for exploiting the possible role of the modulation or switch of receptor status during the neoplastic transformation and tumor progression (12,112,151).

Several open questions remain unsettled but represent exciting perspectives for future basic and translational researches. These investigational issues may be summarized as follows. (1) It is unclear at the present time whether genetic (oncogene activation, tumor suppressor gene inactivation, receptor mutations) and/or epigenetic (gene promoter methylation) alterations can affect—and at what extent—the expression or function of peptide receptors on tumor cells. This knowledge could prove pivotal to get new insights into receptor expression mechanisms and to identify potential options for novel cancer therapy. (2) Previous or concomitant chemotherapy, hormone, or gene therapy may alter the density of receptors on cell membranes, rendering tumor cells much more amenable to treatments with radioligands, analogs, humanized antibodies, or low-molecular weight inhibitors interfering with peptide receptor activity, stability, cell internalization, or immune response. (3) Further investigation is needed on receptor dynamics or trafficking and on in situ activities to explain why the therapeutic and side effects of radioligands or analogs, as well as in vivo scintigraphic detection, are much more evident in tumor than normal cells, despite their both sharing the same receptor status, and to unveil the functional properties of receptors in different tumor conditions, relative to their up- or dowregulation, homo- or heterodimerization, or autocrine loop activation by endogenous peptide excess that can ultimately become useful for diagnosis or therapy. (4) Finally, increasing our knowledge on the co-expression of different peptide receptors by the same tumor cells is one of the most important tasks for the near future, because it allows a more effective use of radiopeptide or analog cocktails in the daily fight against cancer.

REFERENCES

1. Reubi JC. Peptide receptors as molecular targets for cancer diagnosis and therapy. Endocr Rev 2003; 24:389–427.
2. Krenning EP, Bakker WH, Breeman WAP, et al. Localization of endocrine-related tumors with radioiodinated analogue of somatostatin. Lancer 1989; 1:242–244.
3. Serafini AN. From monoclonal antibodies to peptides and molecular recognition units: an overview. J Nucl Med 1993; 34:533–536.
4. Papotti M, Bongiovanni M, Volante M, et al. Expression of somatostatin receptor types 1-5 in 81 cases of gastrointestinal and pancreatic endocrine tumors: a correlative immunohistochemical and reverse-transcriptase polymerase chain reaction analysis. Virchows Arch 2002; 440:461–475.
5. Reubi JC, Waser B. Concomitant expression of several peptide receptors in neuroendocrine tumors: molecular basis for in vivo multireceptor tumor targeting. Eur J Nucl Med Mol Imaging 2003; 30:781–793.
6. Van de Wiele C, Dumont F, Vanden Broecke R, et al. Technetium-99m RP527, a GRP analogue for visualization of GRP receptor-expressing malignancies: a feasibility study. Eur J Nucl Med 2000; 27:1694–1699.
7. de Jong M, Breeman WA, Bernard BF, et al. Tumor response after [^{90}Y-DOTA(0),Tyr(3)]octreotide radionuclide therapy in a transplantable rat tumor model is dependent on tumor size. J Nucl Med 2001; 42:1841–1846.
8. Reubi JC, Gugger M, Waser B. Coexpressed peptide receptors in breast cancers as molecular basis for in vivo multireceptor tumor targeting. Eur J Nucl Med 2002; 29:855–862.

9. Palacios JM, Dietl MM. Regulatory peptide receptors: visualization by autoradiography. Experientia 1987; 43:750–761.
10. Reubi JC, Schaer JC, Waser B. Cholecystokinin(CCK)-A and CCK-B/gastrin receptors in human tumors. Cancer Res 1997; 57:1377–1386.
11. Reubi JC, Läderach U, Waser B, Gebbers J-O, Robberecht P, Laissue JA. Vasoactive intestinal peptide/pituitary adenylate cyclase-activating peptide receptor subtypes in human tumors and their tissues of origin. Cancer Res 2000; 60:3105–3112.
12. Reubi JC, Gugger M, Waser B, Schaer JC. Y1-mediated effect of neuropeptide Y in cancer: breast carcinomas as targets. Cancer Res 2001; 61:4636–4641.
13. Reubi JC, Waser B, Schaer JC, Laissue JA. Somatostatin receptor sst1-sst5 expression in normal and neoplastic human tissues using receptor autoradiography with subtype-selective ligands. Eur J Nucl Med 2001; 28:836–846.
14. Papotti M, Croce S, Bellò M, et al. Expression of somatostatin receptor types 2, 3, and 5 in biopsies and surgical specimens of human lung tumors. Correlatio with preoperative octreotide scintigraphy. Virchows Arch 2001; 439:787–797.
15. Janson ET, Stridsberg M, Gobl A, Weslin J-E, Oeberg K. Determination of somatostatin receptor subtype 2 in carcinoid tumors by immunohistochemical investigation with somatostatin receptor subtype 2 antibodies. Cancer Res 1998; 58:2375–2378.
16. Kimura N, Pilichowska M, Date F, Kimura I, Schindler M. Immunohistochemical expression of somatostatin type 2A receptor in neuroendocrine tumors. Clin Cancer Res 1999; 5:3483–3487.
17. Kulaksiz H, Eissele R, Rossler D, et al. Identification of somatostatin receptor subtypes 1, 2A, 3, and 5 in neuroendocrine tumors with subtype specific antibodies. Gut 2002; 50:52–60.
18. Pelosi G, Pasini F, Pavanel F, Bresaola E, Schiavon I, Iannucci A. Effects of different immunolabeling techniques on the detection of small-cell lung cancer cells in bone marrow. J Histochem Cytochem 1999; 47:1075–1087.
19. Fisher WE, Doran TA, Muscarella P, II, Boros LG, Ellison EC, Schirmer WJ. Expression of somatostatin receptor subtype 1-5 genes in human pancreatic cancer. J Natl Cancer Inst 1998; 90:322–324.
20. Reubi JC, Mazzucchelli L, Hennig I, Laissue JA. Local upregulation of neuropeptide receptors in host blood vessels around human colorectal cancers. Gastroenterology 1996; 110:1719–1726.
21. Pilichowska M, Kimura I, Schindler M, Kobari M. Somatostatin type 2A receptor immunoreactivity in human pancreatic adenocarcinomas. Endocr Pathol 2001; 12:144–155.
22. Pelosi G, Scarpa A, Manzotti M, et al. K-ras gene mutational analysis supports a monoclonal origin of most biphasic pleomorphic carcinoma of the lung. Mod Pathol 2004; 17:538–546.
23. Pinzani P, Orlando C, Raggi CC, et al. Type-2 somatostatin receptor mRNA levels in breast and colon cancer determined by a quantitative RT-PCR assay based on dual label fluorogenic probe and the TaqMan technology. Regul Pept 2001; 99:79–86.
24. Papotti M, Croce S, Macri L, et al. Correlative immunohistochemical and reverse transcriptase polymerase chain reaction analysis of somatostatin receptor type 2 in neuroendocrine tumors of the lung. Diagn Mol Pathol 2000; 9:47–57.

25. Terenghi G, Polak J. Use of comparative in situ hybridization and immunocyto-chemistry for the study of regulatory peptides. In: Coulton GR, de Belleroche J, eds. In situ Hybridization: Medical Applications. 1st ed. Dordrecht: Kluwer Academic Publishers, 1992:37–51.

26. DeLellis RA, Wolfe HJ. Analysis of gene expression in endocrine cells. In: Fenoglio-Preiser CM, Willman CL, eds. Molecular Diagnostic in Pathology. Baltimore: Williams & Wilkins 1991:299–321.

27. Ulrich CD, II, Holtmann M, Miller LJ. Secretin and vasoactive intestinal peptide receptors: members of a unique family of G protein-coupled receptors. Gastroenterology 1998; 114:382–397.

28. O'Dorisio MS. Neuropeptide modulation of the immune response in gut associated lymphoid tissue. Int J Neurosci 1988; 38:189–198.

29. Pozo D, Delgado M, Martinez M, et al. Immunobiology of vasoactive intestinal peptide (VIP). Immunol Today 2000; 21:7–11.

30. Ottaway CA. Insertion and internalization of vasoactive intestinal peptide (VIP) receptors in murine CD4 T lymphocytes. Regul Pept 1992; 41:49–59.

31. Daniel PB, Kieffer TJ, Leech CA, Habener JF. Novel alternatively spliced exon in the extracellular-binding domain of the pituitary adenylate cyclase-activating polypeptide (PACAP) type 1 receptor (PAC1R) selectively increases ligand affinity and alters signal transduction coupling during spermatogenesis. J Biol Chem 2001; 276:12938–12944.

32. Reubi JC. In vitro evaluation of VIP/PACAP receptors in healthy and diseased human tissues: clinical implications. Ann N Y Acad Sci 2000; 921:1–25.

33. Reubi JC, Horisberger U, Kappeler A, Laissue JA. Localization of receptors for vasoactive intestinal peptide, somatostatin, and substance P in distinct compartments of human lymphoid organs. Blood 1998; 92:191–197.

34. Schulz S, Rocken C, Mawrin C, Weise W, Hollt V. Immunocytochemical identification of VPAC1, VPAC2, and PAC1 receptors in normal and neoplastic human tissues with subtype-specific antibodies. Clin Cancer Res 2004; 10:8235–8242.

35. Rettenbacher M, Reubi J. Localization and characterization of neuropeptide receptors in human colon. Naunyn Schmiedebergs Arch Pharmacol 2001; 364:291–304.

36. Rehfeld JF, van Solinge WW. The tumor biology of gastrin and cholecystokinin. Adv Cancer Res 1994; 63:295–347.

37. Kopin AS, Lee Y, McBride EW, et al. Expression, cloning, and characterization of the canine parietal cell gastrin receptor. Proc Natl Acad Sci USA 1992; 89:3605–3609.

38. Wank SA, Pisegna JR, de Weerth A. Brain and gastrointestinal cholecystokinin receptor family: structure and functional expression. Proc Natl Acad Sci USA 1992; 89:8691–8695.

39. Wank SA. Cholecystokinin receptors. Am J Physiol 1995; 269:G628–G646.

40. Singh P, Owlia A, Espeijo R, Dai B. Novel gastrin receptors mediate mitogenic effects of gastrin and processing intermediates of gastrin on Swiss 3T3 fibroblasts. J Biol Chem 1995; 270:8429–8438.

41. Rozengurt E, Walsh JH. Gastrin, CCK signaling, and cancer. Annu Rev Physiol 2001; 63:49–76.

42. Reubi JC, Waser B, Läderach U, et al. Localization of cholecystokinin A and cholecystokinin B/gastrin receptors in the human stomach and gallbladder. Gastroenterology 1997; 112:1197–1205.

43. Moriarty P, Dimaline R, Thompson DG, Dockray GJ. Characterization of cholecystokinin-A and cholecystokinin-B receptors expressed by vagal afferent neurons. Neuroscience 1997; 79:905–913.

44. Noble F, Wank SA, Crawley JN, et al. International Union of Pharmacology. XXI. Structure, distribution, and functions of cholecystokinin receptors. Pharmacol Rev 1999; 51:745–781.

45. Blaker M, Arrenberg P, Stange I, et al. The cholecystokinin2-receptor mediates calcitonin secretion, gene expression, and proliferation in the human medullary thyroid carcinoma cell line, TT. Regul Pept 2004; 118:111–117.

46. Zhang H, Chen J, Waldherr C, et al. Synthesis and evaluation of bombesin derivatives on the basis of pan-bombesin peptides labeled with indium-111, lutetium-177, and yttrium-90 for targeting bombesin receptor-expressing tumors. Cancer Res 2004; 64:6707–6715.

47. Ferris HA, Carroll RE, Lorimer DL, Benya RV. Location and characterization of the human GRP receptor expressed by gastrointestinal epithelial cells. Peptides 1997; 18:663–672.

48. Nock BA, Nikolopoulou A, Galanis A, et al. Potent bombesin-like peptides for GRP-receptor targeting of tumors with 99mTc: a preclinical study. J Med Chem 2005; 48:100–110.

49. Carraway R, Leeman SE. The isolation of a new hypotensive peptide, neurotensin, from bovine hypothalami. J Biol Chem 1973; 248:6854–6861.

50. Vincent JP, Mazella J, Kitabgi P. Neurotensin and neurotensin receptors. Trends Pharmacol Sci 1999; 20:302–309.

51. Evers BM, Izukura M, Chung DH, et al. Neurotensin stimulates growth of colonic mucosa in young and aged rats. Gastroenterology 1992; 103:86–91.

52. Evers BM, Bold RJ, Ehrenfried JA, Li J, Townsend CM, Jr., Klimpel GR. Characterization of functional neurotensin receptors on human lymphocytes. Surgery 1994; 116:134–139.

53. Lemaire I. Neurotensin enhances IL-1 production by activated alveolar macrophages. J Immunol 1988; 140:2983–2988.

54. Chabry J, Labbe-Jullie C, Gully D, Kitabgi P, Vincent JP, Mazella J. Stable expression of the cloned rat brain neurotensin receptor into fibroblasts: binding properties, photoaffinity labeling, transduction mechanisms, and internalization. J Neurochem 1994; 63:19–27.

55. Yamada M, Yamada M, Lombet A, Forgez P, Rostène W. Distinct functional characteristics of levocabastine sensitive rat neurotensin NT2 receptor expressed in Chinese hamster ovary cells. Life Sci 1998; 62:375–380.

56. Mazella J, Zsurger N, Navarro V, et al. The 100-kDa neurotensin receptor is gp95/sortilin, a non-G protein-coupled receptor. J Biol Chem 1998; 273:26273–26276.

57. Beaudet A, Mazella J, Nouel D, et al. Internalization and intracellular mobilization of neurotensin in neuronal cells. Biochem Pharmacol 1994; 47:43–52.

58. Chabry J, Botto JM, Nouel D, Beaudet A, Vincent JP, Mazella J. Thr-422 and Tyr-424 residues in the carboxyl terminus are critical for the internalization of the rat neurotensin receptor. J Biol Chem 1995; 270:2439–2442.

59. Poinot-Chazel C, Portier M, Bouaboula M, et al. Activation of mitogen-activated protein kinase couples neurotensin receptor stimulation to induction of the primary response gene Krox-24. Biochem J 1996; 320:145–151.

60. Hökfelt T, Pernow B, Wahren J. Substance P: a pioneer amongst neuropeptides. J Intern Med 2001; 249:27–40.

61. Hennig IM, Laissue JA, Horisberger U, Reubi JC. Substance P receptors in human primary neoplasms: tumoral and vascular localization. Int J Cancer 1995; 61:786–792.

62. Friess H, Zhu Z, Liard V, et al. Neurokinin-1 receptor (NK-1R) expression and its potential effects on tumor growth in human pancreatic cancer. Lab Invest 2003; 83:731–742.

63. Pedrazzini T, Seydoux J, Künstner P, et al. Cardiovascular response, feeding behavior, and locomotor activity in mice lacking the NPY Y1 receptor. Nat Med 1998; 4:722–726.

64. Michel MC, Rascher W. Neuropeptide Y: a possible role in hypertension? J Hypertens 1995; 13:385–395.

65. Playford RJ, Cox HM. Peptide YY and Neuropeptide Y: two peptides intimately involved in electrolyte homeostasis. Trends Pharmacol Sci 1996; 17:436–438.

66. Sheikh SP. Neuropeptide Y and peptide YY: major modulators of gastrointestinal blood flow and function. Am J Physiol 1991; 261:G701–G715.

67. Wang Z-L, Bennet WM, Wang R-M, Ghatei MA, Bloom SR. Evidence of a paracrine role of neuropeptide-Y in the regulation of insulin release from pancreatic islets of normal and dexamethasone-treated rats. Endocrinology 1994; 135:200–206.

68. Korner M, Waser B, Reubi JC. High expression of neuropeptide y receptors in tumors of the human adrenal gland and extra-adrenal paraganglia. Clin Cancer Res 2004; 10:8426–8433.

69. Michel MC, Beck-Sickinger A, Cox H, et al. XVI International union of pharmacology recommendations for the nomenclature of neuropeptide Y, peptide YY, and pancreatic polypeptide receptors. Pharmacol Rev 1998; 50:143–150.

70. Wong W, Minchin RF. Binding and internalization of the melanocyte stimulating hormone receptor ligand [Nle4, D-Phe7] -MSH in B16 melanoma cells. Int J Biochem Cell Biol 1996; 28:1223–1232.

71. Grundker C, Gunthert AR, Millar RP, Emons G. Expression of gonadotropin-releasing hormone II (GnRH-II) receptor in human endometrial and ovarian cancer cells and effects of GnRH-II on tumor cell proliferation. J Clin Endocrinol Metab 2002; 87:1427–1430.

72. Eidne KA, Flanagan CA, Millar RP. Gonadotropin-releasing hormone binding sites in human breast carcinoma. Science 1985; 229:989–991.

73. Emons G, Schally AV. The use of luteinizing hormone releasing hormone agonists and antagonists in gynaecological cancers. Hum Reprod 1994; 9:1364–1379.

74. Halmos G, Arencibia JM, Schally AV, Davis R, Bostwick DG. High incidence of receptors for luteinizing hormone-releasing hormone (LHRH) and LHRH receptor gene expression in human prostate cancers. J Urol 2000; 163:623–629.

75. Redding TW, Schally AV. Inhibition of mammary tumor growth in rats and mice by administration of agonistic and antagonistic analogs of luteinizing hormone-releasing hormone. Proc Natl Acad Sci USA 1983; 80:1459–1462.

76. Zaidi M, Moonga BS, Bevis PJ, Bascal ZA, Breimer LH. The calcitonin gene peptides: biology and clinical relevance. Crit Rev Clin Lab Sci 1990; 28:109–174.

77. Wang X, Nakamura M, Mori I, et al. Calcitonin receptor gene and breast cancer: quantitative analysis with laser capture microdissection. Breast Cancer Res Treat 2004; 83:109–117.

78. Beaudreuil J, Balasubramanian S, Chenais J, et al. Molecular characterization of two novel isoforms of the human calcitonin receptor. Gene 2004; 343:143–151.

79. Inagami T. Atrial natriuretic factor. J Biol Chem 1989; 264:3043–3046.

80. Sarzani R, Opocher G, Paci MV, et al. Natriuretic peptides receptors in human aldosterone-secreting adenomas. J Endocrinol Invest 1999; 22:514–518.

81. Holz GG, Chepurny OG. Glucagon-like peptide-1 synthetic analogs: new therapeutic agents for use in the treatment of diabetes mellitus. Curr Med Chem 2003; 10:2471–2483.

82. Ranganath L, Sedgwick I, Morgan L, Wright J, Marks V. The ageing entero-insular axis. Diabetologia 1998; 41:1309–1313.

83. Alvarez E, Martinez MD, Roncero I, et al. The expression of GLP-1 receptor mRNA and protein allows the effect of GLP-1 on glucose metabolism in the human hypothalamus and brainstem. J Neurochem 2005; 92:798–806.

84. During MJ, Cao L, Zuzga DS, et al. Glucagon-like peptide-1 receptor is involved in learning and neuroprotection. Nat Med 2003; 9:1173–1179.

85. Brubaker PL, Drucker DJ. Glucagon-like peptides regulate cell proliferation and apoptosis in the pancreas, gut, and central nervous system. Endocrinology 2004; 145:2653–2659.

86. Maggi M, Magini A, Fiscella A, et al. Sex steroid modulation of neurohypophysial hormone receptors in human nonpregnant myometrium. J Clin Endocrinol Metab 1992; 74:385–392.

87. Takemura M, Kimura T, Nomura S, et al. Expression and localization of human oxytocin receptor mRNA and its protein in chorion and decidua during parturition. J Clin Invest 1994; 93:2319–2323.

88. Sapino A, Cassoni P, Stella A, Bussolati G. Oxytocin receptor within the breast: biological function and distribution. Anticancer Res 1998; 18:2181–2186.

89. Gimpl G, Fahrenholz F. The oxytocin receptor system: structure, function, and regulation. Physiol Rev 2001; 81:629–683.

90. Cai L, Wang GJ, Mukherjee K, et al. Endothelins and their receptors in cirrhotic and neoplastic livers of Canadian and Chinese populations. Anticancer Res 1999; 19:2243–2247.

91. Fernandez-Durango R, Rollin R, Mediero A, et al. Localization of endothelin-1 mRNA expression and immunoreactivity in the anterior segment of human eye: expression of ETA and ETB receptors. Mol Vis 2003; 9:103–109.

92. Kopetz ES, Nelson JB, Carducci MA. Endothelin-1 as a target for therapeutic intervention in prostate cancer. Invest New Drugs 2002; 20:173–182.

93. Egidy G, Juillerat-Jeanneret L, Korth P, Bosman FT, Pinet F. The endothelin system in normal human colon. Am J Physiol Gastrointest Liver Physiol 2000; 279:G211–G222.

94. Vaudry D, Gonzalez BJ, Basille M, Yon L, Fournier A, Vaudry H. Pituitary adenylate cyclase-activating polypeptide and its receptors: from structure to functions. Pharmacol Rev 2000; 52:269–324.

95. Moody TW, Walters J, Casibang M, Zia F, Gozes Y. VPAC1 receptors and lung cancer. Ann N Y Acad Sci 2000; 921:26–32.
96. Moody TW, Leyton J, Chan D, et al. VIP receptor antagonists and chemotherapeutic drugs inhibit the growth of breast cancer cells. Breast Cancer Res Treat 2001; 68:55–64.
97. Reubi JC, Korner M, Waser B, Mazzucchelli L, Guillou L. High expression of peptide receptors as a novel target in gastrointestinal stromal tumors. Eur J Nucl Med Mol Imaging 2004; 31:803–810.
98. Oka H, Jin L, Reubi J, et al. Pituitary adenylate-cyclase-activating polypeptide (PACAP) binding sites and PACAP/vasoactive intestinal polypeptide receptor expression in human pituitary adenomas. Am J Pathol 1998; 153:1787–1796.
99. Vertongen P, Devalck C, Sariban E, et al. Pituitary adenylate cyclase activating peptide and its receptors are expressed in human neuroblastomas. J Cell Physiol 1996; 167:36–46.
100. Reubi JC. In vitro identification of vasoactive intestinal peptide receptors in human tumors: implications for tumor imaging. J Nucl Med 1995; 36:1846–1853.
101. Mailleux P, Vanderhaeghen JJ. Cholecystokinin receptors of A type in the human dorsal medulla oblongata and meningiomas, and of B type in small cell lung carcinomas. Neurosci Lett 1990; 117:243–247.
102. Schaer JC, Reubi JC. High gastrin and cholecystokinin (CKK) gene expression in human neuronal, renal and myogenic stem cell tumors: comparison with CCK-A and CCK-B receptor content. J Clin Endocrinol Metab 1999; 84:233–239.
103. Blaker M, de Weerth A, Tometten M, et al. Expression of the cholecystokinin 2-receptor in normal human thyroid gland and medullary thyroid carcinoma. Eur J Endocrinol 2002; 146:89–96.
104. Reubi JC, Koefoed P, Hansen TO, et al. Procholecystokinin as marker of human Ewing sarcomas. Clin Cancer Res 2004; 10:5523–5530.
105. Fleischmann A, Läderach U, Friess H, Buechler M, Reubi JC. Bombesin receptors in distinct tissue compartments of human pancreatic diseases. Lab Invest 2000; 80:1807–1817.
106. Sun B, Halmos G, Schally AV, Wang X, Martinez M. Presence of receptors for bombesin/gastrin-releasing peptide and mRNA for three receptor subtypes in human prostate cancers. Prostate 2000; 42:295–303.
107. Carroll RE, Carroll R, Benya RV. Characterization of gastrin-releasing peptide receptors aberrantly expressed by non-antral gastric adenocarcinomas. Peptides 1999; 20:229–237.
108. Moody TW, Zia F, Venugopal R, Fagarasan M, Oie H, Hu V. GRP receptors are present in non small cell lung cancer cells. J Cell Biochem Suppl 1996; 24:247–256.
109. Kim S, Hu W, Kelly DR, Hellmich MR, Evers BM, Chung DH. Gastrin-releasing peptide is a growth factor for human neuroblastomas. Ann Surg 2002; 235:621–629.
110. Pansky A, de Weerth A, Fasler-Kan EV, et al. Gastrin releasing peptide-preferring bombesin receptors mediate growth of human renal cell carcinoma. J Am Soc Nephrol 2000; 11:1409–1418.
111. Gugger M, Reubi JC. GRP receptors in non-neoplastic and neoplastic human breast. Am J Pathol 1999; 155:2067–2076.
112. Markwalder R, Reubi JC. Gastrin-releasing peptide receptors in the human prostate: relation to neoplastic transformation. Cancer Res 1999; 59:1152–1159.

113. Reubi JC, Wenger S, Schmuckli-Maurer J, Schaer JC, Gugger M. Bombesin receptor subtypes in human cancers: detection with the universal radioligand (125)I-[D-TYR(6), β-ALA(11), PHE(13), NLE(14)] bombesin(6–14). Clin Cancer Res 2002; 8:1139–1146.

114. Krenning EP, Kwekkeboom DJ, Valkema R, Pauwels S, Kvols LK, De Jong M. Peptide recptor radionuclide therapy. Ann N Y Acad Sci 2004; 1014:234–245.

115. Przedborski S, Levivier M, Cadet JL. Neurotensin receptors in human meningiomas. Ann Neurol 1991; 30:650–654.

116. Reubi JC, Waser B, Schaer JC, Laissue JA. Neurotensin receptors in human neoplasms: High incidence in Ewing sarcomas. Int J Cancer 1999; 82:213–218.

117. Reubi JC, Waser B, Friess H, Büchler MW, Laissue JA. Neurotensin receptors: a new marker for human ductal pancreatic adenocarcinoma. Gut 1998; 42:546–550.

118. Moody TW, Chiles J, Casibang M, Moody E, Chan D, Davis TP. SR48692 is a neurotensin receptor antagonist which inhibits the growth of small cell lung cancer cells. Peptides 2001; 22:109–115.

119. Dal Farra C, Sarret P, Navarro V, Botto JM, Mazella J, Vincent JP. Involvement of the neurotensin receptor subtype NTR3 in the growth effect of neurotensin on cancer cell lines. Int J Cancer 2001; 92:503–509.

120. Korner M, Waser B, Reubi JC. Neuropeptide Y receptor expression in human primary ovarian neoplasms. Lab Invest 2004; 84:71–80.

121. Magni P, Motta M. Expression of neuropeptide Y receptors in human prostate cancer cells. Ann Oncol 2001; 12:S27–S29.

122. Siegrist W, Solca F, Stutz S, et al. Characterization of receptors for melanocyte-stimulating hormone on human melanoma cells. Cancer 1989; 49:6352–6358.

123. Gunthert AR, Grundker C, Bongertz T, Nagy A, Schally AV, Emons G. Induction of apoptosis by AN-152, a cytotoxic analog of luteinizing hormone-releasing hormone (LHRH), in LHRH-R positive human breast cancer cells is independent of multidrug resistance-1 (MDR-1) system. Breast Cancer Res Treat 2004; 87:255–264.

124. Schally AV, Comaru-Schally AM, Redding TW. Antitumor effects of analogs of hypothalamic hormones in endocrine-dependent cancers. Proc Soc Exp Biol Med 1984; 175:259–281.

125. Frendo JL, Delage-Mourroux R, Cohen R, et al. Calcitonin receptor mRNA expression in TT cells: effect of dexamethasone. Mol Cell Endocrinol 1998; 139:37–43.

126. Suzuki K, Uchii M, Nozawa R. Expression of calcitonin receptors on human myeloid leukemia cells. J Biochem (Tokyo) 1995; 118:448–452.

127. Lelievre V, Pineau N, Hu Z, et al. Proliferative actions of natriuretic peptides on neuroblastoma cells. Involvement of guanylyl cyclase and non-guanylyl cyclase pathways. J Biol Chem 2001; 276:43668–43676.

128. Cassoni P, Fulcheri E, Carcangiu ML, Stella A, Deaglio S, Bussolati G. Oxytocin receptors in human adenocarcinomas of the endometrium: presence and biological significance. J Pathol 2000; 190:470–477.

129. Cassoni P, Sapino A, Stella A, Fortunati N, Bussolati G. Presence and significance of oxytocin receptors in human neuroblastomas and glial tumors. Int J Cancer 1998; 77:695–700.

130. Bussolati G, Cassoni P, Ghisolfi G, Negro F, Sapino A. Immunolocalization and gene expression of oxytocin receptors in carcinomas and non-neoplastic tissues of the breast. Am J Pathol 1996; 148:1895–1903.

131. Morita T, Shibata K, Kikkawa F, Kajiyama H, Ino K, Mizutani S. Oxytocin inhibits the progression of human ovarian carcinoma cells in vitro and in vivo. Int J Cancer 2004; 109:525–532.

132. Novak JF, Judkins MB, Chernin MI, et al. A plasmin-derived hexapeptide from the carboxyl end of osteocalcin counteracts oxytocin-mediated growth inhibition [corrected] of osteosarcoma cells. Cancer Res 2000; 60:3470–3476.

133. Cassoni P, Sapino A, Munaron L, et al. Activation of functional oxytocin receptors stimulates cell proliferation in human trophoblast and choriocarcinoma cell lines. Endocrinology 2001; 142:1130–1136.

134. Cassoni P, Sapino A, Deaglio S, et al. Oxytocin is a growth factor for Kaposi's sarcoma cells: evidence of endocrine-immunological cross-talk. Cancer Res 2002; 62:2406–2413.

135. Pequeux C, Breton C, Hendrick JC, et al. Oxytocin synthesis and oxytocin receptor expression by cell lines of human small cell carcinoma of the lung stimulate tumor growth through autocrine/paracrine signaling. Cancer Res 2002; 62:4623–4629.

136. Bussolati G, Chinol M, Chini B, Nacca A, Cassoni P, Paganelli G. 111In-labeled 1,4,7,10-tetraazacyclododecane-N,N$'$,N$''$,N$'''$-tetraacetic acid-lys(8)-vasotocin: a new powerful radioligand for oxytocin receptor-expressing tumors. Cancer Res 2001; 61:4393–4397.

137. Chini B, Chinol M, Cassoni P, et al. Improved radiotracing of oxytocin receptor-expressing tumors using the new [111In]-DOTA-Lys8-deamino-vasotocin analogue. Br J Cancer 2003; 89:930–936.

138. Pagotto U, Arzberger T, Hopfner U, et al. Expression and localization of endothelin-1 and endothelin receptors in human meningiomas. Evidence for a role in tumoral growth. J Clin Invest 1995; 96:2017–2025.

139. Lahav R, Suva ML, Rimoldi D, Patterson PH, Stamenkovic I. Endothelin receptor B inhibition triggers apoptosis and enhances angiogenesis in melanomas. Cancer Res 2004; 64:8945–8953.

140. Ahmed SI, Thompson J, Coulson JM, Woll PJ. Studies on the expression of endothelin, its receptor subtypes, and converting enzymes in lung cancer and in human bronchial epithelium. Am J Respir Cell Mol Biol 2000; 22:422–431.

141. Alanen K, Deng DX, Chakrabarti S. Augmented expression of endothelin-1, endothelin-3, and the endothelin-B receptor in breast carcinoma. Histopathology 2000; 36:161–167.

142. Bagnato A, Salani D, Di Castro V, et al. Expression of endothelin 1 and endothelin A receptor in ovarian carcinoma: evidence for an autocrine role in tumor growth. Cancer Res 1999; 59:720–727.

143. Wulfing P, Gotte M, Sonntag B, et al. Overexpression of Endothelin-A-receptor in breast cancer: Regulation by estradiol and cobalt-chloride induced hypoxia. Int J Oncol 2005; 26:951–960.

144. Wulfing C, Eltze E, Piechota H, et al. Expression of endothelin-1 and endothelin-A and -B receptors in invasive bladder cancer. Oncol Rep 2005; 13:223–228.

145. Boukerche H, Su ZZ, Kang DC, Fisher PB. Identification and cloning of genes displaying elevated expression as a consequence of metastatic progression in human melanoma cells by rapid subtraction hybridization. Gene 2004; 343:191–201.

146. Donckier J, Michel L, Delos M, Van Beneden R, Havaux X. Endothelin axis expression in medullary thyroid carcinoma: a potential therapeutic target. Clin Endocrinol (Oxf) 2004; 61:282–284.

147. Spinella F, Rosano L, Di Castro V, Nicotra MR, Natali PG, Bagnato A. Inhibition of cyclooxygenase-1 and -2 expression by targeting the endothelin a receptor in human ovarian carcinoma cells. Clin Cancer Res 2004; 10:4670–4679.

148. Nilsson S, Reubi JC, Kalkner K, et al. Metastatic hormone-refractory prostatic adenocarcinoma expresses somatostatin receptors and is visualized in vivo by (111-In)-labeled DTPA-D-(Phe-1)-octreotide scintigraphy. Cancer Res 1995; 55:S5805–S5810.

149. De Pas T, Pelosi G, de Braud F, et al. The epidermal growth factor receptor (EGFR) status of non-small cell lung cancer can shift from negative to positive after systemic chemotherapy. J Clin Oncol 2004; 22:4966–4970.

150. Visser-Wisselaar HA, Hofland LJ, van Uffelen CJ, van Koetsveld PM, Lamberts SW. Somatostatin receptor manipulation. Digestion 1996; 57:7–10.

151. Buscail L, Saint-Laurent N, Chastre E, et al. Loss of sst2 somatostatin receptor gene expression in human pancreatic and colorectal cancer. Cancer Res 1996; 56:1823–1827.

8

Peptide Receptor Therapy with ^{90}Y-Dotatoc: The Emerging Experience in Chile

Horacio Amaral

*Nuclear Medicine Center, Clinica Alemana and A. Lopez Perez
Foundation, and Faculty of Medicine, Universidad del
Desarrollo, Santiago, Chile*

INTRODUCTION

Most neuroendocrine tumors (NT) and a few others, such as small cell lung cancer, hepatomas, lymphomas, breast cancer, and meningiomas, have a variable degree of over-expression of somatostatin receptors (SSTRs) on their cellular surface (1–4). Somatostatin is a tetradecapeptide produced by the hypothalamus and pancreas with a very short biological half-life. It is possible to recognize five different sub-types (5) of SSTRs, with the SSTR2 sub-type as the most prevalent. The synthetic variant of the human somatostatin with a chain of 8 peptides, named Octreotide, has the advantage of a prolonged "in vivo" half-life retaining its specificity for the cellular receptors. These characteristics allow the detection of both primary tumors and their metastases by diagnostic scintigraphic images with this polypeptide labeled with ^{111}In (6–7).

Patients with inoperable, residual, or metastatic NT have typically a poor response to conventional external radiotherapy or systemic chemotherapy. A new valid option for therapeutic purposes in such cases is the use of a similar peptide like DOTA-D-Phe-Tyr-Octreotide labeled with Yttrium-90 (^{90}Y-DOTATOC) (8–13). This radiopharmaceutical is a pure beta emitter with specific affinity for subtype 2 SSTRs, allowing a high radiation dose to cellular level in NT.

In collaboration with the European Institute of Oncology, Milano (Italy), we have successfully introduced this therapy in Chile including both the local labeling of the radiopharmaceutical and the design of the clinical protocols.

At the moment our experience is limited, however, the trials are ongoing. This chapter illustrates some of our cases and their follow-up.

PATIENT POPULATION AND METHODS

Since January 2004 we have treated 23 patients, 11 men and 12 women (average 46.6 years old, range 12–70), 22 with histologically confirmed residual or metastatic NT and 1 hepatoma. All of them had positive SSTRs demonstrated by ^{111}In-Octreotide whole body and SPECT scintigraphy in a dual head camera. The primary tumor was located in the pancreas in 10 (one glucagon-producing neuroendocrine tumor with necrolytic migratory erythema and nine non-functioning pancreatic endocrine tumors), intestine in five, medullary thyroid carcinoma in two, thymus in one, bronchial one and of unknown origin in three.

All patients received renal protection with amino acids immediately before the radiopharmaceutical administration. The ^{90}Y-DOTATOC was administered intravenously in single doses between 0.925–8,9 GBq (25–240 mCi). The maximum cumulative individual dose was 19.8 GBq (537) mCi. The whole group received 66 single therapy cycles. So far, 16 patients have received more than one cycle, two cycles in six of them, three in two, four in two, five in four, six in one and seven in one. Only this sub-group is considered for evaluation of treatment response.

RESULTS

The treatment was well tolerated in all the 23 patients except in one in whom, although the quality control of the injected material showed a radiochemical purity greater than 98%, by causes not yet determined the "in vivo" biodistribution of ^{90}Y-DOTATOC was altered showing mainly bone marrow uptake (non-tumor) and presenting a severe but reversible hematological toxicity. The other patients showed mild (grade 1–2 WHO) hematological toxicity spontaneously recovered after four to six weeks, none of them requiring further support. In the sub-group of 16 patients with more than one cycle, there has been complete remission of the tumor activity in one, significant partial remission in 10, partial remission with further relapse in three and progression in two of them.

SELECTED CASES

Case A

A 55-year-old man suffering from metastatic pancreatic tumor with portal vein thrombosis and portal hypertension syndrome was declared non-operable five years ago after a surgical exploration assuming an adenocarcinoma. After four years of evolution the patient presented a relative stable disease, but symptomatic with severe abdominal pain and diarrhea. Due to the atypical progression of the disease a biopsy was indicated. This revealed a pancreatic endocrine tumor. The ^{111}In-Octreotide showed a strongly positive tumor uptake of the radiopharmaceutical. Therefore, the patient received 5 cycles of ^{90}Y-DOTATOC, with a total cumulative activity of 14.54 GBq (393 mCi) at 8 to 10 week intervals. The patient showed a marked reduction of the primary and metastatic foci and is now clinically asymptomatic. Comparative whole body images acquired 24 hours after the first and fifth administration of ^{90}Y-DOTATOC using the Bremsstrahlung radiation from the β particles (Fig. 1) demonstrated the almost complete disappearance of both the primary pancreatic tumor and liver metastases.

Case B

This is the youngest patient in our series, a 12-year-old boy in medical control for a tricuspid valve disease with functional class II of the NYHA. The patient presented several episodes of cyanosis accompanied by arterial hypertension, flushing of the

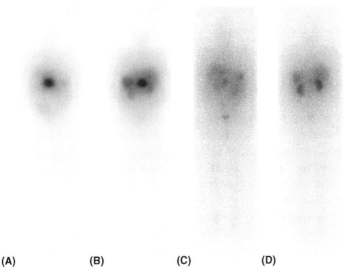

(A)   (B)   (C)   (D)

Figure 1 Comparative whole body images of patient A acquired 24 hours after the administration of ^{90}Y-DOTATOC using the Bremsstrahlung radiation from the β⁻ particles. (**A, B**) AP and PA images were obtained after the first dose and (**C, D**) AP and PA images after the fifth one. Note the remarkable change of radiopharmaceutical uptake in both the primary pancreatic tumor and liver metastases between the first and the latest treatment.

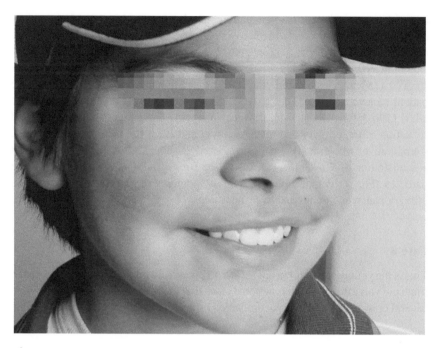

Figure 2 Patient B showing typical changes in his cheeks produced by the carcinoid tumor.

skin, and red plaques in the cheeks (Fig. 2). Further screening with abdominal ultrasound revealed a multinodular liver disease suggesting metastases. Liver biopsy confirmed a metastatic carcinoid tumor and laboratory test showed a marked elevation of 5-hydroxyndolacetic acid in urine. Cardiac involvement associated with carcinoid tumors is a well-recognized clinical entity associated with increased levels of serotonin produced by this type of tumor (14,15). A diagnostic ^{111}In-Octreotide imaging showed several liver nodes and a focal uptake in the small intestine. After surgical removal of the primary tumor, the histopathology and immunohistochemical analysis confirmed the diagnosis of a carcinoid tumor of the intestine. Subsequently, the patient received five cycles of ^{90}Y-DOTATOC with a total cumulative activity of 9.14 GBq (247 mCi), with a good partial response from a clinical and morphological point of view. Comparative whole body images acquired 24 hours after the administration of ^{90}Y-DOTATOC using the Bremsstrahlung radiation from the β particles (Fig. 3) show the significant reduction of the tumor mass. The tumor/background (lung) ratio of the main lesion was reduced by 63% from 11.7 at the beginning to 4.3 after the fifth dose.

The patient is still in good physical condition, waiting for a tricuspid valve replacement and further ^{90}Y-DOTATOC doses. His hematological parameters, liver, and renal functions are within normal limits.

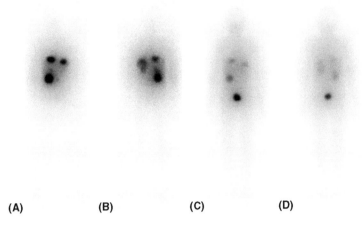

(A)   **(B)**   **(C)**   **(D)**

Figure 3 Comparative (**A, C**) AP and (**B, D**) PA whole body images from Bremsstrahlung radiation after ^{90}Y-DOTATOC acquired after the first and fifth administration. The tumor/background (lung) ratio in the inferior liver mass diminished from (**A, B**) 11.7 (**C, D**) to 4.3 a decrease of 63%.

Case C

This is a 36-year-old female patient suffering in the last nine years from a progressive endocrine pancreatic tumor with multiple metastases, including the skeleton with severe bone pain, lungs, and a diffuse bone marrow involvement. During this long period of time she received systemic chemotherapy and external radiotherapy with no response. Due to her progressive disease and being refractory to standard treatments, a ^{90}Y-DOTATOC was recommended. Since this type of treatment was, at that time, not yet available in Chile, the patient was referred to the European Institute of Oncology (Milano, Italy), where she received the first dose 3.03 GBq (82 mCi) of ^{90}Y-DOTATOC, and four months later a second one of 2.4 GBq (65 mCi). Afterward she received five more cycles, now dispensed in Chile, with an excellent palliative response. Due to the persistence of bone marrow involvement, the administered activities were small, in the range of 924 MBq (25 mCi). Serial bone scans performed during her follow-up revealed that most of the bone lesions disappeared in coincidence with bone pain release and significant improvement on her quality of life.

Unfortunately, she relapsed a few months later with multiple new bone metastases (Fig. 4), bone marrow tumor spread, and diffuse lung involvement. The patient presented a rapid deterioration and was in critical condition. Under these life-threatening circumstances a high dose of ^{90}Y-DOTATOC followed by autologous stem cells transplantation was considered. After an adequate stem cell harvest, 8.88 GBq (240 mCi) of ^{90}Y-DOTATOC were administered divided in two administrations of 4.44 GBq each six hours apart, followed by a successful

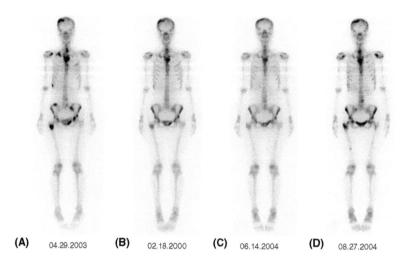

(A) 04.29.2003   **(B)** 02.18.2000   **(C)** 06.14.2004   **(D)** 08.27.2004

Figure 4 Sequential images of anterior bone scans from (**A**) April 2003 to (**D**) August 2004 in patient C. The sequence demonstrated (**C**) the excellent response to ^{90}Y-DOTATOC treatments in bone metastasis and (**D**) further relapse of new bony lesions.

autologous stem cell transplantation one week later. After three months the patient presented a significant clinical response with no pain and marked improvement of her pulmonary function, from oxygen dependency to no current support. Anecdotally, the patient presented a temporary alopecia areata limited to the extension of the skull metastasis demonstrating the high local radiation dose. As far as we know this is the first communicated case of autologous stem cell transplantation administered to a patient with severe bone marrow involvement generated by a neuroendocrine tumor after a high dose of ^{90}Y-DOTATOC.

CONCLUSION

These preliminary data indicate that the treatment with ^{90}Y-DOTATOC, now available in Chile, is a valuable therapeutic option for these tumor types that frequently do not respond to conventional treatments like systemic chemotherapy or external radiotherapy. Peptide receptor therapy should be considered as a first line treatment in well-differentiated NT and potentially in other over-expressing SSTR tumors.

It is also worthy to highlight the very rewarding example of collaboration and technology transfer between institutions improving the technical level of our specialty by incorporating new applications, which are now available to more patients in this part of the world.

REFERENCES

1. Reubi JC, Kvols LK, Waser B, et al. Detection of somatostatin receptors in surgical and percutaneous needle biopsy samples of carcinoid and islet cell carcinomas. Cancer Res 1990; 50:5969–5977.
2. Reubi JC, Lamberts SW, Maurer R. Somatostatin receptors in normal and tumoral tissues. Horm Res 1988; 29:65–69.
3. Papoti M, Macri L, Bussolati G, Reubi JC. Correlative study on neuro-endocrine differentiation and presence of somatostatin receptors in breast carcinomas. Int J Cancer 1989; 43:365–369.
4. Hofland LJ, van Hagen PM, Lamberts SW. Functional role of somatostatin receptors in neuroendocrine and immune cells. Ann Med 1999; 31:23–27.
5. Kubota A, Yamada Y, Kagimoto S, et al. Identification of somatostatin receptor subtype and an implication for the efficacy of somatostatin analogue SMS 201-995 in treatment of human endocrine tumors. J Clin Invest 1994; 93:1321–1325.
6. Lamberts SW. Somatostatin-receptor imaging in the localization of endocrine tumors. N Engl J Med 1990; 323:1246–1249.
7. Krenning EP, Kwekkeboom DJ, Pauwels EK, Kvols LK, Reubi JC. Somato-statin receptor scintigraphy. Nuclear Medicine Annual. New York: Raven Press, 1995:1–50.
8. Chinol M, Bodei L, Cremosi M, et al. Receptor-mediated radiotherapy with ^{90}Y-DOTA-$_D$Phe^1-Tyr^3-octreotide: the experience of the European Institute of Oncology. Semin Nucl Med 2002; 32:141–147.
9. Virgolini I, Britton K, Buscombe J, Moncayo R, Paganelli G, Riva P. ^{111}In and ^{90}Y-DOTA-lanreotide: results and implications of the MAURITIUS trial. Semin Nucl Med 2002; 23:148–155.
10. Bodei L, Cremonesi M, Grana C, et al. Receptor radionuclide therapy with 90Y-[DOTA]0-Tyr3-Octreotide (90Y-DOTATOC) in neuroendocrine tumors. Eur J Nucl Med 2004; 31:1038–1046.
11. Lewington VJ. Targeted radionuclide therapy for neuroendocrine tumors. Endocr Relat Cancer 2003; 10:497–501.
12. Waldherr C, Pless M, Maecke HR, et al. Tumor response and clinical benefit in neuroendocrine tumors after 7.4 GBq (90)Y-DOTATOC. J Nucl Med 2002; 43:610–616.
13. Valdes Olmos RA, Hoefnagel CA, Bais E, et al. Therapeutic advances of nuclear medicine in oncology. Rev Esp Med Nucl 2001; 20:547–557.
14. Narine KK, Dohmen PM, Daenen W. Tricuspid and pulmonary valve involvement in carcinoid disease. Tex Heart Inst J 2000; 27:405–407.
15. Jian B, Xu J, Connolly J, Savani RC, Narula BL, Levy RJ. Serotonin mechanisms in heart valve disease I. Am J Pathol 2002; 161:2111–2121.

9

Therapeutic Potential of Radiolabeled Peptides: The Basel Experience

Christian Waldherr

Institute of Nuclear Medicine, University Hospital Basel, Basel, and Department of Diagnostic Radiology, University Hospital Bern, Bern, Switzerland, and Department of Molecular and Medical Pharmacology, Ahmanson Biological Imaging Center, David Geffen School of Medicine, University of California, Los Angeles, California, U.S.A.

Jan Müller-Brand

Institute of Nuclear Medicine, University Hospital Basel, Basel, Switzerland

Human neuroendocrine tumor cells internalize the radioligand $[^{111}\text{In-DTPA}^0]$octreotide (OctreoScan) and therefore, it is widely used for diagnostic purposes (1,2). However, this radiopharmaceutical is not a suitable compound to carry out peptide receptor radionuclide therapy (PRRT), firstly because the Auger electrons emitter ^{111}In has a low tissue penetration, and secondly, a stable coupling of α- or β-emitting isotopes to $[\text{DTPA}^0]$octreotide could not be achieved. This initiated the development of novel octreotide compounds, and in 1996 Helmut R. Maecke of Basel and co-workers were finally able to synthesize a series of octreotide analogs that could tightly chelate beta-emitting rare earths (e.g., ^{90}Y). Among these compounds was [DOTA-D-Phe1, Tyr3]octreotide (DOTATOC or SMT 487) (3–6), which, labeled with ^{111}In or ^{90}Y, showed excellent binding to somatostatin receptors with nanomolar affinity and advantageous properties in tumor models (3,7). In early 1997, the Basel group was able for the first time to study ^{111}In-DOTATOC and ^{90}Y-DOTATOC in patients.

The aim of our clinical research was twofold:

1. Clinical evaluation (phase I-III) of PRRT with ^{90}Y-DOTATOC in patients with somatostatin receptor overexpressing tumors (neuro-endocrine tumors and thyroid cancer).
2. Clinical evaluation (phase I-III) of locoregional PRRT with ^{90}Y-DOTATOC in patients with glioma.

PRRT WITH ^{90}Y-DOTATOC IN PATIENTS WITH NEUROENDO-CRINE TUMORS AND WITH THYROID CANCER

First Description of Use

Our first clinical publication presented the first successful use of DOTATOC, labeled with the beta-emitting ^{90}Y, for the treatment of a patient with somatostatin receptor-positive abdominal metastases of a neuroendocrine carcinoma of unknown localization. Tumor response and symptomatic relief were achieved. In addition, DOTATOC was labeled with the diagnostic chemical analog ^{111}In and studied in three patients with histopathologically verified neuroendocrine abdominal tumors for its diagnostic sensitivity and compared with the commercially available [^{111}In-DTPA^0]octreotide. In all patients the kidney-to-tumor uptake ratio was on average 1.9-fold lower with ^{111}In-DOTATOC than with [^{111}In-DTPA^0] octreotide (Tables 1 and 2) (4,8).

Phase I–II, Dose Escalation Study

To determine a safe dose for a phase II trial and to define acute effects on normal tissues, a phase I-II study was conducted in 29 patients with advanced somatostatin receptor-positive tumors who had no other treatment option. The dose was increased gradually until a level was found that produced limiting but tolerable adverse events and/or clear signs of therapeutic activity. The patients received four or more single doses of ^{90}Y-DOTATOC with escalating activity at intervals of approximately six weeks (cumulative dose 6.12 ± 1.35 GBq/m^2). Twenty of the 29 patients showed a disease stabilization, two a partial remission, four a minor response and three a progression of tumor growth. Investigating the maximum tolerated dose (MTD), five patients who received a cumulative dose of >7.4 GBq/m^2 without Hartmann-Hepa 8% solution (this solution of aminoacids inhibits peptide renal reabsorption) developed renal and/or haematological toxicity. Two of these patients showed stable renal insufficiency and two required haemodialysis. Two of the patients exhibited anemia (both grade 3) and thrombocytopenia (grade 2 and 4, respectively) (9).

Table 1 Phase I-II, Dose Escalation Study: Patient Data

Patient year of birth	Sex	Treatments	Injected activity (GBq)	Diagnosis
C.A. 1954	M	4	1.85 2.59 2.775 2.96	Thymic carcinoid
D.M. 1959	M	5	1.48 2.22 2.96 3.7 4.44	Malignant thymoma
D.L. 1931	F	4	1.665 2.035 2.59 2.96	Medullary thyroid carcinoma
D.W. 1951	M	5	2.22 2.96 3.7 3.33 2.96	Thymic carcinoid
E.A. 1971	F	5	1.48 2.22 3.33 2.96 2.96	Thymic carcinoid
G.J. 1943	M	4	2.22 2.96 2.96 2.96	Presacral teratoma
G.E. 1943	F	4	1.48 1.665 2.035 2.405	Ileal carcinoid
H.W. 1925	M	5	1.48 2.22 2.96 3.7 4.07	Aesthesioneuroblastoma
K.J. 1947	F	4	1.48 2.22 2.96 2.96	Small gut carcinoid

(Continued)

Table 1 Phase I-II, Dose Escalation Study: Patient Data (*Continued*)

Patient year of birth	Sex	Treatments	Injected activity (GBq)	Diagnosis
K.F. 1939	M	4	1.48	Meningioma
			2.22	
			2.2	
			2.22	
K.E. 1936	F	4	1.665	Medullary thyroid carcinoma
			2.22	
			2.775	
			2.96	
K.G. 1944	M	4	1.665	Islet cell carcinoma
			2.405	
			2.96	
			2.96	
K.M. 1980	F	4	1.48	Small gut carcinoid
			2.22	
			2.775	
			2.96	
M.A. 1947	M	4	1.665	Carcinoid with hepatic metastases
			2.405	
			2.96	
			2.96	
M.F. 1921	F	4	1.665	Small gut carcinoid
			2.22	
			2.775	
			2.96	
M.M. 1951	F	4	1.665	Small gut carcinoid
			2.405	
			2.96	
			2.96	
N.J. 1948	F	5	1.48	Neuroendocrine hepatic metastases of unknown primary
			2.22	
			2.96	
			3.515	
			3.885	
P.G. 1939	F	4	1.48	Endocrine pancreatic tumor
			1.85	
			2.22	
			2.96	

(Continued)

Table 1 Phase I-II, Dose Escalation Study: Patient Data (*Continued*)

Patient year of birth	Sex	Treatments	Injected activity (GBq)	Diagnosis
R.P. 1957	M	4	1.665	Duodenal carcinoid
			2.405	
			3.145	
			3.145	
R.R. 1952	M	8	0.925	Neuroendocrine metastases of unknown primary
			0.74	
			1.48	
			1.85	
			1.85	
			2.22	
			2.96	
			2.96	
S.E. 1957	F	5	1.48	Neuroendocrine hepatic metastases of unknown primary
			2.22	
			2.775	
			3.145	
			3.77	
S.M. 1961	M	4	1.665	Phaeochromocytoma
			2.22	
			2.775	
			2.96	
S.J. 1937	M	4	1.665	Pituitary adenoma
			2.405	
			2.96	
			2.96	
S.J. 1952	M	4	1.85	Neuroendocrine metastases of unknown primary
			2.59	
			3.33	
			2.96	
ST.E. 1945	F	4	1.11	Endocrine pancreatic tumor
			1.665	
			2.22	
			2.775	
T.R. 1960	M	4	1.665	Neuroendocrine metastases of unknown primary
			1.665	

(*Continued*)

Table 1   Phase I-II, Dose Escalation Study: Patient Data (*Continued*)

Patient year of birth	Sex	Treatments	Injected activity (GBq)	Diagnosis
T.F. 1946	F	4	2.96 2.96 1.48 1.85 2.22	Meningeoma
V.E. 1945	F	5	2.775 1.48 2.22 2.96 3.515	Neuroendocrine paraganglioma with osseous infiltration
v.S.H. 1914	F	4	4.07 2.331 2.96 3.33 2.96	Meningeoma

Pathologic Determination of Nephrotoxicity

To determine the cause of chronic renal failure after PRRT, which was observed in our phase I trial, we conducted a retrospective collaboration study with the Department of Pathology of the University of Basel (10).

Twenty-nine patients (14 men, 15 women) with normal renal function before therapy had been treated with divided intravenous doses of ^{90}Y-DOTATOC approximately six weeks apart (mean normalized cumulative dose, $6.12 +/- 1.18$ GBq/m^2). Twenty-two of the 29 patients had been administered a normalized cumulative dose of 7.4 GBq/m^2 without side effects. Among the seven patients (six women, one man) administered a normalized cumulative dose greater than 7.4 GBq/m^2 without kidney protection of a Hartmann-Hepa 8% solution, five patients (four women, one man) developed renal failure. Increasing serum creatinine levels were observed within three months after the last ^{90}Y-DOTATOC injection. The evolution was rapidly progressive in three patients, resulting in end-stage renal failure within six months. The remaining two patients developed chronic renal insufficiency (mean serum creatinine level, 300 micromol/L an average 16 months after the end of treatment). Renal biopsies were performed in three patients and showed typical signs of thrombotic microangiopathy (TMA) involving glomeruli, arterioles, and small arteries. The

Table 2 Phase I-II, Dose Escalation Study: Patient Data and Tumor Response

Patient	Body surface (m2)	Normalized cumulative dose (GBq/m2)	Hartmann-hepa-aminoacid-solution 8%	Tumor response
C.A 1954	1.7	5.985	Sometimes	SD
D.M. 1959	2.2	6.727	Never	SD
D.L. 1931	1.6	5.781	Sometimes	SD
D.W. 1951	1.7	8.924	Never	PD
E.A. 1971	1.65	7.848	Sometimes	SD
G.J. 1943	2.02	5.495	Never	PD
G.E. 1943	1.6	4.741	Always	SD
H.W. 1925	2.0	7.215	Never	Remission
K.J. 1947	1.6	6.013	Never	SD
K.F 1939	2.05	3.971	Sometimes	SD
K.E. 1936	1.62	5.938	Sometimes	SD
K.G. 1944	1.85	5.4	Never	SD
K.M. 1980	1.52	6.207	Sometimes	SD
M.A 1947	1.81	5.519	Never	SD
M.F. 1921	1.7	5.659	Sometimes	SD
M.M. 1951	1.92	5.203	Never	SD
N.J. 1948	1.6	8.788	Never	PD
P.G. 1939	1.4	6.079	Always	SD
R.P. 1957	2.16	4.796	Sometimes	SD
R.R. 1952	2.93	5.114	Never	SD for 2 years
S.E. 1957	1.75	7.611	Never	Remission
S.M. 1961	1.75	5.497	Sometimes	SD
S.J. 1937	2.0	4.995	Sometimes	SD
S.J. 1952	1.8	5.961	Sometimes	Remission
ST.E. 1945	1.65	4.709	Sometimes	SD
T.R. 1960	1.9	4.868	Sometimes	SD
T.F. 1946	1.7	4.897	Never	Remission
V.E. 1945	1.6	8.903	Never	PR of metastases SD of primary
v.S.H. 1914	1.55	7.472	Never	SD

Abbreviations: PD, progressive disease; SD, stable disease; PR, partial remission.

histopathologic lesions were identical to those found after external radiotherapy, which suggests a causal relationship between ^{90}Y-DOTATOC and renal TMA.

Thus, we concluded that patients treated with a cumulative dose > 7.4 GBq/m^2 ^{90}Y-DOTATOC without Hartmann-Hepa 8% solution are at high risk to develop severe renal failure caused by TMA lesions. To conduct a safe phase II study, totals were therefore reduced to 6 GBq/m^2 and ever since, all patients received 500 mL Hartmann-HEPA 8% amino acid solution (Ringer's lactated Hartmann solution, Proteinsteril [B. Braun Medical AG, Sempach,

Switzerland] HEPA 8%, Mg 5-Sulfat [B. Braun Medical AG]) to inhibit tubular reabsorption of the radiopeptide thirty minutes before the injection of each treatment dose, followed by an additional 2,000 mL within 2.5 hours after ^{90}Y-DOTATOC bolus injection.

Phase II, Escalating Dose Scheme, 6 GBq

To determine the antitumor activity of ^{90}Y-DOTATOC and to estimate the response rate in a homogeneous patient population with gastroenteropancreatic and bronchial neuroendocrine tumors, we treated 41 patients with these tumor entities. Eighty-two percent of the patients had a therapy-resistant and progressive disease (PD). The treatment consisted of four intravenous injections of a total of 6 GBq/m^2 ^{90}Y-DOTATOC, administered at intervals of six weeks. All patients received aminoacid solutions as described above. The overall response rate was 24%. For endocrine pancreatic tumors, it was 36%. With a median follow up of nine months (range two months to 26 months), responses were ongoing in all patients. The 24-month survival time calculated by Kaplan-Meier method was $76 \pm 16\%$. Eighty-three percent of the patients suffering from malignant carcinoid syndrome achieved a significant reduction of symptoms. The treatment was well tolerated. All patients (5/41) with morphine dependent tumor-associated pain were able to change to NSAID or stopped any pain relief medication completely. Side effects were grade 3 pancytopenia in 5% of patients and vomiting shortly after injection in 23%. We did not observe any severe renal toxicity grade 3, 4 (Tables 3 and 4) (Figure 1**A** and **B**) (11).

Thus we concluded that ^{90}Y-DOTATOC had the potential to induce complete tumor remission in patients with neuroendocrine tumors with calculable radiotoxicity to the kidneys. After reports of Bernard et al. and others that intravenous D-lysine reduces the renal uptake of ^{90}Y-DOTATOC by 65%, we decided to increase the total to 7.4 GBq/m^2 in a second phase II trial (6,12).

However, the outlook for a patient diagnosed with an advanced neuroendocrine tumor still remained gloomy in terms of prognosis and survival, and the roles of chemotherapy and other treatments remained a source of debate. Any benefit in terms of gain in survival time and alleviation of symptoms must be balanced against the costs of treatment toxicity and any deterioration in quality of life. Therefore, there was an overwhelming consensus in our group that a standardized quality of life assessment was required in our next study.

Phase II, Constant Dose Scheme, 7.4 GBq

To determine the antitumor activity of a total of 7.4 GBq/m^2 ^{90}Y-DOTATOC and the benefit of life quality in a homogeneous patient population with gastroenteropancreatic and bronchial neuroendocrine tumors, we treated thirty-nine patients with these tumor entities. All patients had a therapy-resistant and PD. The treatment consisted of four equal intravenous injections of 7.4 GBq/m^2 ^{90}Y-DOTATOC, administered at intervals of six weeks. All patients received

Table 3 Phase II, Escalating Dose Scheme, 6 GBq: Patient Data

Patient	Location of primary/histology	Resection	Chemotherapy	Octreotide	Interferone-α	External radiotherapy	Liver transplantation
1	Pancreas/EPT		5FU			x	
2	Pancreas/EPT	x	DACT,5FUSTZ				
3	Pancreas/islet cell	x					
4	NETUP						
5	Pancreas/EPT	x					
6	Lung/carcinoid	x		x	x		
7	Paravertebral/neuro-ecto-dermal		(VAIA), (VIA)			x	
8	Pancreas/EPT	x					
9	Liver/NETUP						
10	Colon/Int. NET	x	CMP, DACT, ETO				
11	Pancreas/EPT		GEM				
12	Small bowel/carcinoid	x					
13	Abdominal lymph nodes/carcinoid	x					
14	Small bowel/carcinoid	x		x	x		

(Continued)

Table 3 Phase II, Escalating Dose Scheme, 6 GBq: Patient Data (*Continued*)

Patient	Location of primary/histology	Resection	Chemotherapy	Octreotide	Interferone-α	External radiotherapy	Liver transplantation
15	Pancreas/islet cell	x	CDDP, ETO, GEM				
16	Liver/bone/carcinoid		5FU				
17	Liver/NETUP	x		x			
18	Paravertebral/paraganglioma	x	DACT, IFO, CDDP			x	
19	Lung/liver/carotid body	x					
20	Liver/NETUP	x					
21	Coecum/carcinoid	x					
22	Pancreas/islet cell		CDDP, GEM				
23	Pancreas/EPT	x					
24	Pancreas/EPT						
25	Duodenum/Int. NET	x		x	x		
26	Ileum/Int. NET	x	STZ, 5FU				
27	Pancreas/gastrinoma		x*				x
28	Pancreas/EPT	x				x	
29	Liver/NETUP	x	x*			x	x

30	Pancreas/EPT	x					
31	Pancreas/EPT	x					
32	Abdomen/phaeo-chromo-cytoma						x
33	Lung/carcinoid	x					
34	Liver/NETUP		x* DACT, ADM, STZ, CDDP, ETO	x		x	
35	Rectum/Int. NET						x
36	Small bowel/Int. NET		5FU			x	
37	Lung/carcinoid	x					
38	Lung/carcinoid	x					
39	Lung/carcinoid	x			x		
40	Lung/carcinoid	x					
41	Lung/carcinoid	x					
41		27 (66%)	15 (37%)	5 (12%)	3 (7%)	7 (17%)	3 (7%)

Abbreviations: DACT, actinomycine D; ADM, adriablastine; CMP, cyclo-phosphamide; CDDP, cisplatine; ETO, etoposide; 5FU, 5-fluorouracil; GEM, gemcitabine; IFO, ifosfamide; STZ, streptozotocin; VCR, vincristine; x*, not specified combinations; VAIA, vincristine, adriamycine, ifosfamide, actinomycine D; VIA, vincristine, ifosfamide, adriamycine; EPT, endocrine pancreatic tumor; NETUP, neuroendocrine tumor with unknown origin; int. NET, intestinal NET.

Table 4 Phase II, Escalating Dose Scheme, 6 GBq: Tumor Response

	Progression before treatment %/(n)	Complete remissions (CR) n	Partial remissions (PR) n	Stable disease (SD) n	Progressive disease within or after treatment	Overall tumor response %	CR, PR, SD n (%)
EPT (n=14)	71% (10)	–	5	7	2	36%	12 (86%)
Intestinal NET (n=8)	88% (7)	1	1	6	1	13%	7 (88%)
Bronchial NET (n=7)	100% (7)	1	1	5	–	29%	7 (100%)
NET of unknown origin (n=8)	50% (4)	–	2	5	1	25%	7 (89%)
Others (n=4)	100% (4)	–	–	2	2	0%	2 (50%)
All (n=41)	82% (34)	1	9	25	6	24%	35 (85%)

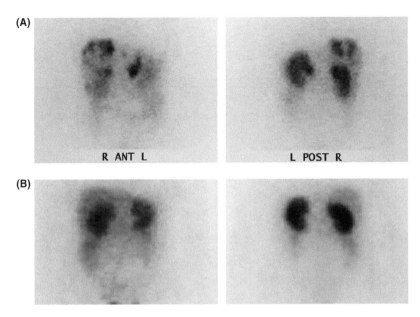

Figure 1 (**A**) ^{111}In-DOTATOC scintiscan of the abdomen in a 43-year-old female with a recurrence of endocrine pancreatic tumor and multiple liver metastases before DOTATOC-treatment. (**B**) After DOTATOC treatment ^{111}In-DOTATOC scintiscan of the abdomen revealed no enhancement in the pancreas region and in the liver. MRI assessed a CR.

aminoacid solutions as described earlier. After each treatment cycle, we performed a life quality assessment according to the National Cancer Institute Grading Criteria (NCI-CTC). The overall objective response rate was 21% and 38% for endocrine pancreatic tumors. These responses have been maintained up to a median of six months (median duration of follow up, range two months to 12 months). A significant reduction of clinical features was found in 83% of patients with diarrhea, in 46% of patients with flushes, in 63% of patients with wheezing, and in 75% of patients with pellagra. The overall clinical response was 63%. Side effects were grade 3/4 lymphocytopenia in 23% of patients, anemia grade 3 in 3%, and renal insufficiency grade 2 in 3% (Tables 5 and 6) (Figure 2**A** and **B**) (13).

Phase II, 2 Treatment Sessions, 7.4 GBq (Abstract EANM Vienna 2002)

Suggestions that lowering the number of treatment sessions at constant injected dose would increase the rate of tumor responses were addressed in this study.

Table 5 Phase II, Constant Dose Scheme, 7.4 GBq: Patient Data

Patient	Histology	Localization and number of lesions	Onset of diagnosis/time to treatment (months)	Pretreatments	Pre DOTATOC medication	Tumor response to DOTATOC
1	EPT	Pancreas 1, liver >10	8/99/6 months	None	None	SD
2	EPT	Liver >10	9/98/13 months	Chemotherapies (STZ, 5FU, x) chemoembolisations	Octreotide	PD
3	EPT	Liver 2	11/98/4 months	Operations	None	PR
4	EPT	Pancreas 1, liver >10	2/95/60 months	Chemotherapies (CDDP, 5FU) octreotide	None	PR
5	EPT	Pancreas 1, liver >10	1/99/7 months	Operations, octreotide	Octreotide	CR
6	EPT	Pancreas 1, liver 3	3/99/5 months	None	None	SD
7	EPT	Abdomen 4, lymph node 1	4/98/18 months	Operations	None	PD
8	EPT	Pancreas 1, liver 6	9/96/38 months	Operations	None	SD
9	EPT	Liver >10, bone 10	12/93/72 months	Chemoembolisations, octreotide	Octreotide	PR
10	EPT	Liver >10, bone 1	7/96/32 months	Operations	None	SD
11	EPT	Liver >10	9/97/9 months	Operations, octreotide, interferon	None	SD
12	EPT	Liver >10, abdomen 4	3/99/2 months	None	None	PR
13	EPT	Liver >10, pancreas 1	7/97/31 months	Chemotherapies (x), octreotide, interferon	Octreotide	SD
14	int. NET	Abdomen 5, liver >10	5/99/3 months	None	None	SD
15	int. NET	Liver > 10, bowel 1	11/99/2 months	None	None	PR

16	int. NET	Liver > 10, bone > 10	3/96/44 months	Chemotherapies (STZ, 5FU, doxorubicin), chemoembolisations	Octreotide	SD
17	int. NET	Bowel 1, bone > 10, lymph 5	7/99/7 months	Operations	None	SD
18	int. NET	Bowel 1, lymph nodes 2	2/97/33 months	Operations, chemotherapies (5FU, x)	Octreotide	SD
19	int. NET	Liver >10, abomen 7, bowel 1	2/00/3 months	Octreotide	Octreotide	SD
20	int. NET	Liver 2	12/99/4 months	Operations	None	SD
21	int. NET	Liver 1, abdomen 1	12/99/3 months	Operations	None	SD
22	int. NET	Bowel 1, liver 10	12/97/8 months	Octreotide, interferon	Octreotide	SD
23	int. NET	Liver 2	11/98/24 months	Operations, interferon, octreotide	None	SD
24	int. NET	Liver >10, lymph nodes 5	11/90/112 months	Chemotherapies (x), chemo-embolisations, operations, octreotide	Octreotide	SD
25	int. NET	Liver >10, bowel >10, lymph nodes 4	8/99/5 months	Octreotide	Octreotide	SD
26	bronch. NET	Bone 1, mediastinal 4	7/99/3 months	Operations	None	SD
27	bronch. NET	Liver >10, mediastinum 1	7/87/152 months	Chemotherapies (x), chemoembolisations, radiatio, operations, interferon, octreotide	Octreotide	SD
28	bronch. NET	Liver 5, bone >10	1/98/23 months	Operations, radiatio, interferon	None	SD
29	NETup	Liver >10, heart 2, rectum 4	4/96/26 months	Octreotide, interferon	None	PD

(Continued)

Table 5 Phase II, Constant Dose Scheme, 7.4 GBq: Patient Data (*Continued*)

Patient	Histology	Localization and number of lesions	Onset of diagnosis/time to treatment (months)	Pretreatments	Pre DOTATOC medication	Tumor response to DOTATOC
30	NETup	Liver >10, mediastinal 6, abdomen 4	1/98/16 months	I-MIBG-therapy	None	SD
31	NETup	Liver >10	8/95/52 months	Operations, octreotide, interferon, chemotherapy (dacarbacin)	Octreotide	SD
32	NETup	Liver >10	9/96/42 months	Chemoembolisations, octreotide, interferon	Octreotide	PR
33	NETup	Liver >10, bone >10	7/99/6 months	Chemotherapies (ETO, CDDP)	None	PR
34	NETup	Liver >10, lymph nodes 2	8/99/1 month	None	None	SD
35	NETup	Liver >10, lymph node 1	12/99/5 months	Octreotide	Octreotide	SD
36	NETup	Liver >10, bone 10, lymph nodes 3	8/94/63 months	Chemotherapies (x), chemoembolisations, interferon	None	SD
37	NETup	Bowel 1, lymph nodes 2	9/99/2 months	None	None	SD
38	Other	Liver 1	7/99/6 months	None	None	CR
39	Other	Liver 8, abdomen 4	8/93/11 months	Operations, radiatio	None	SD

Abbreviations: CDDP, cisplatine; ETO, etoposide; 5FU, 5-fluorouracil; STZ, streptozotocin; x*, combinations not specified; EPT, endocrine pancreatic tumor; NETup, neuroendocrine tumor with unknown origin; int. NET, intestinal NET; bronch. NET, bronchial NET.

Table 6 Phase II, Constant Dose Scheme, 7.4 GBq: Tumor Response

	Progression before treatment	CR	PR	SD	PD	Overall tumor response	CR, PR, SD
EPT (n=13)	100% (13)	1	4	6	2	38%	11 (85%)
Intestinal NET (n=12)	100% (12)	–	1	11	–	8%	12 (100%)
Bronchial NET (n=3)	100% (3)	–	–	3	–	0%	3 (100%)
NET of unknown origin (n=9)	100% (9)	–	2	6	1	22%	8 (89%)
Others (n=2)	100% (2)	1	–	1	–	50%	2 (100%)
All (n= 39)	100% (39)	2	7	27	3	23%	36 (92%)

A total of 7.4 GBq/m^2 ^{90}Y-DOTATOC divided into two equal intravenous injections was administered at intervals of eight weeks. In addition, a life quality assessment using the European Life Quality questionnaire QLQ-C30 was performed. Thirty-six consecutive patients (mean age 54.7 year, female: 17, male: 19) with progressive neuroendocrine tumors were included. CT, MRI, and ultrasound assessed tumor response. After each treatment session, the patients answered a QLQ-C30 questionnaire. The overall objective response rate was 33%. Complete remissions (CR) were found in 6% (2/36), Partial remissions (PR) in 28% (10/36), a stable disease (SD) in 54% (20/36), and PD in 12% (4/36). A significant increase of life quality was found. All response (both clinical benefit and response) was ongoing for the duration of follow-up (median 10.5 months, range 4–18 months). Side effects were grade 1/2 lymphocytopenia in 17%,

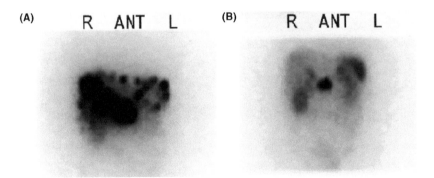

Figure 2 (**A**) ^{111}In-DOTATOC scintiscan of the abdomen in a female patient with a endocrine pancreatic tumor and multiple liver metastases before DOTATOC-treatment. (**B**) After DOTATOC treatment ^{111}In-DOTATOC scintiscan of the abdomen revealed a partial remission, which was confirmed by CT.

anemia grade 1/2 in 33%, thrombocytopenia 1/2 in 11%, grade 3 in 3%, grade 1–2 leucopoenia in 19% and renal insufficiency grade 1 in 3%, grade 4 in 3%. Thus, compared to previous trials, lowering the number of treatment sessions at constant injected dose seems to increase the objective response rate. However, the occurrence of renal insufficiency in patients with kidney protection was concerning. We concluded that individual pretherapeutic dosimetry for ^{90}Y-DOTATOC therapy is necessary considering the large differences in organ doses between individual patients. According to Forster et al, dosimetry based on [86]Y-DOTATOC and ^{111}In-DTPA-octreotide yields similar organ doses, but if possible, dosimetry should be performed with the chemically identical tracer [86]Y-DOTATOC (14). Its availability is still a problem (Table 7).

Pilot Study, Medullary and Differentiated Thyroid Cancer

Only two thirds of patients with differentiated thyroid carcinoma concentrate iodine in their metastases and, during the course of disease, uptake disappears in a

Table 7 Pilot Study, Medullary and Differentiated Thyroid Cancer. Patient Characteristics, Tumor Classification, and Pretreatment

Patients	Sex	Age	Tumor classification	Pretreatment
1	M	72	MTC	TT, ND, EN
2	M	62	MTC	TT, R, BP, BT, C
3	M	69	MTC	TT, EN
4	F	24	MTC/MEN 2A	TT, EN, C
5	M	41	MTC	TT, EN
6	F	58	MTC	TT, R, C
7	F	50	MTC	TT
8	F	64	MTC	TT, RIT, EN, BT
9	M	70	MTC	TT
10	M	49	MTC	TT, ND
11	F	69	MTC	TT, R, EN, C
12	M	42	MTC	TT
13	M	56	FC	TT, RIT
14	M	44	FC	TT, RIT, R, EN
15	F	74	FC	TT, ND, RIT
16	F	66	PC	TT, R, EN
17	F	70	PC	TT, RIT, EN
18	M	54	PC	TT, R, RIT, EN
19	F	60	PC	TT, R, EN
20	F	57	AC	TT, C

Abbreviations: MTC, medullary thyroid carcinoma; FC, follicular carcinoma; PC, papillary carcinoma; AC, anaplastic carcinoma; TT, total thyroidectomy; ND, neck dissection; EN, enucleation of metastases; RIT, radioiodine therapy; C, chemotherapy; R, external irradiation; BP, biphosphonate therapy; BT, biotherapy with octreotide.

further significant proportion (16). However, multiple somatostatin receptor subtypes are known to be present in various densities in medullary thyroid cancer and in the majority of differentiated thyroid tumors (17). Thus, we selected medullary and differentiated xthyroid cancer as target for PRRT with ^{90}Y-DOTATOC (Tables 7 and 8) (15).

Table 8 Pilot Study, Medullary and Differentiated Thyroid Cancer. Treatment Data, Uptake Score, and Tumor Response

Patients	Number of cycles	Total dose in GBq	Tumor uptake score	Tumor response	TTP/months
1	3	6.1	1	SD	11
2	2	14.0	3	SD	3
3	3	11.1	1	PD on/during therapy	
4	2	6.2	1	PD on/during therapy	
5	4	10.0	2	PD on/during therapy	
6	2	3.7	1	PD on/during therapy	
7	1	1.7	1	PD on/during therapy	
8	4	9.1	2	SD	14
9	2	9.3	2	SD	3
10	4	13.2	2	PD on/during therapy	
11	4	9.1	3	SD	10
12	2	3.3	1	PD on/during therapy	
13	4	14.8	3	SD	8
14	4	12.4	1	PD on/during therapy	
15	1	1.7	2	PD on/during therapy	
16	2	5.6	2	PD on/during therapy	
17	4	9.1	2	SD	8
18	2	4.5	2	PD on/during therapy	
19	3	6.1	1	PD on/during therapy	
20	3	7.4	1	PD on/during therapy	

Abbreviations: SD, stable disease; PD, progressive disease; TTP, time to progression.

To determine the antitumor activity of ^{90}Y-DOTATOC and to estimate the response rate in a homogeneous patient population with differentiated or medullary thyroid cancer, we treated 20 patients with these tumor entities. All patients had been in a therapy-resistant and PD before ^{90}Y-DOTATOC therapy. The dose applied was between totals of 1.7 to 7.4 GBq/m^2 ^{90}Y-DOTATOC, administered in one to four injections at intervals of six weeks. Eleven patients had no renal reabsorption protection, nine received a Hartmann-Hepa 8% solution. The objective response rate was 0%. A SD was achieved in 35% (7/20), and a PD was observed in 65% (13/20). The median time to progression (TTP) was eight months, and the median follow up 15 months. The treatment was well tolerated. There were no grade 3/4 haematological or renal toxicities. However, by looking on the objective response rate, we had to conclude that our PRRT treatment protocol with ^{90}Y-DOTATOC was ineffective in metastasizing medullary and differentiated thyroid cancer.

Value of chromogranin A (CgA), (Abstract SGNM Aarau 2002)

Diagnosis and staging of neuroendocrine tumors were significantly improved by the introduction of the chromogranin A (CgA)assay in plasma or serum as a tumor marker. However, the clinical role of the CgA assay compared with PRRT in the management of neuroendocrine tumors had not been elucidated. The aim of this study was therefore to investigate the diagnostic and prognostic value of plasma CgA, specified with a new solid-phase two site immunoradiometric assay, in therapeutic follow-up after PRRT. The study included 55 selected patients with advanced neuroendocrine tumors and high standardized uptake values (SUV). All patients underwent PRRT with different totals of ^{90}Y-DOTATOC. CgA plasma samples were obtained from each patient before starting irradiation and after therapy termination. CgA plasma levels were measured using a radioimmuno-assay kit (CGA-RIACT, CIS bio international, Cedex/France). The objective response was identified by CT, MRI or ultrasound. All 55 patients (100%) had elevated basal CgA level before treatment, median 824 ng/ml (68–1968 ng/ml). According to conventional imaging, the objective response rate after PRRT was 35% (CR 6%, PR 29%, SD 53%, PD 13%). The CgA level in patients with CR decreased median 45.8%±50.9, in patients with PR median 22.9%±42.7, in patients with SD, CgA increased median 1.3%±20.4, and finally in patients with PD, CgA decreased median 18.9%±39.2. In 65% of the patients, CgA levels showed intratherapeutically the later achieved objective response. The results also showed a positive correlation between CgA levels and tumor volume: in patients with less than 10 metastases, CgA was median 284.5±646.9 ng/ml, in patients with >10<20 metastases 654.5±480.5 ng/ml, in patients with >20<30 metastases 1404±582.3 ng/ml, and in patients >30 metastases 1704± 898.1 ng/ml. In conclusion, CgA levels correlate well with tumor volume and thus, CgA appears to be a good marker for treatment follow-up. But despite being clearly affected by PRRT, the magnitude of decrease of intratherapeutically measured CgA cannot predict PRRT outcome.

LOCOREGIONAL PRRT WITH ^{90}Y-DOTATOC IN PATIENTS WITH GLIOMA

Most glioma are not curable by surgery, radiotherapy, or chemotherapy, and residual tumor of variable extent is left to adjuvant measures of limited efficacy (18). In the vast majority of patients, the long-term prognosis is grim (19,20).

Direct intratumoral administration of radioimmunoconjugates, toxin compounds, and gene-expressing viral vectors is supposed to lead to high intratumoral doses or drug concentrations with reduced systemic toxicity. Since human glioma, especially of low-grade type, were shown to express high-affinity somatostatin receptor type 2 (21), we regarded ^{90}Y-DOTATOC as a prototypical highly diffusible vector to target infiltrative disease.

Pilot Study

To determine the antitumor activity of locoregional PRRT and to define acute effects on normal tissues, Dr. A. Merlo of Basel enrolled seven low-grade and four anaplastic glioma patients in a pilot study using ^{90}Y-DOTATOC for receptor targeting. The radiopharmakon was locoregionally injected into a stereotactically inserted Port-a-cath. Diagnostic ^{111}In-labeled DOTATOC-scintigraphy following local injection displayed homogeneous to nodular intratumoral vector distribution. The cumulative activity of regionally injected peptide-bound ^{90}Y amounted to 0.37–3.3 GBq, which is equivalent to an effective dose range between 60 ± 15 and 550 ± 110 Gy. The activity was injected in one to four fractions according to tumor volumes; 1.11 GBq of ^{90}Y-labeled DOTATOC was the maximum activity per single injection. Six disease stabilizations and shrinking of a cystic low-grade astrocytoma component were observed. The only toxicity seen was secondary perifocal edema. We concluded that SR-positive human glioma, especially of low-grade type, can be successfully targeted by intratumoral injection of the metabolically stable DOTATOC (Table 9 and 10) (22).

Pilot Study, Long-Term Follow-Up

In this study, we reported on the four-year follow-up after initiation of locoregional PRRT to treat PD in a patient with a complex eleven year history of fibrillary low-grade astrocytoma. ^{90}Y-DOTATOC was repeatedly injected via catheters placed into the resection cavity or into tumor nodules. The radiopharmakon was not only locally injected into the resection cavity following debulking surgery, but also administered by slow infusion technique to target recurrent and infiltrative tumor zones in the subventricular region around the inferior and posterior horns (23).

Table 9 Locoregional PRRT with ^{90}Y-DOTATOC in Patients with Glioma: Clinical Data, and Response Rates (Pilot Study)

Patient	Age, gender	Histology, location	Previous therapies	KPS	Auto-radi-ography	Activity (MBq), fractions	Volume (mL)	Effective dose (Gy)	Dose ratio (MBq/Gy)	Response	Progression free/overall survival
1	30,m	CAII-Rf	B-Dr-R*	90	ND	370, 2	20	100±20	3.7	CR	+4/+4
2	31,m	AII-Rf	S	90	NA	555, 1	15	380±75	1.5	SD	+15/+15
3	43,f	OII-Bf	B	100	ND	2405, 4	36	550±110	4.4	SD	18/18
4	30,m	OII-Rf	S	100	++	555, 1	12	208±21	2.7	SD	+14/+14
5	42,f	AII-Lf	B-R	100	ND	1100, 2	30	280±40	3.9	SD	+6/+6
6	39,m	AII-Lf	B-R	60	ND	740, 3	30	60±15	12.3	sDet	0/8
7	43,m	AII,Lft	B-R	50	–	2200, 3	79	99±24	22.2	sDet	0/13

Table 10 Locoregional PRRT with ^{90}Y-DOTATOC in Patients with Glioma: Clinical Data, and Response Rates (Pilot Study)

Patient	Age, Gender	Histology, Location	Previous Therapies	KPS	Auto-radiography	Activity (MBq), fractions	Volume (mL)	Effective dose (Gy)	Dose ratio (MBq/Gy)	Response	Progression free/overall survival
1	63, f	OIII-RfP	S	100	++	1110, 2	20	480±55	2.3	SD	+10/+10
2	43, m	GBM-Rto	S-R	100	+++	3330, 3	130	335±40	9.8	SDet	0/6
3	37, f	GBM-Lt	S-R	80	–	2405, 4	77	496±100	4.8	SD	10/15
4	28, M	GBM-Rto	S-R-C	90	ND	2035, 3	47	147±30	13.8	Sdet	0/9

Abbreviations: C, cystic; AII, fibrillary astrocytoma; OII, oligodendroglioma grade II; AIII, anaplastic astrocytoma; GBM, glioblastoma multiforme; R, right; L, left; f, frontal; t, temporal; o, occipital; B, biopsy; R*, brachytherapy with 125I seeds, Dr: cyst drainage; R, external beam radiotherapy; S, surgery; C, chemotherapy; KPS, Karnofsky score at time of enrollment; ND, not done; NA, not accessible; +, SR-positive; −, SR-negative; CR, complete remission; SD, stable disease; PD, pogressive disease; sDet, slow deterioration; Survival, in months.

Table 11 Locoregional PRRT with ^{90}Y-DOTATOC in Patients with Glioma: Clinical Data and Response Rates (Extended Pilot Study)

Patient, location[a]	Age, gender	Histology[b]	Previous therapy[c]	KPS (pre-/post-brachytherapy)[d]	Autoradiography[e]	Toxicity[f] (WHO grades I-IV)	Response[g]	Progression-free survival (months)[h]
PD								
1, fR	31, M	AII	Seed, S	80/80	NA	None	R	+45
2, fL	42, F	OAII	RT, S	70/60	ND	pN(II)*	R	+33/+38
3, fL	35, M	AIII	B	90/90	+(+)	pN(II)*	R	+28
4, tR	36, F	AIII	S, RT, Ch	100/100	ND	None	R	+13/25
5, fR	65, F	aOIII	S	100/100	+(+)	None	R	24**
Resection								
6, pL	43, M	OAII	S	100/100	+(+)	None	SD	+15
7, fR	33, M	OAII	S	100/100	+(+)	None	SD	+10
8, fR	30, M	OII	S	100/90	+(+)	None	SD	+45
9, pL	43, M	OII	S	100/90	+(+)	tN(II)	SD	+20
10, fL	43, M	AII	S	100/90	(+)	None	SD	+18

[a] f, Frontal; t, temporal; p, parietal; L, left; R, right.

[b] AII, Fibrillary astrocytoma, WHO grade II; OAII, oligo-astrocytoma, grade II; AIII, anaplastic astrocytoma, grade III; aOIII, anaplastic oligodendroglioma, grade III; OII, oligodendroglioma, grade II.

[c] S, Surgery; B, biopsy; RT, external beam radiotherapy; Ch, chemotherapy.

[d] KPS, Karnofsky Performance Score.

[e] ND, Not done; NA, not assessible; +(+), low to moderate somatostatin receptor density; (+), weak staining.

[f] N, Neurological; p, permanent; t, transient; *Pre-existing neurological deficit.

[g] SD, Stable disease; R, response defined as halting of tumor progression, see Materials and methods.

[h] +, Alive; **Non-tumor-related death (heart attack).

In conclusion, we found locoregional PRRT to be safe, of mild and transitory toxicity, and effective in long-term tumor control.

Extended Pilot Study

In this study, we were focusing on locoregional PRRT of low-grade and anaplastic glioma. Five progressive glioma of WHO grades II and III and five extensively debulked low-grade glioma were treated with varying fractions of ^{90}Y-DOTATOC. The vectors were locally injected into the resection cavity or into solid tumor. The activity per single injection ranged from 0.555 to 1.875 GBq, and the cumulative activity from 0.555 to 7.030 GBq, according to tumor volumes and eloquence of the affected brain area, yielding dose estimates from $76+/-15$ to $312+/-62$ Gy. Response was assessed by the clinical status, by steroid dependence and, every 4–6 months, by magnetic resonance imaging and fluorine-18 fluorodeoxyglucose positron emission tomography. In five patients with progressive glioma, lasting responses were obtained for at least 13–45 months without the need for steroids. Locoregional PRRT with ^{90}Y-DOTATOC had been the only modality applied to counter tumor progression. Interestingly, we observed the slow transformation of a solid, primarily inoperable anaplastic astrocytoma into a resectable multi-cystic lesion two years after PRRT. Based on these observations, we also assessed the feasibility of local PRRT following extensive debulking, which was well tolerated (Table 11 and 12) (24).

Thus, we finally concluded that locoregional PRRT with ^{90}Y-DOTATOC is a promising modality for the treatment of malignant glioma.

Table 12 Locoregional PRRT with ^{90}Y-DOTATOC in Patients with Glioma: Dose Rates (Extended Pilot Study)

Patient, location	Activity (MBq) (fractions)	Volume (tumor/ cavity) (ml)	Effective therapeutic volume (ml)[a]	Dose (Gy)
PD				
1, fR	3663 (5)	105	271	76 ± 15
2, fL	2960 (3)	30	105	163 ± 33
3, fL	7030 (5)	155	335	227 ± 45
4, tR	1480 (2)	14	90	219 ± 44
5, fR	2960 (4)	20	81	312 ± 62
Resection				
6, pL	2220 (4)	14	65	262 ± 52
7, fR	2960 (2)	52	157	111 ± 22
8, fR	555 (1)	12	59	42 ± 8
9, pL	1850 (2)	16	70	206 ± 41
10, fL	1850 (5)	51	154	114 ± 23

[a] Volume of cavity or tumor including a 1-cm margin.

DISCUSSION

In conclusion, the results of our clinical studies of antitumor effects and benefit of quality of life in patients with neuroendocrine tumors and glioma after PRRT with ^{90}Y-DOTATOC are most encouraging.

The use of a combination of ^{90}Y- and ^{177}Lu-labeled DOTATOC as well as the combination of standard radiosensitizing chemotherapy regimen plus ^{90}Y- and ^{177}Lu-labeled DOTATOC is supposed to improve future results significantly (25). Trials are in preparation at Basel and elsewhere. Special care has to be taken of patients who were pretreated with the standard agent streptozotocin, which is known to be nephrotoxic (26).

However, in PRRT of neuroendocrine tumors, the radiosensitive kidney is the dose-limiting organ because of high tubular reuptake of the peptide analogs after glomerular filtration and retention of the radionuclides in the tubular cells. This reuptake process can be inhibited by positively charged amino acids such as lysine and arginine.

In our studies, we have aimed at a maximum kidney radiation dose of 23–27 Gy. On the basis of experience with external-beam radiation, this dose is expected to produce clinically significant nephrotoxicity in 5–50% of subjects by five years of follow-up (27). The radiation dose that can be administered safely to the kidneys during PRRT still remains to be established. A certain dose received from external-beam radiation can be expected to be different from that after PRRT, because of differences in the nature of the radiation (radiation period and dose rate), in localization, and in path length (27).

However, the occurrence of renal insufficiency in patients with kidney protection is still of great concern. Thus, we encourage individual pretherapeutic dosimetry for all patients and the exclusion of patients who are pretreated with streptozotocin. In patients with accurate kidney protection by positively charged amino acids and individual pretherapeutic dosimetry and without streptozotocin pretreatment, ^{90}Y-DOTATOC is a very well tolerated treatment with clear antitumor effects and palliation both concerning the malignant carcinoid syndrome and tumor-associated pain. The combination of ^{90}Y- and ^{177}Lu-labeled DOTATOC with radiosensitizing chemotherapies appears to be very promising.

REFERENCES

1. Hofland LJ, Lamberts SW. The pathophysiological consequences of somatostatin receptor internalization and resistance. Endocr Rev 2003; 24:28–47.
2. Krenning EP, Kwekkeboom DJ, Bakker WH, et al. Somatostatin receptor scintigraphy with [111In-DTPA-D-Phe1]- and [123I-Tyr3]-octreotide: the Rotterdam experience with more than 1000 patients. Eur J Nucl Med 1993; 20:716–731.
3. de Jong M, Bakker WH, Krenning EP, et al. Yttrium-90 and indium-111 labelling, receptor binding and biodistribution of [DOTA0,d-Phe1,Tyr3]octreotide, a promising somatostatin analogue for radionuclide therapy. Eur J Nucl Med 1997; 24:368–371.

4. Otte A, Jermann E, Behe M, et al. DOTATOC: a powerful new tool for receptor-mediated radionuclide therapy. Eur J Nucl Med 1997; 24:792–795.

5. Smith-Jones PM, Stolz B, Albert R, Knecht H, Bruns C. Synthesis, biodistribution and renal handling of various chelate-somatostatin conjugates with metabolizable linking groups. Nucl Med Biol 1997; 24:761–769.

6. Bernard BF, Krenning EP, Breeman WA, et al. D-lysine reduction of indium-111 octreotide and yttrium-90 octreotide renal uptake. J Nucl Med 1997; 38:1929–1933.

7. Stolz B, Weckbecker G, Smith-Jones PM, Albert R, Raulf F, Bruns C. The somatostatin receptor-targeted radiotherapeutic [90Y-DOTA-DPhe1, Tyr3]octreotide (90Y-SMT 487) eradicates experimental rat pancreatic CA 20948 tumors. Eur J Nucl Med 1998; 25:668–674.

8. Otte A, Mueller-Brand J, Dellas S, Nitzsche EU, Herrmann R, Maecke HR. Yttrium-90-labelled somatostatin-analogue for cancer treatment. Lancet 1998; 351:417–418.

9. Otte A, Herrmann R, Heppeler A, et al. Yttrium-90 DOTATOC: first clinical results. Eur J Nucl Med 1999; 26:1439–1447.

10. Moll S, Nickeleit V, Mueller-Brand J, Brunner FP, Maecke HR, Mihatsch MJ. A new cause of renal thrombotic microangiopathy: yttrium 90-DOTATOC internal radiotherapy. Am J Kidney Dis 2001; 37:847–851.

11. Waldherr C, Pless M, Maecke HR, Haldemann A, Mueller-Brand J. The clinical value of [90Y-DOTA]-D-Phe1-Tyr3-octreotide (90Y-DOTATOC) in the treatment of neuroendocrine tumors: a clinical phase II study. Ann Oncol 2001; 12:941–945.

12. Rosch F, Herzog H, Stolz B, et al. Uptake kinetics of the somatostatin receptor ligand [86Y]DOTA-DPhe1-Tyr3-octreotide ([86Y]SMT487) using positron emission tomography in non-human primates and calculation of radiation doses of the 90Y-labelled analogue. Eur J Nucl Med 1999; 26:358–366.

13. Waldherr C, Pless M, Maecke HR, et al. Tumor response and clinical benefit in neuroendocrine tumors after 7.4 GBq (90)Y-DOTATOC. J Nucl Med 2002; 43:610–616.

14. Forster GJ, Engelbach MJ, Brockmann JJ, et al. Preliminary data on biodistribution and dosimetry for therapy planning of somatostatin receptor positive tumors: comparison of (86)Y-DOTATOC and (111)In-DTPA-octreotide. Eur J Nucl Med 2001; 28:1743–1750.

15. Waldherr C, Schumacher T, Pless M, et al. Radiopeptide transmitted internal irradiation of non-iodophil thyroid cancer and conventionally untreatable medullary thyroid cancer using. Nucl Med Commun 2001; 22:673–678.

16. Schlumberger M, Challeton C, De Vathaire F, et al. Radioactive iodine treatment and external radiotherapy for lung and bone metastases from thyroid carcinoma. J Nucl Med 1996; 37:598–605.

17. Forssell-Aronsson EB, Nilsson O, Bejegard SA, et al. 111In-DTPA-D-Phe1-octreotide binding and somatostatin receptor subtypes in thyroid tumors. J Nucl Med 2000; 41:636–642.

18. Walker MD, Green SB, Byar DP, et al. Randomized comparisons of radiotherapy and nitrosoureas for the treatment of malignant glioma after surgery. N Engl J Med 1980; 303:1323–1329.

19. Black PM. Brain tumor. Part 2. N Engl J Med 1991; 324:1555–1564.

20. Black PM. Brain tumors. Part 1. N Engl J Med 1991; 324:1471–1476.

21. Reubi JC, Horisberger U, Lang W, Koper JW, Braakman R, Lamberts SW. Coincidence of EGF receptors and somatostatin receptors in meningiomas but inverse, differentiation-dependent relationship in glial tumors. Am J Pathol 1989; 134:337–344.

22. Merlo A, Hausmann O, Wasner M, et al. Locoregional regulatory peptide receptor targeting with the diffusible somatostatin analogue 90Y-labeled DOTA0-D-Phe1-Tyr3-octreotide (DOTATOC): a pilot study in human gliomas. Clin Cancer Res 1999; 5:1025–1033.

23. Hofer S, Eichhorn K, Freitag P, et al. Successful diffusible brachytherapy (dBT) of a progressive low-grade astrocytoma using the locally injected peptidic vector and somatostatin analogue [90Y]-DOTA0-D-Phe1-Tyr3-octreotide (DOTATOC). Swiss Med Wkly 2001; 131:640–644.

24. Schumacher T, Hofer S, Eichhorn K, et al. Local injection of the 90Y-labelled peptidic vector DOTATOC to control gliomas of WHO grades II and III: an extended pilot study. Eur J Nucl Med Mol Imaging 2002; 29:486–493.

25. de Jong M, Breeman WA, Bernard BF, et al. [177Lu-DOTA(0),Tyr3] octreotate for somatostatin receptor-targeted radionuclide therapy. Int J Cancer 2001; 92:628–633.

26. Fjallskog ML, Granberg DP, Welin SL, et al. Treatment with cisplatin and etoposide in patients with neuroendocrine tumors. Cancer 2001; 92:1101–1107.

27. de Jong M, Krenning E. New advances in peptide receptor radionuclide therapy. J Nucl Med 2002; 43:617–620.

10

Somatostatin Receptor-Mediated Radionuclide Therapy for Cancer: Therapy with ^{90}Y-DOTA-Lanreotide

Irene Virgolini, Tatjana Traub-Weidinger, Michael Gabriel, Dirk Heute, and Margarida Rodrigues

Department of Nuclear Medicine, Innsbruck Medical University, Innsbruck, Austria

SUMMARY

Somatostatin (SST) receptor (R) (SSTR) scintigraphy has improved the ability to diagnose and detect, stage disease, and review the response to therapy in patients with neuroendocrine tumors. Many other tumor entities are also candidates for SSTR mediated therapy, including thyroid cancer, brain tumors, melanoma, breast cancer, and thymoma. The biodistribution of ^{111}In-DTPA-D-Phe^1-octreotide as well as of ^{111}In-/^{90}Y-DOTA-D-Phe^1-Tyr^3-octreotide differs from that of ^{111}In-/^{90}Y-DOTA-lanreotide in terms of higher liver and kidney, and less bone marrow uptake. The MAURITIUS (Multicenter Analysis of a Universal Receptor Imaging and Treatment Initiative, a European Study) trial was initiated in 1997 at the University of Vienna, and several centers throughout Europe have treated tumor patients with ^{90}Y-DOTA-lanreotide. Data reported here are based on results from studies in Cesena, London, Milano, Innsbruck, and Vienna. At most centers, comparative scintigraphy with ^{111}In-DTPA-D-Phe^1-octreotide or ^{111}In-DOTA-D-Phe^1-Tyr^3-octreotide was performed for tumor evaluation. Dosimetric studies were performed to predict individual tumor doses and doses for the critical organs. Patients (n$=$235) with neuroendocrine tumors, thymoma, thyroid cancer, brain tumors, lymphoma, intestinal adenocarcinoma, or other rare tumors, received up to a total of 8.5 GBq of ^{90}Y-DOTA-lanreotide in up to seven treatment applications. The therapeutic agent of ^{90}Y-DOTA-lanreotide was given either intravenously (121 patients), intraarterially (21 patients), or by local intratumoral injection (93 patients). Patients were at a stage of progressive disease when entering treatment. During the follow-up period, disease was evaluated by repeated scintigraphy and computer tomography/magnetic resonance imaging, documenting the response to therapy (in terms of stable disease, progressive disease, partial remission, or complete remission), as well as by documenting the time of progression of disease and quality of life parameters. Overall results indicate that beneficial effects can be suspected from therapy with ^{90}Y-DOTA-lanreotide. An update of the five years follow-up period indicated that 37% (40/109) of the patients treated with ^{90}Y-DOTA-lanreotide had stable disease and 17% (18/109) partial remission of tumor lesions. Objective response of quality of life measurements was documented in 10–20% of patients, and subjective response was found in 30–50% of patients. So far, results of the MAURITIUS trial indicate that radiolabeled SST analogs may be considered in patients with SSTR-positive tumors for size reduction and improvement of quality of life paramaters.

INTRODUCTION

The high-level expression of peptide receptors (Rs) on various tumor cells as compared with normal tissues or normal blood cells (1,2) has provided the molecular basis for sucessful use of radiolabeled peptide analogs as tumor tracers in nuclear medicine. Receptor scintigraphy using radiolabeled peptide ligands, in particular somatostatin (SST) analogs, is nowadays established in clinical practice. First treatment results (3,4) encouraged the implementation of therapeutic attempts to specifically target SSTR.

The vast majority of human tumor entities seem to overexpress one or the other of the five distinct known human (h) SSTR subtypes (hSSTR1-5). Whereas neuroendocrine tumors frequently overexpress hSSTR2 (5), intestinal adenocarcinomas and a variety of other tumor types seem to overexpress mainly hSSTR3 and/or hSSTR4 (6,7). On thyroid cancer cells, the existence of hSSTR 2, 3 and 5 has been identified (8,9).

In contrast, ^{111}In-DTPA-D-Phe^{1}-octreotide (Octreoscan$^{®}$) and ^{111}In-DOTA-D-Phe^{1}-Tyr^{3}-octreotide (^{111}In-DOTA-TOCT), which both bind to hSSTR2 and hSSTR5 with very high affinity, to hSSTR3 with moderate affinity, and do not bind to hSSTR1 and hSSTR4 (10,11), ^{111}In-/^{90}Y-DOTA-lanreotide binds to hSSTR2-5 with high affinity, and to hSSTR1 with lower affinity (11,12). Based on this hSSTR binding profile, ^{111}In-DOTA-lanreotide may be a potential radioligand for tumor diagnosis, and ^{90}Y-DOTA-lanreotide for SSTR-mediated radionuclide therapy.

When directly compared in patients with neuroendocrine tumors, discrepancies concerning both the tumor uptake and the detection of tumor lesions were found between ^{111}In-DOTA-lanreotide and ^{111}In-DTPA-D-Phe^1-octreotide or ^{111}In-DOTA- D-Phe^1-Tyr^3-octreotide in about one third of the patients (13). This divergency is most probably based on a different SSTR binding profile.

The first study (Phase I/IIa trial) applying ^{90}Y-DOTA-lanreotide for SSTR-mediated receptor-mediated radionuclide therapy was initiated in 1997 and conducted in Austria at the Universities of Vienna and Innsbruck. First experience obtained in this Vienna-Innsbruck Multicenter Study suggested a significant potential for ^{90}Y-DOTA-lanreotide therapy. Preliminary treatment results of the European study "MAURITIUS" (Multicenter Analysis of a Universal Receptor Imaging and Treatment Initiative, a European Study), confirmed the potential usefulness of ^{90}Y-DOTA-lanreotide for diagnosis and therapy in 154 patients with different tumor entities expressing hSSTR (11).

Here, we review the MAURITIUS trial [for review of principles and previous preliminary data obtained in 154 patients see (11)], and present the clinical data obtained with the update of the trial performed in May 2003, after almost five years of follow-up.

SELECTION OF PATIENTS

In principal, all patients with tumors known to express hSSTR are eligible for the application of high dose labeled SST analogs, provided the tumors demonstrate sufficient uptake of radiolabeled peptide on scintigraphy. However, most of the patients treated so far with radiolabeled peptides had no other treatment option, were refractory to conventional treatment strategies and/or were at a progressive stage at the time of the first treatment application of these radiopharmaceuticals.

A positive scintigraphic study and a dosimetric evaluation are a prerequisite for the initiation of treatment with radiolabeled peptides. In general, the clinical protocols available are designed such that tumor uptake is controlled by dosimetry, or at least by repeated scintigraphic studies which score the tumor uptake during the whole treatment and follow-up period. Usually, patients who were included in therapeutical trials had multiple sites of disease evidenced by scintigraphic and dosimetric evaluation with ^{111}In-/^{99m}Tc-labeled peptides and/or by imaging with positron emission tomography (PET) performed with ^{86}Y-/^{68}Ga-labeled peptide analogs.

In our trials, substances known to block hSSTRs such as octreotide or lanreotide had to be withdrawn at least seven days prior to a planned dosimetric study and each treatment cycle. However, there are conflicting data on withdrawal of pre-existing therapy with long-acting SST analogs (14,15).

In the Vienna-Innsbruck Multicenter Study, only tumor patients refractory to conventional therapy with tumors who had previously been shown to express hSSTR2-5 subtype receptors were included. Approximately 150 MBq (10 µg peptide) ^{111}In-DOTA-lanreotide were administered intravenously and subsequent dosimetry measurements were performed using a standard protocol.

If the calculated tumor uptake exceeded more than 10 Gy/GBq, treatment with ^{90}Y-DOTA-lanreotide with 1 GBq (30 μg peptide) was initiated. Additional doses of 1 GBq ^{90}Y-DOTA-lanreotide each were administered every four weeks. Disease, safety evaluations, and dosimetry measurements were performed prior to treatment, and every two months thereafter. Treatment was discontinued if the patient showed progressive disease under treatment with ^{90}Y-DOTA-lanreotide or in case of dose-limiting toxicity.

In the MAURITIUS trial, which included centers in Vienna, Innsbruck, London, Milan, and Cesena, therapy inclusion criteria were as follows:

1. Positive ^{111}In-DOTA-lanreotide scintigraphy with a calculated tumor uptake > 10 Gy/GBq ^{90}Y-DOTA-lanreotide
2. Progressive tumor disease under conventional therapy
3. Life expectancy > 3 months, Karnofsky score > 60, age > 18 years (females of child bearing age had to practice efficient birth control)
4. Laboratory tests: granulocytes > 1500/mm^3, platelets > 100.000/mm^3, liver and kidney function < grade I toxicity according to World Health Organization (WHO)-criteria
5. Written informed consent from each patient to his/her participation in the study.

Therapy exclusion criteria of the MAURITIUS trial were pregnancy, breast-feeding females, severe concomitant illness including severe psychiatric disorder, and absence of the inclusion criteria.

A total of 235 patients with different tumor entities expressing hSSTR were included in the MAURITIUS trial. Complete documentation of follow-up was possible in 109 patients.

PREPARATION OF ^{111}IN-/^{90}Y-DOTA-LANREOTIDE

DOTA-lanreotide was synthesized using the commercially available lanreotide [Somatuline® (Bioipsen, Paris, France)] as described previously (12), and radiolabeled as mentioned elsewhere (11).

DIAGNOSTIC AND DOSIMETRIC EVALUATION

For diagnostic and dosimetric evaluation, serial whole-body scintigraphies, in anterior and posterior view, up to 48 hours after intravenous injection of ^{111}In-DOTA-lanreotide were performed. The dosimetry protocol for each patient followed standard nuclear medicine procedures which included these whole-body scintigraphies and also blood and urinary collections. For organ and tumor dose calculations, regions of interest (ROIs) were drawn on the whole-body scintigram at each acquisition time. The mean of anterior and posterior counts were calculated for large ROIs of the liver, spleen, kidneys, and urinary bladder. In addition, ROIs were drawn for all tracer accumulations regarded as tumor sites and background regions using the software written for the camera analyzing system. The background and decay were corrected to the time of injection. The derived residence times were used for organ dose calculation on the basis of the medical internal radiation dose (MIRD) concept for the organ dose calculation, and the "Nodule Module" option of the program for estimating the self-s values of spherical tumors for tumor dose calculation, as described previously (16). The effective dose, as defined by the International Commission on radiological protection, was calculated (17). For assessment of tumor volume, conventional radiological techniques such as computer tomography (CT) and/or magnetic resonance imaging (MRI) were used.

The primary critical organ with radiopeptide therapy is the kidney because small peptides are filtered through the glomerular capillaries and are reabsorbed by the proximal tubular cells (18). From external beam radiation, the critical dose to the kidneys was set in most protocols to about 30 Gy accumulative dose of the radiopeptide. Some groups have recommended infusion of positively charged amino acids such as L-lysin or L-arginine to reduce renal uptake of peptide tracers (11). However, because the administration of amino acids may cause considerable discomfort to the patient and no consistent effect for kidney uptake or radiolabeled peptides was shown, no kidney protection with amino acid was foreseen in the MAURITIUS trial.

DOSE AND ADMINISTRATION OF ^{90}Y-DOTA-LANREOTIDE

Therapeutic doses of ^{90}Y-DOTA-lanreotide were given as infusion over a 30-minute period, and were applied every four weeks using a standard dose of 1 GBq each in the first study (i.e., Vienna-Innsbruck Multicenter Study). Therapeutic applications were repeated only if the patient did not have dose-limiting toxic reactions (i.e., WHO-grade IV haematologic toxicity or grade III nonhaematologic toxicity), had stable disease or tumor regression with measurable persistent disease, and if the blood count, levels of hepatic and renal function, and performance status were in the range of that originally required for patient entry in the study.

^{90}Y-DOTA-lanreotide therapy was continued until a maximum of eight cycles of administration unless there was evidence of progression of tumor disease.

Therapy was terminated if severe adverse side effects according to WHO standard criteria occured, or if the calculated kidney dose exceeded 30 Gy/Gq, no therapeutic success (i.e., progressive disease), and/or a diminished ^{111}In-DOTA-lanreotide tumor uptake was observed.

So far, in the MAURITIUS trial ^{90}Y-DOTA-lanreotide was applied via intra-venous injection in 121 patients (0.8–8.5 GBq, in 1–7 cycles) and via intraarterial in 21 patients (2 GBq, in 1–3 cycles). Ninety-three patients received intratumoral injections of ^{90}Y-DOTA-lanreotide of lower doses (0.6–2 GBq, in 1–6 cycles).

EVALUATION OF THERAPEUTIC RESPONSE

Tumor Disease Evaluation

Evaluation of the tumor disease response was performed according to WHO standard criteria. Accordingly, disease was classified as complete remission (disappearance of all tumor masses for a minimum of four weeks), partial remission (decrease of all tumor masses by at least 50% without appearance of new lesions for a duration of at least four weeks), stable disease [no significant regression (i.e., >50% of all lesions) or increase (i.e., <25% of measurable tumor masses, no new lesions)] or progressive disease (increase of known tumor masses by >25%, or appearance of any new lesions). CT and/or MRI were performed after each further second dose of ^{90}Y-DOTA-lanreotide.

In addition to evaluation of response to treatment, the time to disease progression and the survival time were recorded.

Tumor markers most commonly used for following treatment of respective tumor entities were measured immediately before and every four weeks under therapy with ^{90}Y-DOTA-lanreotide.

Quality of Life

To determine the quality of life, we evaluated in our patients the pain intensity by quantitative measurement of a visual analog score prior, immediately after, and every four weeks following therapy (two cycles), and by recording the use of analgesics. The Karnofsky score and vegetative symptoms such as appetite, weight, bowel movement, miction, and sleep were recorded before and every four weeks under therapy. The general well-being (from comfortable feeling to discomfort) was evaluated by interviewing the patient.

RESULTS

Tumor Disease Response

Update of treatment results obtained in 109 patients indicated partial regressive tumor disease in 17% (18 of 109) of patients (Fig. 1), stable disease in 37% (40 of 109) of patients, and progressive disease under therapy in 47% (51 of 109) of patients. For further details see Table 1. Complete remission has not been reported.

A tumor size dose-response relationship was documented in most centers. In general, the smaller the tumor lesions in the patients treated with radiolabeled peptides, the better was the response observed for these particular lesions.

Time of Progression of Disease

Overall long-term and survival statistics are not yet available. The follow-up of patients until death will probably give further information about the usefulness of ^{90}Y-DOTA-lanreotide therapy.

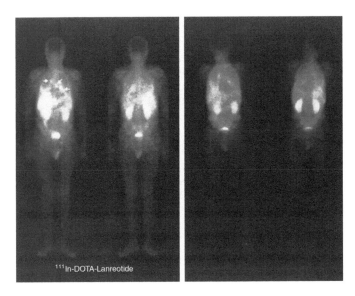

Figure 1 Patient with Hurthle cell carcinoma prior to (*left panel*) and after (*right panel*) several cycles of therapy with ^{90}Y-DOTA-lanreotide (each cycle 1 GBq). Whereas the smaller lung metastases (*arrow*) showed regressive disease under therapy, the larger metastases did not respond to therapy with ^{90}Y-DOTA-lanreotide.

Quality of Life

Improvement in the quality of life for some months up to two years was reported in all MAURITIUS centers.

Objective response of quality of life measurement documented improvement in the quality of life in 10–20% of patients, and subjective improvement was

Table 1 Tumor Disease Response in the MAURITIUS Trial

	Total	PR	SD	P+D
Carcinoids	38	6	14	18
Other GEP tumors	6	3	2	1
Thyroid cancer/MTC	28	5	12	11
NSCLC/SCLC	12	0	5	7
Thymoma	11	4	3	4
Lymphoma	5	0	2	3
Hepatoma	2	0	0	2
Intestinal adenocarcinoma	7	0	2	5
Summary	109	18	40	51

Abbreviations: PR, partial regressive disease; SD, stable disease; PD, progressive disease; GEP, Gastroenteropancreatic; MTC, medullary thyroid cancer; NSCL, non-small-cell lung cancer; SCLC, small-cell lung cancer.

reported in 30–50% of patients. Reduction of general pain, bone pain reduction or relief, reduction of headache, and improvement of sleeping behavior, appetite, weight, and general well-being were found. Most patients with subjective improvement reported this after single injections of therapy.

The response of improved quality of life was not dependent on the tumor response, and was observed also in patients with progressive disease.

Biochemical Parameters

Changes in laboratory parameters such as in serotonin, gastrin, or thyroglobulin serum levels have been found. However, no conclusions can be made yet on the general behavior of hormone values in hormone-producing tumor patients undergoing therapy with ^{90}Y-DOTA-lanreotide.

Side Effects

Side effects of receptor-mediated radionuclide therapy concern mainly the critical organs, which are bone marrow and kidney.

None of the patients treated with ^{90}Y-DOTA-lanreotide developed any severe acute or chronic haematologic side effect, or had significant changes in renal or liver function parameters caused by this type of radiopeptide therapy under the doses administered.

Transient thrombocytopenia or leucopenia grade 1–2 was found in 17 patients, grade 2 in four patients, grade 3 in three patients and grade 4 in one patient who had received intravenous infusion of ^{90}Y-DOTA-lanreotide, and grade 3 in two patients and grade 4 in two patients who were treated via intraarterial.

Total accumulated kidney doses ranged between 5 and 64 Gy/GBq and reduced creatinine clearance was seen in only two patients (with an accumulative kidney dose of 18 Gy/GBq and 64 Gy/GBq) in the follow-up period.

TUMOR UPTAKE OF ^{111}IN-DOTA-LANREOTIDE COMPARED WITH OCTREOTIDE DERIVATES

In about two thirds of patients with neuroendocrine tumors, ^{111}In-DOTA-lanreotide tumor uptake was found to be lower than that with other octreotide derivates, mainly ^{111}In-DOTA-D-Phe^1-Tyr^3-octreotide. Therefore, ^{90}Y-DOTA-D-Phe^1-Tyr^3-octreotide should be considered the first choice for experimental SSTR-based therapy in patients with neuroendocrine tumors. Evaluation of the type of radiotracer to be used for SSTR-targeted radiotherapy, based on scintigraphic pattern and dosimetric studies, should, however, always be performed for the individual patient, because of the discrepancies concerning both the tumor uptake and the detection of tumor lesions between the different radiopharmaceuticals available.

Potential indications for ^{90}Y-DOTA-lanreotide remain radioiodine-negative thyroid cancer, hepatocellular cancer, lung cancer, brain tumors, and possibly malignant melanomas.

DRAWBACKS

One of the major problems is still the lack of these radiopeptides in general, and the request for new and cheaper therapeutic radionuclides in particular.

So far, only patients with an advanced stage of tumor disease have been treated with peptide receptor-mediated radionuclide therapy. Future therapeutic trials should discuss the possibility of inclusion of patients at an earlier stage of disease and therefore be able to evaluate the possible potential of radiopeptide therapy at an earlier stage of tumor disease.

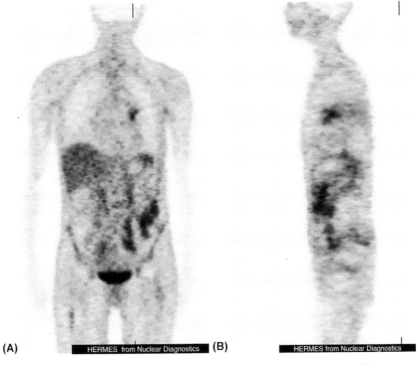

(A)   HERMES from Nuclear Diagnostics   (B)   HERMES from Nuclear Diagnostics

Figure 2 (**A**) Coronal and (**B**) sagittal PET study after injection of 100 MBq of ^{68}Ga-DOTA-lanreotide to a patient with lung cancer who had a negative ^{68}Ga-DOTA-Tyr^3-octreotide PET scan.

CONCLUSIONS

Results with ^{90}Y-DOTA-lanreotide therapy have pointed out the clinical potential of SSTR-targeted radiotherapy in patients with tumor sites expressing hSSTR. In particular, the MAURITIUS trial documented the possibility to image and treat specifically (receptor-mediated) cancer patients in an advanced stage of the disease, with only mild side effects. Although all patients included in this trial started ^{90}Y-DOTA-lanreotide therapy when tumor disease was progressive, disease control at a cost much less than that of conventional chemotherapy was achieved in several patients. Reduction of tumor size and improvement in quality of life was found in a significant number of patients, even in patients with progressive disease.

FUTURE OUTLOOK

In recent months, first applications of ^{68}Ga-DOTA-lanreotide to patients with negative ^{68}Ga-DOTA-Tyr^3-octreotide PET-scans were performed (Fig. 2). These applications demonstrated high uptake of ^{68}Ga-DOTA-lanreotide in patients with metastasized disease and provided successful information in patients prior to therapy with the ^{90}Y-DOTA- or ^{177}Lu-labeled lanreotide analogue.

REFERENCES

1. Reubi JC, Maurer K, vonWerder K, Torhost J, Klijn GM, Lamberts SWJ. Somatostatin receptors in human endocrine tumors. Cancer Res 1987; 47:551–558.
2. Virgolini I, Yang Q, Li S, et al. Cross-competition between vasoactive intestinal peptide and somatostatin for binding to tumor cell membrane receptors. Cancer Res 1994; 54:690–700.
3. Krenning EP, Kwekkeboom DJ, Bakker WH, et al. Somatostatin receptor scintigraphy with [^{111}In-DTPA-D-Phe1]- and [^{123}I-Tyr3]-octreotide: the Rotterdam experience with more than 1000 patients. Eur J Nucl Med 1993; 20:716–731.
4. Otte A, Jermann E, Behe M, et al. DOTATOC—a powerful new pool for receptor-mediated radionuclide therapy. Eur J Nucl Med 1997; 24:792–795.
5. Reubi J, Schaer JC, Waser B, Mengod G. Expression and localization of somatostatin receptor SSTR1, SSTR2 and SSTR3 mRNAs in primary human tumors using in situ hybridization. Cancer Res 1994; 54:3455–3459.
6. Virgolini I, Pangerl T, Bischof C, Smith-Jones P, Peck-Radosavljevic M. Somatostatin receptor subtype expression in human tissues: a prediction for diagnosis and treatment of cancer? Eur J Clin Invest 1997; 27:645–647.
7. Virgolini I, Traub T, Novotny C, et al. New trends in peptide receptor radioligands. Q J Nucl Med 2001; 45:153–159.
8. Ain KB, Taylor KD, Tofiq S, Venkataraman G. Somatostatin receptor subtype expression in human thyroid and thyroid carcinoma cell lines. J Clin Endocr Metab 1997; 82:1857–1862.

9. Kölby L, Wängberg B, Ahlman H, et al. Somatostatin receptor subtypes, octreotide scintigraphy, and clinical response to octreotide treatment in patients with neuroendocrine tumors. World J Surg 1998; 22:679–683.

10. Reubi JC, Schar JC, Waser B, et al. Affinity profiles for human somatostatin receptor subtypes SST1-SST5 of somatostatin radiotracers selected for scintigraphic and radiotherapeutic use. Eur J Nucl Med 2000; 27:273–282.

11. Virgolini I, Britton K, Buscombe J, Moncayo R, Paganelli G, Riva P. ^{111}In- and ^{90}Y-DOTA-lanreotide: results and implications of the MAURITIUS trial. Semin Nucl Med 2002; 32:148–155.

12. Smith-Jones PM, Bischof C, Leimer M, et al. DOTA-lanreotide: a novel somatostatin analog for tumor diagnosis and therapy. Endocrinology 1999; 140:5136–5148.

13. Virgolini I, Traub T, Novotny C, et al. Experience with indium-111 and yttrium-90-labeled somatostatin analogs. Curr Pharm Design 2002; 8:1781–1807.

14. Dorr U, Wurm K, Horing E, Guzman G, Rath U, Bihl H. Diagnostic reliability of somatostatin receptor scintigraphy during continuous treatment with different somatostatin analogs. Horm Metab Res 1993; 27:36–43.

15. Soresi E, Invernizzi G, Boffi R, et al. Intensification of ^{111}In-DTPA-octreotide scintigraphy by means of pretreatment with cold octreotide in small cell lung cancer. Lung Cancer 1997; 17:231–238.

16. Stabin MG. MIRDOSE. Personal computer software for internal dose assessment in nuclear medicine. J Nucl Med 1996; 37:538–546.

17. Johansson L, Mattson S, Nosslin B, Svegborn SR. Effective dose from radio-pharmaceuticals. Eur J Nucl Med 1993; 19:933–938.

18. Morgensen CE, Solling K. Studies on renal tubular protein reabsorption: partial and near complete inhibition by certain amino acids. Scand J Clin Lab Invest 1977; 37:477–486.

11

Receptor Radionuclide Therapy with ^{90}Y-[DOTA^0]-Tyr^3-Octreotide (^{90}Y-DOTATOC): The IEO Experience

Lisa Bodei and Giovanni Paganelli

Division of Nuclear Medicine, European Institute of Oncology, Milan, Italy

INTRODUCTION

High concentrations of subtype 2 somatostatin tumor receptors (sst$_2$) are expressed in numerous tumors, enabling primary and metastatic masses to be localized by scintigraphy after injecting ^{111}In-labeled somatostatin analogue octreotide. In addition to neuroendocrine tumors, somatostatin receptors have also been identified on cancers of the central nervous system, breast, lung, and lymphatic tissue, and the use of radionuclide-labelled somatostatin analogs appeared promising for therapy as well as for diagnosis of such malignancies (1–3).

Neuroendocrine tumors are rare and may be sporadic or part of hereditary syndromes. Despite the single definition, these tumors form a heterogeneous group including, as an example, gastroenteropancreatic neuroendocrine tumors, medullary thyroid carcinomas and bronchial neuroendocrine tumors. They may present to the physician at different stages of disease, with or without associated hormonal syndromes. Functioning tumors are usually detected in earlier stages, due to hormone secretion rather than tumor bulk. Non-functioning tumors are usually diagnosed for the presence of a mass, along with distant metastases. Neuroendocrine tumors are frequently slow-growing, and this allows several different therapeutic approaches to be attempted. Therefore, a therapeutic pathway involving different disciplines, alias a multidisciplinary approach, must be outlined, and frequently tailored to each patient. This approach is the procedure we adopted in our institution. The first step is the symptomatic control of hypersecretory syndromes in functioning tumors by biotherapy with somatostatin analogs and/or interferon alpha-2b. Surgery is the therapy of choice, especially in localized disease, where it may be curative. Cytoreduction, by means of trans-arterial chemoembolization (TACE) and/or surgery of the primary tumor and/or its metastases, should always be attempted in metastatic disease, when feasible, in order to reduce the amount of tumor to be subsequently treated. Receptor radionuclide therapy with radiolabelled somatostatin analogs is a recently developed option to treat neuroendocrine tumors by selective irradiation of the masses. We indicate this treatment within a multidiciplinary approach, after debulking with chemoembolization or surgery, along with somatostatin analogs and/or interferon alpha-2b. While this seems appropriate for slow-growing tumors, for those which have randomly progressed in disease because of poorly differentiated histology or measured clinical evidence of rapid growth, chemotherapy schemes, such as carboplatin + etoposide or epidoxorubicin + cisplatin + 5-fluorouracyl, are currently used in our institution.

Receptor radionuclide therapy consists in the intravenous administration of a peptide, such as octreotide, labelled with a therapeutic radionuclide (Fig.1). The basis for receptor radionuclide therapy with radiolabelled octreotide in

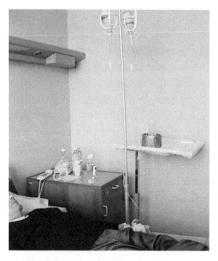
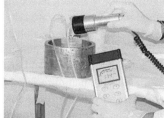

Figure 1 *Patient administration.* The radiopharmaceutical is administered through a patented infusion system (*left*). The infusion begins by allowing the saline solution to drip into the vial, thus forcing the radiopharmaceutical out to the patient IV port. This method was developed to avoid the handling of syringes, and hence reduce the radiation burden to the physician. The termination of the infusion is checked by measuring the dose rate outside the vial (*right*).

somatostatin receptor rich tissues is the receptor-mediated endocytosis of the radiopeptide that is trapped inside the cytoplasm, thus allowing the irradiation of the cell. Labels currently used are the Auger electron emitter [111]In ([^{111}In-DTPA[0]]-octreotide), the pure beta emitter [90]Y ([^{90}Y-DOTA][0]-Tyr[3]-Octreotide or ^{90}Y-DOTATOC), and the beta-gamma emitter [177]Lu ([^{177}Lu-DOTA[0]]-Tyr[3]-octeotate or ^{177}Lu-DOTATATE) (4–6). The total amount of radioactivity is fractionated in several cycles, up to a cumulative activity sufficient to irradiate the tumor but below the kidney or the bone marrow dose-threshold.

We chose Yttrium-90 as label for its high beta energy (E_{max} 2.27 MeV) and long penetration in tissues (R_{max} 11 mm), that may allow a "cross-fire" effect on surrounding receptor-negative cells. Our experience of receptor radionuclide therapy with ^{90}Y-DOTATOC began in 1997, first with the dosimetric studies, then with two phase I studies (with and without renal protection with amino acids), followed by the evaluation of the response to therapy and the evaluation of kidney protection (7–11).

SAFETY ASPECTS

With the pharmacokinetic and dosimetric studies we established that ^{90}Y-DOTATOC gives a short-term total body irradiation and that the organs with the highest absorbed dose were the spleen and the kidney. The tumor receives a high irradiation (1.4-31 Gy/GBq, mean 10), while the bone marrow receives a low dose (0.04 ± 0.02 Gy/GBq; Cremonesi et al. see chapter). The spleen and kidney, in contrast, receive a relatively high dose (7.2 ± 5.2, and 3.8 ± 2.0 Gy/GBq, respectively), but, given its threshold of dose-related toxicity, the kidney represents the dose-limiting organ.

Possible toxicity deriving from ^{90}Y-DOTATOC therapy may be divided in to acute and delayed. Acute toxicity almost exclusively consists of a transient reduction in blood figures, with a nadir occurring 3–5 weeks after therapy, and is determined by blood circulating activity and, to a lesser extent, by specific bone marrow uptake. Acute effects such as nausea and vomiting sometimes occur and appear to be related to the co-administration of renal protective agents, such as positively charged amino acids.

We evaluated acute toxicity of ^{90}Y-DOTATOC in a first phase I study including 30 patients, divided in six groups, affected by sst_2-expressing tumors, free from any chemo- or radiotherapy for at least the month before and two months after therapy. Patients were in good general condition and had preserved blood, liver, and renal parameters. Three equivalent activity doses were administered to each patient, eight weeks apart. Amino acid co-administration was not performed, in order to have a "clean" phase I study. The activity was escalated from 1.11 to 2.59 GBq of ^{90}Y, by 0.37 GBq steps in each group. No major acute reactions, such as skin reaction, allergy, or fever, were observed after ^{90}Y-DOTATOC injection up to 2.59 GBq per cycle, although five patients had moderate gastrointestinal toxicity. Major haematological toxicity (grade 3 or 4) did not occur, except for a transient reduction in lymphocytes (grade 3, and 4 in almost all patients); up to 5.55 GBq cumulative activity, most patients had haematological toxicity in the 0–1 range.

We continued studying acute toxicity of ^{90}Y-DOTATOC and the effect of amino acid co-administration in a second phase I trial including 40 patients with sst_2-expressing tumors, with the same characteristics as the previous one. Patients were divided in eight groups and received two cycles of ^{90}Y-DOTATOC eight weeks apart. The activity was escalated from 2.96 to 5.55 GBq per cycle, by 0.37 GBq steps in each group. All patients received lysine ± arginine infusion immediately before and after therapy. Forty-eight percent developed acute grade 1–2 gastrointestinal toxicity (nausea and vomiting) after amino acid infusion, whereas no acute adverse reactions occurred after ^{90}Y-DOTATOC injection up to 5.55 GBq/cycle. Grade 3 haematological toxicity occurred in three of seven (43%) patients receiving 5.18 GBq, which was defined as the maximum tolerable activity per cycle.

Since no spleen toxicity was ever found after therapy, the kidneys represent undoubtedly the critical organs in repeated cycles, due to the renal interstitial irradiation deriving from tubular peptide reabsorption. The cumulative absorbed dose to the kidney may, in fact, cause renal damage above the conventional threshold dose of 23–25 Gy (12). Since the 23–25 Gy limit was derived from external radiotherapy, the real threshold dose for kidney toxicity with internal emitters appears questionable, possibly higher than the one established for external radiotherapy, owing to the different kinetics of irradiation exposure that typically decrease with time. Nevertheless, concern about possible renal failure when dose threshold is trespassed is fully justified. We therefore started to protect the kidney by the co-administration of positively charged amino acids, e.g., L-lysine and/or L-arginine, that have demonstrated to competitively inhibit the proximal tubular reabsorption of the radiopeptide, resulting in potential reduction of the renal dose. We tested various combinations in 40 patients in the mentioned study. Renal protection with amino acids included three schemes: L.A.: 20 g lysine in 1000 ml + 40 g arginine in 1000 ml over 3–4 hours before therapy; L.A.L.: 10 g lysine in 500 ml + 20 g arginine in 500 ml over 1–2 hours before therapy and 10 g lysine in 500 ml over 2–3 hours after therapy; L.L.: 10 g lysine in 500 ml over 1 hour before therapy and 15 g lysine in 750 ml over 2 hours after therapy. The reduction in renal dose ranged from 18 to 26%, in six patients who underwent dosimetric studies with ^{111}In-DOTATOC. Forty-eight percent developed acute grade 1–2 gastrointestinal toxicity (nausea and vomiting) after amino acid infusion.

In order to enhance the renal protection and to reduce side effects in patients, we performed another study aimed at evaluating different combinations of lysine, arginine, and other positively charged molecules, such as avidin and dextran. We studied 16 patients, treated with 2–8 cycles of ^{90}Y-DOTATOC (4.1–14.0 GBq cumulative activity) and undergone a dosimetry study with and without kidney protection. The combination of lysine and arginine (lysine 15 g and arginine 20 g before ^{111}In-DOTATOC and 10 g after) was frequently associated with gastrointestinal toxicity (nausea and vomiting) and allowed a mean 37% reduction of kidney dose. The combination of lysine with the positively charged molecule of avidin (10 g and 2 mg/Kg before ^{111}In-DOTATOC, respectively) yielded a reduction of the dose up to 50%. Nevertheless, native avidin was slightly immunogenic, as already reported, and induced an allergic reaction (bronchospasm and flushing) in one patient (13). Therefore, this molecule was not used anymore. On the other hand, the combination of lysinated dextran with lysine (2–8 mg/Kg and 10 g before ^{111}In-DOTATOC, respectively), was well tolerated and gave the highest protection, with a mean 55% dose reduction.

In another study we evaluated the effect of the duration of the infusion; prolonging the lysine infusion, 20 g per day divided in two administrations of four hours each, up to two days after the therapy, induced a consistent reduction (up to 65%) in two pilot cases (14).

These patients were followed up as regards the course of main toxicity parameters for a period of 6 to 50 months. Resulting from the dosimetric studies performed in this group of patients, the estimate of the cumulative absorbed dose to the kidneys ranged from 6.6 to 47.1 Gy (mean 28.3). Slight but permanent renal toxicity, with a rise in creatinine and a decrease in GFR, were observed in 7/16 (44%) patients (maximum grade 2 WHO). When considering renal toxicity compared with the absorbed dose to the kidneys, the alteration of creatinine and GFR occurred when more than 25 Gy had been delivered to the kidneys.

Our studies confirm that high activities of ^{90}Y-DOTATOC can be administered without causing serious toxicity. Accurate renal protection schemes, based on amino acid co-administration, are strongly recommended, in order to give an average of 10–15 GBq cumulative activity, with low risk of permanent renal toxicity. Whether or not this amount of activity should be hyper- or hypofractionated is still to be clarified in controlled randomized phase II studies.

No endocrine disfunction of pituitary axes (thyroid, adrenals, gonads) nor diabetes mellitus was observed after ^{90}Y-DOTATOC, except for a transient impairment in spermatogenesis, revealed by a > 80 decrease in serum inhibin B and a correspondent raise in FSH (5). Regarding cumulative bone marrow toxicity, the possibility of a mild but progressive impoverishment in bone marrow reserves, in repeated cycles, has also to be considered.

EFFICACY

Dosimetric studies indicate that ^{90}Y-DOTATOC is suitable for efficient receptor radiotherapy. Residence times (τ) in tumors can yield variable absorbed doses (1.4-31 Gy/GBq, mean 10.1, Cremonesi et al. see chapter), depending on tumor volume, interstitial pressure, receptor density heterogeneity on the tumor surface and, possibly, tissue viability.

As resulting from previous animal and human studies, high absorbed doses to tumor lesions (> 80–100 Gy) may result in a high percentage of cure (15).

Accordingly, this range of doses should be reached in humans for administered activities of at least 7.4 GBq (5,11).

We therefore evaluated, from 1997 to 2002, the objective response of 141 patients (67 females, 74 males), treated with cumulative activities of 7.4-26.4 GBq of ^{90}Y-DOTATOC, divided in 2–16 cycles, administered 4-6 weeks apart. Patients were affected mainly (114/141 patients, 81%) by neuroendocrine tumors, 42% (59/141) of which were of gastro-entero-pancreatic origin and 39% from other sites. We observed a 26% objective response [PR + CR; (Fig. 2A)]. The majority of patients were progressing at the time of the enrollment (113/141 patients or 80.1% progressing). Considering the progressive patients, an overall clinical benefit (CR + PR + SD) was observed in 76% of cases (Fig. 2B). Stable patients showed a response (CR + PR) in 32% of cases (Fig. 2C). The duration of responses ranged between 2 and 59 months (median 18). In progressing patients, the time to treatment failure (TTF) was 2–49 months (median 13), while in stable patients was 6-33 months (median 16). Patients who responded were affected mainly (69.7% of cases) by gastro-entero-pancreatic neuroendocrine tumors.

Figure 3 reports an example of objective response in a patient affected by non-functioning pancreatic endocrine carcinoma, treated with 9.6 GBq of ^{90}Y-DOTATOC.

We must emphasise that these results derive from designed phase I-II trials, thus not specifically addressed to evaluate the efficacy. To date, the parameters determining the response have to be extrapolated from these available "broad-spectrum" studies. According to the literature, typical neuroendocrine tumors of the gastro-entero-pancreatic area seem to respond better than the whole series of

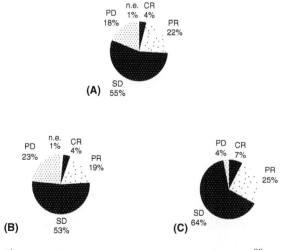

Figure 2 (A) Response in 141 patients treated with ^{90}Y-DOTATOC (MCA ≥ 7.4 GBq), (B) Response in progressing patients (113/141) and (C) response in stable patients (28/141).

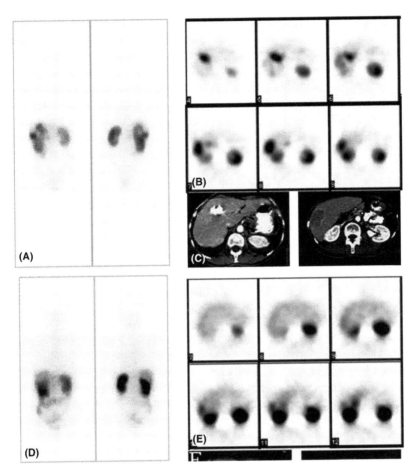

Figure 3 Best objective response in a patient affected by liver metastases from non-functioning endocrine pancreatic carcinoma, treated with 9.6 GBq of ^{90}Y-DOTATOC. At the enrollment the patient had progressed to Trans-Arterial Chemo-Embolization, performed six months before radionuclide therapy (**A, B** and **C**: basal whole-body scan, anterior and posterior view, SPECT sections and CT sections, respectively; **D, E** and **F**: whole-body scan, anterior and posterior view, SPECT sections and CT sections after therapy).

tumors simply expressing somatostatin receptors as demonstrated at OctreoScan (16). In addition, the tumor bulk, especially in the liver, as well as performance status, must be considered as important parameters determining the response and the outcome (6). Therefore early treatment would be recommended rather than a "wait and see" approach. Anyway, we definitely need pathology-oriented phase II trials to assess the potential of ^{90}Y-DOTATOC therapy in each class of disease. Nevertheless, we tried to address some of these open questions with retrospective studies in small cohorts of patients affected by medullary thyroid carcinoma, small cell lung carcinoma and meningioma (17). Studies aimed at evaluating the efficacy of ^{90}Y-DOTATOC in single classes of neuroendocrine tumors are ongoing.

Metastatic medullary thyroid cancer usually shows a progressive course. Surgery represents to date the only curative treatment. In advanced disease, chemo- and radiotherapy schemes have been attempted with poor results. Following our experience of receptor radionuclide therapy with ^{90}Y-DOTATOC in neuroendo- crine tumors, we started evaluating the efficacy of ^{90}Y-DOTATOC therapy in metastatic patients affected by sst_2-positive medullary thyroid carcinoma. We studied 21 patients, progressing after conventional treatments, receiving a cumulative activity of 7.5–19.2 GBq of ^{90}Y-DOTATOC, divided in 2–8 cycles. We observed a complete response in two patients (10%), as evaluated by CT, MRI, and/or ultrasound, and a stabilization of disease in 12 patients (57%). Seven patients (33%) did not respond to therapy. The duration of the response ranged between 3-40 months. Using biochemical parameters, such as calcitonin and CEA, a complete response was observed in one patient (5%), while partial response in five (24%) and stabilization in three (14%). Twelve patients had progression (57%). Complete responses were observed in patients with lower tumor burden and calcitonin values at the time of the enrollment. This retrospective analysis is consistent with the literature, regarding a low response rate in medullary thyroid cancers treated with ^{90}Y-DOTATOC (18). Nevertheless, patients with smaller tumors and higher uptake of the radiopeptide tended to respond better. Studies with ^{90}Y-DOTATOC administered in earlier phases of the disease will help to evaluate the ability of this treatment to enhance survival. We believe that other and more specific peptides, such as gastrin derivatives, and possibly new isotopes, such as the beta-gamma emitter Lutetium-177, will also represent an option of a better treatment of this tumor, especially in minimal residual disease.

Small cell lung cancer is extremely chemosensitive, with an objective response to poly-chemotherapy ranging from 70% to 90%. Still, relapse is a rule and median survival of patients is nine months (six months in advanced disease), with a rate of long-survivors less than 20% in limited disease and anecdotal in extensive disease. However, small cell lung cancer is extremely radiosensitive and a combination of radio- and chemotherapy appears therefore justified by their synergistic effect and by the need to increase survival. We hypothesized that receptor radionuclide therapy could be advantageous, compared to external radiotherapy, since it allows the selective delivery of very high doses to the tumor, while sparing normal tissues. To evaluate the efficacy, in terms of objective response and survival, of ^{90}Y-DOTATOC therapy associated with chemotherapy with carboplatin and etoposide, we enrolled five patients affected by sst_2- expressing small cell lung cancer, as seen on OctreoScan, pre-treated with a maximum of three cycles of chemotherapy. Patients had locally advanced disease and distant metastases in the liver (four patients), bone (three patients) and brain (one patient). After appropriate preparation and hydration with amino acids, patients received 1.11 GBq of ^{90}Y-DOTATOC on day one, followed by carboplatin (Calvert AUC 3) and etoposide (120 mg/sqm) on day two, and etoposide alone (120 mg/sqm) on day three and four. The schedule included three combined treatments. All the five patients died for disease progression, with an interval ranging from 15 days to eight months from the beginning of the therapy. Only two patients could accomplish the programmed schedule, with three cycles of combined therapy. The first of these patients had a minor response after the third cycle lasting two months. The second patient, despite three cycles of combined therapy, had a systemic progression of disease, with brain, lymph node, and adrenal metastases. The other patients could perform only one cycle of combined therapy, due to disease progression. Despite this small series of patients, we can conclude that we possibly selected particularly aggressive tumors by the expression of somatostatin receptors.

Meningiomas are rare, accounting for about 20% of intracranial and 25% of intraspinal tumors. They are generally slow-growing but they can behave quite differently, from small and indolent lesions to very aggressive masses, encasing or compressing vital structures, thus causing major morbidity and even mortality. The large majority of meningiomas are benign, 5% are called atypical, and 2–3% are malignant. Total surgical excision, when feasible, is the best treatment option for benign meningiomas, since sub-totally resected lesions have a high tendency to progress with time. The use of fractionated radiotherapy or stereotactic radiosurgery is increasing for lesions not entirely or not at all removed, as well as for recurrent, atypical, or anaplastic meningiomas (19).

Following this trend and since meningiomas express somatostatin receptors subtype 2 in virtually all cases (20), from 1998 to 2004, 29 patients (20 females, nine males, aged 18–75 years) affected by meningioma were enrolled for radiopeptide therapy with ^{90}Y-DOTATOC. Patients were progressing after conventional therapies at the time of enrolment. According to WHO classification, the group included 14 patients with a grade 1 meningioma, nine with a grade 2, and six with a grade 3. Twenty-six patients had previously undergone to surgery (radical in only seven cases), and 18 of them received also radiotherapy. The median Karnofsky score was 80. Patients received a cumulative activity ranging from 5 to 20 GBq of ^{90}Y-DOTATOC, divided in 2–8 cycles, with amino acid co-administration.

Clinical and neuroradiological evaluation performed before, during, and at the end of treatments showed that stabilization of disease was achieved in 19 patients (66%), while progression continued in the remaining 10 patients. Response appeared related to the grade of disease. Specifically, the 14 patients (86%) with benign grade 1 meningioma had stabilization of disease, while stabilization was achieved only in 40% of the 15 patients with malignant meningiomas (grade 2 and 3). The treatment was well tolerated in all patients, either from clinical or neurological point of view, and gave valuable results. Therefore, we propose receptor radionuclide therapy with ^{90}Y-DOTATOC in earlier stages of disease.

CONCLUSIONS

^{90}Y-DOTATOC therapy has proven to be a safe and effective treatment. The present knowledge and the experience carried out so far would indicate that it is possible to deliver high activities, and therefore high absorbed doses, to tumors expressing sst_2 receptors, with objective therapeutic responses in 26% patients. In almost a decade of clinical use many things have been done. Nevertheless, the ideal study has yet to be performed. New prospective controlled randomized trials will define the exact role of ^{90}Y-DOTATOC in sst_2-positive tumors.

Recently, pre-clinical studies in rats demonstrated excellent responses dependent on tumor size at therapy start. ^{90}Y-DOTATOC would seem able to give higher response rate in bigger lesions (optimal diameter 3.4 cm), while Lutetium-DOTA-Tyr[3]-octreotate (a newer analogue labelled with a beta-gamma emitter) in smaller tumors (optimal diameter 2 cm) (5). Probably the radius of beta emission of the radioisotope has to fit the tumor dimension. Therefore, the administration of combinations of radioisotopes for different sized lesions should be evaluated in future studies.

REFERENCES

1. Reubi JC, Schar JC, Waser B, et al. Affinity profiles for human somatostatin receptor subtypes SST1-SST5 of somatostatin radiotracers selected for scintigraphic and radiotherapeutic use. Eur J Nucl Med 2000; 27:273–282.
2. Krenning EP, Kwekkeboom DJ, Bakker WH, et al. Somatostatin receptor scintigraphy with [111In-DTPA-D-Phe1]- and [123I-Tyr3]-octreotide: the rotterdam experience with more than 1000 patients. Eur J Nucl Med 1993; 20:716–731.
3. Reubi JC, Waser B, Schaer JC, Laissue JA. Somatostatin receptor sst1-sst5 expression in normal and neoplastic human tissues using receptor autoradiography with subtype-selective ligands. Eur J Nucl Med 2001; 28:836–846.
4. Valkema R, De Jong M, Bakker WH, et al. Phase I study of peptide receptor radionuclide therapy with [In-DTPA]octreotide: the rotterdam experience. Semin Nucl Med 2002; 32:110–122.
5. De Jong M, Valkema R, Jamar F, et al. Somatostatin receptor-targeted radionuclide therapy of tumors: preclinical and clinical findings. Semin Nucl Med 2002; 32:133–140.
6. Kwekkeboom DJ, Teunissen JJ, Bakker WH, et al. Radiolabeled somatostatin analog [177Lu-DOTA0,Tyr3]octreotate in patients with endocrine gastroenteropancreatic tumors. J Clin Oncol 2005; 23:2754–2762.
7. Cremonesi M, Ferrari M, Zoboli S, et al. Biokinetics and dosimetry in patients administered with (111)In-DOTA-Tyr(3)-octreotide: implications for internal radiotherapy with (90)Y-DOTATOC. Eur J Nucl Med 1999; 26:877–886.
8. Paganelli G, Zoboli S, Cremonesi M, et al. Receptor-mediated radiotherapy with 90Y-DOTA-D-Phe1-Tyr3-octreotide. Eur J Nucl Med 2001; 28:426–434.
9. Chinol M, Bodei L, Cremonesi M, Paganelli G. Receptor-mediated radiotherapy with 90Y-DOTA-D-Phe1-Tyr3-octreotide: the experience of the European Institute of Oncology group. Semin Nucl Med 2002; 32:141–147.

10. Bodei L, Cremonesi M, Zoboli S, et al. Receptor-mediated radionuclide therapy with (90)Y-DOTATOC in association with amino acid infusion: a phase I study. Eur J Nucl Med Mol Imaging 2003; 30:207–216.

11. Bodei L, Cremonesi M, Grana C, et al. Receptor radionuclide therapy with 90Y-[DOTA0]-Tyr3 -octreotide (90Y-DOTATOC) in neuroendocrine tumors. Eur J Nucl Med Mol Imaging 2004; 7:1038–1046.

12. Bodei L, Chinol M, Cremonesi M, Paganelli G. Facts and myths about radiopeptide therapy: Scylla. Charybdis and Sibyl. Eur J Nucl Med 2002; 29:1099–1100.

13. Chinol M, Casalini P, Maggiolo M, et al. Biochemical modifications of avidin improve pharmacokinetics and biodistribution, and reduce immunogenicity. Br J Cancer 1998; 78:189–197.

14. Cremonesi M, Bodei M, Rocca P, Stabin M, Maecke H, Paganelli G. Kidney protection during receptor-mediated radiotherapy with ^{90}Y-[DOTA^{0},Tyr^{3}]octreotide. Cancer Biother Radiopharm 2002; 17:344.

15. Pauwels S, Barone R, Walrand S, et al. Practical dosimetry of peptide receptor radionuclide therapy with (90)Y-labeled somatostatin analogs. J Nucl Med 2005; 46:92S–98S.

16. Kwekkeboom DJ, Mueller-Brand J, Paganelli G, et al. An overview of the results of peptide receptor radionuclide therapy with 3 different radiolabeled somatostatin analogues. J Nucl Med 2005; 46:62S–66S.

17. Bodei L, Handkiewicz-Junak D, Grana C, et al. Receptor radionuclide therapy with 90Y-DOTATOC in patients with medullary thyroid carcinomas. Cancer Biother Radiopharm 2004; 19:65–71.

18. Waldherr C, Schumacher T, Pless M, et al. Radiopeptide transmitted internal radiation of non-iodophil thyroid cancer and conventionally untreatable medullary thyroid cancer using [90Y]-DOTA-D-Phe1-Tyr3-octreotide: a pilot study. Nucl Med Comm 2001; 22:673–678.

19. Whittle IR, Smith C, Navoo P, Collie D. Meningiomas. Lancet 2004; 363:1535–1543.

20. Dutour A, Kumar U, Panetta R, et al. Expression of somatostatin receptor subtypes in human brain tumors. Int J Cancer 1998; 76:620–627.

12

New Clinical Studies with ^{177}Lu-Labelled Somatostatin Analogs

Dik J. Kwekkeboom

Department of Nuclear Medicine, Erasmus MC Rotterdam, Rotterdam, The Netherlands

Eric P. Krenning

Department of Nuclear Medicine, and Department of Internal Medicine, Erasmus MC Rotterdam, Rotterdam, The Netherlands

Neuroendocrine gastro-entero-pancreatic (GEP) tumors, which comprise pancreatic islet-cell tumors, non-functioning neuroendocrine pancreatic tumors, and carcinoids, are usually slow-growing. When metastasized, treatment with somatostatin analogs results in reduced hormonal overproduction and symptomatic relief in most cases. Treatment with somatostatin analogs, whether or not in combination with Interferon-alpha, is, however, seldom successful in terms of CT or MRI assessed tumorsize reduction (1).

A new treatment modality for inoperable or metastasized GEP tumors is the use of radiolabelled somatostatin analogs. The majority of GEP tumors possess somatostatin receptors and can therefore be visualized in vivo using the radiolabelled somatostatin analogue [^{111}In-DTPA^0]octreotide (Octreoscan®). A logical sequence to this tumor visualization in patients was therefore to also try to treat these patients with radiolabelled somatostatin analogs.

Initial studies with high dosages of [^{111}In-DTPA^0]octreotide in patients with metastasized neuroendocrine tumors were encouraging, although partial remissions (PRs) were exceptional (2). However, ^{111}In-coupled peptides are not ideal for peptide receptor radionuclide radiotherapy (PRRT) because of the small particle range and therefore short tissue penetration.

Therefore, another radiolabelled somatostatin analogue, [^{90}Y-DOTA^0, Tyr^3]octreotide (^{90}Y-DOTATOC; OctreoTher$^®$) was developed. Using this compound, different phase-1 and phase-2 PRRT trials have been performed. Chinol et al. from the European Institute of Oncology (Milan, Italy) (3) described dosimetric and dose-finding studies with ^{90}Y-DOTATOC, with and without the administration of kidney-protecting agents. No major acute reactions were observed up to an administered dose of 150 mCi per cycle. Reversible grade 3 haematological toxicity was found in 43% of patients injected with 140 mCi, which was defined as the maximum tolerated dose per cycle. None of the patients developed acute or delayed kidney nephropathy, although follow-up was short. Partial and complete remissions (CRs) were reported by the same group in 28% of 87 patients with neuroendocrine tumors (4).

Waldherr et al. (University Hospital Basel, Switzerland) (5) reported different phase-2 studies in patients with neuroendocrine GEP tumors. Thirty-nine patients received four doses of ^{90}Y-DOTATOC, up to a total dose of 200 mCi/m^2, at intervals of approximately six weeks. Renal or haematological toxicity observed was $\leq$ grade 3 according to the National Cancer Institute grading criteria. Complete and PRs occurred in 23% of patients. Later, the same group compared these results to those in which a group of 36 patients were treated with two injections of 100 mCi/m^2, instead of four injections of 50 mCi/m^2, administered at an eight week interval (6). Complete and PRs were found in 34% of patients, versus 23% in the first study. It should be emphasized, however, that this was not a randomized trial comparing two dosing schemes.

Another study with ^{90}Y-DOTATOC (OctreoTher$^®$) is a multicenter phase-1 study which was performed in Rotterdam, Brussels, and Tampa, in which 60 patients received escalating doses up to 250 mCi/m^2, without reaching the maximum tolerated single dose (7). The cumulative radiation dose to kidneys was limited to 27 Gy. All received amino acids concomitant with ^{90}Y-DOTATOC for kidney protection. Three patients had dose-limiting toxicity: 1 liver toxicity grade 3, 1 thrombocytopenia grade 4, and 1 myelodysplastic syndrome. Four out of 54 (8%) patients who had received their maximum allowed dose had a PR, and seven (13%) had a minor response (25–50% tumor volume reduction).

Despite differences in protocols used, complete plus PRs in most of the different studies with ^{90}Y-DOTATOC are in the same range, between 10% and 25%, and therefore better than those obtained with [^{111}In-DTPA^0]octreotide.

Recently, it was reported that [DTPA^0,Tyr^3]octreotate, if compared with [DTPA^0,Tyr^3]octreotide, the difference being only that the C-terminal threoninol is replaced with threonine, shows an improved binding to somatostatin receptor positive tissues in animal experiments (8). Also, its DOTA-coupled counterpart, [DOTA^0,Tyr^3]octreotate, labelled with the beta and gamma emitting radionuclide ^{177}Lu, was reported very successful in terms of tumor regression and animal survival in a rat model (9). Reubi et al. (10) reported a nine-fold increase in affinity for the somatostatin receptor subtype 2 for [DOTA^0,Tyr^3]octreotate if compared with [DOTA^0,Tyr^3]octreotide, and a six to seven-fold increase in affinity for their Yttrium-loaded counterparts.

In a comparison in patients, we found that the uptake of radioactivity, expressed as percentage of the injected dose of [^{177}Lu-DOTA^0,Tyr^3]octreotate (^{177}Lu-octreotate), was comparable to that after [^{111}In-DTPA^0]octreotide for kidneys, spleen, and liver, but was 3- to 4-fold higher for four of five tumors (Fig 1) (11). Therefore, we concluded that ^{177}Lu-octreotate potentially represents an important improvement because of the higher absorbed doses that can be achieved to most tumors with about equal doses to potentially dose-limiting organs and because of the lower tissue penetration range of ^{177}Lu if compared with ^{90}Y, which may be especially important for small tumors.

The first treatment effects of ^{177}Lu-octreotate therapy were described in 35 patients with neuroendocrine GEP tumors, who had a follow-up of three to six months after receiving their final dose (12). Patients were treated with dosages of 100, 150, or 200 mCi ^{177}Lu-octreotate, up to a final cumulative dose of 600-800 mCi, with treatment intervals of six to nine weeks.

The effects of the therapy on tumor size were evaluable in 34 patients. Three months after the final administration, a CR was found in one patient (3%), PR in 12 (35%), stable disease (SD) in 14 (41%), and progressive disease (PD) in seven (21%), including three patients who died during the treatment period. Tumor response was positively correlated with a high uptake on the octreoscan, limited hepatic tumor mass, and high Karnofsky Performance Score. The side effects of treatment with ^{177}Lu-octreotate were few and mostly transient, with mild bone marrow depression as the most common finding.

In a more recent update of this treatment in 76 patients with GEP tumors (13), CR was found in one patient (1%), PR in 22 (29%), minor remission (MR) in nine (12%), SD in 30 (40%), and PD in 14 patients (18%) (Table 1). Six out of 32 patients who had initially SD or tumor regression after the therapy and were also evaluated after 12 months (mean 18 months from therapy start) became progressive; in the other 26 the tumor response was unchanged. Median time to progression was not reached at 25 months from therapy start.

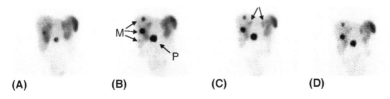

(A)   **(B)**   **(C)**   **(D)**

Figure 1 Anterior abdominal images in a patient with a neuroendocrine pancreatic tumor with liver metastases. (**A**) Octreoscan, 24 hours after injection of 6 mCi [^{111}In-DTPA]octreotide; (**B–D**) post-therapy scans 1, 3, and 10 days after injection of 200 mCi ^{177}Lu-octreotate. (**B**) Note the higher uptake in the primary tumor (P) and metastases (M) after ^{177}Lu-octreotate. (**C**) Also, the adrenals are visualized after ^{177}Lu-octreotate (*arrows*). Physiologic uptake in the liver, spleen, and kidneys is seen on all scans.

Table 1   Tumor Responses in 76 Patients, Three Months After the Final Administration of ^{177}Lu-octreotate. Six Patients with PD Died Before Reaching Their Intended Cumulative Dose

Tumor type	Response					
	Complete remission	Partial remission	Minor remission	Stable disease	Progress-ive disease	Total
Carcinoid		8 (22%)	4 (11%)	17 (47%)	7 (19%)	36
NE pancreas, nonfunction-ing	1 (5%)	4 (19%)	3 (14%)	10 (48%)	3 (14%)	21
NE unknown origin		5 (42%)	1 (8%)	3 (25%)	3 (25%)	12
Insulinoma					1 (100%)	1
Gastrinoma		5 (83%)	1 (17%)			6
Total	1 (1%)	22 (29%)	9 (12%)	30 (40%)	14 (18%)	76

Abbreviation: NE, neuroendocrine.

PERSPECTIVE

The treatment with radiolabelled somatostatin analogs is a promising new tool in the management of patients with inoperable or metastasized neuroendocrine tumors. The results that we obtained with ^{177}Lu-octreotate are very encouraging, yet a direct, randomized comparison with ^{90}Y-DOTATOC treatment is lacking. Also, the reported percentages of tumor remission after ^{90}Y-DOTATOC treatment vary. This may have several causes: 1.The administered doses and dosing schemes differ; some studies use dose-escalating schemes, whereas others use fixed doses; 2.There are several patient and tumor characteristics that determine treatment outcome, such as amount of uptake on the octreoscan, the estimated total tumor burden, and the extent of liver involvement. Therefore, differences in patient selection may play an important role in determining treatment outcome. For these reasons we planned a multicenter randomized trial comparing the effects of treatment with ^{90}Y-labelled somatostatin analogs with those of ^{177}Lu-octreotate. Because in animal experiments ^{90}Y-labelled somatostatin analogs are more effective for larger tumors, and ^{177}Lu-labelled somatostatin analogs are more effective for smaller tumors, but their combination was found to be most effective (14), a third treatment arm will consist of sequential ^{90}Y-labelled and ^{177}Lu-labelled somatostatin analogue treatment.

Apart from the combination of analogs labelled with different radio-isotopes, future directions to improve this therapy may also include efforts to upregulate the somatostatin receptor expression on the tumors, as well as studies to the effects of the use of radiosensitizers.

REFERENCES

1. Janson ET, Oberg K. Long-term management of the carcinoid syndrome. Treatment with octreotide alone and in combination with alpha-interferon. Acta Oncol 1993; 32:225–229.
2. Valkema R, de Jong M, Bakker WH, et al. Phase I study of peptide receptor radionuclide therapy with [^{111}In-DTPA^0]octreotide: the rotterdam experience. Semin Nucl Med 2002; 32:110–122.
3. Chinol M, Bodei L, Cremonesi M, Paganelli G. Receptor-mediated radiotherapy with Y-DOTA-DPhe-Tyr-octreotide: the experience of the European Institute of Oncology Group. Semin Nucl Med 2002; 32:141–147.
4. Paganelli G, Bodei L, Handkiewicz Junak D, et al. 90Y-DOTA-D-Phe1-Tyr3-octreotide in therapy of neuroendocrine malignancies. Biopolymers 2002; 66:393–398.
5. Waldherr C, Pless M, Maecke HR, et al. Tumor response and clinical benefit in neuroendocrine tumors after 7.4 GBq (90)Y-DOTATOC. J Nucl Med 2002; 43:617–620.
6. Waldherr C, Schumacher T, Maecke HR, et al. Does tumor response depend on the number of treatment sessions at constant injected dose using 90Yttrium-DOTATOC in neuroendocrine tumors? Eur J Nucl Med 2002; 29:S100.
7. Valkema R, Pauwels S, Kvols L, et al. Long-term follow-up of a phase 1 study of peptide receptor radionuclide therapy (PRRT) with [90Y-DOTA0,Tyr3]octreotide in patients with somatostatin receptor positive tumors. Eur J Nucl Med Mol Imaging 2003; 30:S232.
8. De Jong M, Breeman WA, Bakker WH, et al. Comparison of (111)Inlabeled somatostatin analogues for tumor scintigraphy and radionuclide therapy. Cancer Res 1998; 58:437–441.
9. Erion JL, Bugaj JE, Schmidt MA, Wilhelm RR, Srinivasan A. High radiotherapeutic efficacy of [Lu-177]-DOTA-Y(3)-octreotate in a rat tumor model. J Nucl Med 1999; 40:223.
10. Reubi JC, Schar JC, Waser B, et al. Affinity profiles for human somatostatin receptor subtypes SST1-SST5 of somatostatin radiotracers selected for scintigraphic and radiotherapeutic use. Eur J Nucl Med 2000; 27:273–282.
11. Kwekkeboom DJ, Bakker WH, Kooij PP, et al. [177Lu-DOTA0Tyr3]octreotate: comparison with [111In-DTPA0]octreotide in patients. Eur J Nucl Med 2001; 28:1319–1325.
12. Kwekkeboom DJ, Bakker WH, Kam BL, et al. Treatment of patients with gastro-entero-pancreatic (GEP) tumors with the novel radiolabelled somatostatin analogue [177Lu-DOTA^0,Tyr^3]octreotate. Eur J Nucl Med Mol Imaging 2003; 30:417–422.
13. Kwekkeboom DJ, Bakker WH, Teunissen JJM, Kooij PPM, Krenning EP. Treatment with Lu-177-DOTA-Tyr3-octreotate in patients with neuroendocrine tumors: interim results. Eur J Nucl Med Mol Imaging 2003; 30:S231.
14. De Jong M, Valkema R, Jamar F, et al. Somatostatin receptor-targeted radionuclide therapy of tumors: preclinical and clinical findings. Semin Nucl Med 2002; 32:133–140.

13

Radiation Dosimetry Methods for Therapy

Michael G. Stabin

Department of Radiology and Radiological Sciences,
Vanderbilt University, Nashville, Tennessee, U.S.A.

INTRODUCTION

A variety of therapeutic agents are under evaluation in nuclear medicine practice or clinical trials. The basic goal of radiation therapy (internal or external) is to ensure that enough radiation-absorbed dose is delivered to tumor without causing undesired effects in healthy tissues. Generally, patient-individualized dose calculations are applied in the optimization of this process with external beam therapy, but are not done for internal emitter therapy. Many physicians administer about the same activity to all patients, expecting that this will probably provide an effective dose to any existing tumors while not delivering a radiation dose that could cause deleterious side effects to normal organs (usually the most concern is with active bone marrow).

Many new therapeutic agents, particularly monoclonal antibodies, peptides, and other molecules for radioimmunotherapy (RIT), often have relatively low tumor-to-normal tissue absorbed dose ratios, and ideally should be administered using a patient-specific treatment planning strategy based on radiation-absorbed dose, in which activity administration is optimized to maximize treatment efficacy while minimizing the risk of toxicity to bone marrow and other normal tissues. The dose-limiting toxicity for these agents is usually myelosuppression (1–4), but not all patients' bone marrows are equally radiosensitive. Many RIT patients have compromised bone marrow due to marrow infiltration by tumor as well as by effects of prior chemotherapy or radiotherapy, so these patients' marrows may not be able to tolerate the radiation dose that a normal, previously untreated bone marrow could. It has been shown that the variability in tumor uptake and retention half-time among different patients may vary by factors of five or more (5,6). A "one-dose-fits-all" approach to radiation therapy with internal emitter treatments is not ideal (due to the narrow range between tumor ablation and bone marrow toxicity). In hyperthyroidism and thyroid cancer therapy, wide variations are observed in the methods used to calculate dose to patients (6). Application of activity without performing any dose calculations may result in more activity being given than is needed for some patients, causing the delivery of potentially unnecessary radiation. In RIT, the tendency is to cautiously underdose the patients, resulting in poor efficacy. RIT patients have usually failed other treatments, and may enter radiotherapy with compromised marrow due to these other treatments. Thus, their therapies should be optimized, taking into account individual parameters of radionuclide kinetics, bone marrow reserve, and sensitivity as much as is possible. Several authors have advocated a patient-specific approach to hyperthyroidism and thyroid cancer therapy as well, to provide an optimized therapeutic approach without the need for extensive imaging and measurement protocols (6,7).

If one were to approach the radiation oncologist or medical physicist in an external beam therapy program and suggest that all patients with a certain type of cancer should receive the exact same protocol (beam type, energy, beam exposure time, geometry, etc.), the idea would certainly be rejected as not being in the best interests of the patient. Instead, a patient-specific treatment plan would be implemented in which treatment times are varied to deliver the same radiation dose to all patients. Patient-specific calculations of doses delivered to tumors and normal tissues have been routine in external beam radiotherapy and brachytherapy for decades. The routine use of a fixed GBq/kg, GBq/m^2, or simply GBq, administration of radionuclides for therapy is equivalent to treating all patients in external beam radiotherapy with the same protocol. Varying the treatment time to result in equal absorbed dose for external beam radiotherapy is equivalent to accounting for the known variation in patients' uptake and retention half-time of activity of radionuclides to achieve equal tumor-absorbed dose for internal-emitter radiotherapy. It has been suggested that fixed activity-administration protocol designs provide little useful information about the variability among patients relative to the normal organ dose than can be tolerated without dose-limiting toxicity compared to radiation dose-driven protocols (8).

Given knowledge of the target dose needed to treat individual cancers, modern radiation oncology practice uses patient-specific administration approaches. However, at present, there are a number of problems impeding the acceptance of routine dosimetry calculations for therapy patients receiving internal emitters. The accuracy of the activity measurements and dose calculation models are perceived to be low. There is no uniformity of opinion among physicians prescribing internal-emitter therapy as to what radiation dose should be delivered to tumors of different types, sizes, and locations. The variability of individual patients' responses to similar levels of radiation dose is high, and the reasons for this are not well understood. These issues should be addressed, and patient-specific dose calculations should be applied in most forms of cancer therapy, especially in the use of the newer radionuclide therapies, particularly RIT. It remains to be seen if patient-specific treatment planning will improve cancer patient outcomes; this should be systematically evaluated. Nonetheless, RIT patients clearly will benefit from a patient-specific dose assessment which takes into account individual kinetics and physical characteristics, if tumor and marrow response parameters can be determined and applied.

INTERNAL DOSIMETRY METHODS

Concepts

A number of quantities have been studied for many years to relate radiation exposure to safety and risk evaluations. For exposure to internally deposited radionuclides, the concept of "exposure" (charge per unit mass of air) is not applicable, and we start with "absorbed dose," which is the energy deposited per unit mass of matter (with units of J/kg, 1 J/kg = 1 Gy) (9). Other quantities have been derived by various scientific and advisory bodies, for example the concepts of equivalent dose and effective dose, as defined by the international commission on radiological protection (ICRP) (10). Such quantities are not applicable in radiation therapy, however, and we remain with the concept of absorbed dose to relate a quantity of radiation exposure to risk (to normal tissues) and desired effect (to tumor tissue). Absorbed dose is very easy to understand, and is just what it appears, the total energy absorbed in a unit quantity of tissue divided by the mass of that tissue. In therapeutic studies, the response of tissues is mostly proportional to absorbed dose. It is interesting that significant nonlinearities between dose and effect exist at lower doses, necessitating the definition of other quantities, such as Relative Biological Effectiveness, RBE, weighting factors (radiation weighting factors, tissue weighting factors), etc. This suggests that energy absorbed per unit mass does not predict response at all levels, and some other factors must be at work. We know that damage to cells is due primarily to indirect effects of radiation (formation of free radicals in water, with their diffusion, and subsequent interaction with cellular components, mostly DNA), and to some degree to direct effects (direct damage to DNA from radiation interaction) (11). We also know that different tissues and different individuals have different abilities to respond to and repair this damage. Thus, linking of physical quantities like absorbed dose must be made to radiobiological quantities to completely understand and be able to predict effects in a system. At present, our understanding of how to do this is limited, but it is evolving. Two recent papers showed significant improvements in correlations between calculated radiation dose and patients' biological response to the radiation when patient-specific physical and biological factors were considered (12,13).

Equations

Internal dose can be calculated by the following simple equation (14):

$$D = N \times DF \tag{1}$$

where D=absorbed dose in a target organ (Gy), N is the number of nuclear transitions that occur in source region S, and DF is a "dose factor." The factor DF contains a number of components; basically it depends on combining decay data with absorbed fractions (AFs), which are derived generally using Monte Carlo simulation of radiation transport in models of the body and its internal structures (organs, tumors, etc.):

$$DF = \frac{k \sum_i n_i E_i \phi_i}{m} \tag{2}$$

n_i = the number of radiations with energy E_i emitted per nuclear transition, E_i = the energy per radiation (MeV), ϕ = the absorbed fraction (AF, fraction of radiation energy emitted in a source that is absorbed in the target), m = the mass of target region (g or kg), and k = a proportionality constant (Gy kg/MBq sec MeV).

As written, equation 1 gives only the dose from one source region to one target region, but it can be generalized easily to multiple source and target regions.

When the components of the various published internal dose calculational schemes are carefully studied, they can all be reduced to this single generic equation. For example, the dose equation used by the Medical Internal Radiation Dose (MIRD) Committee of the Society of Nuclear Medicine is (15):

$$D = \tilde{A} \cdot S = A_0 \cdot \tau \cdot S \tag{3}$$

where $\tilde{A}$=cumulated activity (sum of all nuclear transitions that occurred) in a source organ (MBq-s), τ is the residence time, which is simply equal to $\tilde{A}/A_0$, the cumulated activity divided by the patient's administered activity (A_0), and, S is given by:

$$S = \frac{k \sum_i n_i E_i \phi_i}{m} \tag{4}$$

The MIRD concept of "residence time" (15) has often caused confusion, because of its apparent units of time (even though it really expresses the number of nuclear transitions that occur in a source region) and because of the use of this term to represent the "mean life" of atoms in biological or engineering applications.

In the ICRP system of radiation protection for workers (10), the dose equation is:

$$H = U_S \cdot SEE \tag{5}$$

Here, H is the dose equivalent (the absorbed dose, D multiplied by a radiation weighting factor w_R, formerly known as a quality factor, Q), U_S is the number of nuclear transitions that occur in source region S, and SEE is:

$$SEE = \frac{k \sum_i n_i E_i \phi_i w_{R_i}}{m} \tag{6}$$

Available Models

Current technology for estimating the AF (ϕ) in the above equations rests on the use of anthropomorphic phantoms. The first well defined phantom was the Fisher/Snyder phantom (16). This phantom used a combination of geometric shapes—spheres, cylinders, cones, etc.,—to create a reasonably anatomically accurate representation of the body, with the organ masses based on data provided in the ICRP report on Reference Man (17). This report provided various anatomical data assumed to represent the average working adult male in the Western hemisphere. Although this was most often applied to adult males, this phantom also contained regions representing organs specific to the adult female. This phantom was used with Monte Carlo computer programs which simulated the creation and transport of photons through these various structures in the body. Using this phantom and the equations defined above, radiation doses could be calculated for adults based on activity residing in any organ and irradiating any other organ. AFs at discrete photon energies were calculated and published by the MIRD Committee (18). In addition, S values (defined above), were calculated for 20 source and target regions in the phantom for over 100 radionuclides (19).

Cristy and Eckerman (20) then developed a series of phantoms permitting dose calculations for different individuals of different size and age. Six phantoms were developed, which were assumed to represent children and adults of both genders. AFs for photons at discrete energies were published for these phantoms, which contained approximately 25 source and target regions. Tables of S values were made available in the MIRDOSE computer software (21), and were later published for over 800 radionuclides by Stabin and Siegel (14). Stabin et al. (22) developed phantoms for the nonpregnant adult female and the adult female at three stages of pregnancy. These phantoms attempted to model the changes to the uterus, intestines, bladder, and other organs that occur during pregnancy, and included specific models for the fetus, fetal soft tissue, fetal skeleton, and placenta. S values for these phantoms were also made available through the MIRDOSE software and in the recent Stabin and Siegel article (14).

Input Data Needed

If a standardized model such as was discussed in the previous section is used, the main input data needed for evaluation of radiation dose are the biokinetic data that characterize the distribution and retention of the radiopharmaceutical throughout the biological system. Enough data need to be obtained to model all phases of uptake and excretion. Some knowledge of the expected biokinetics is needed to plan and design an appropriate study to collect the necessary data. Normally, initial understanding is gained through studies involving experimental animals. Even here, however, one needs to know approximately how the compound will be taken up and cleared from the various organs and the whole body, to collect samples at the appropriate times. Most therapeutic agents have a relatively fast phase of organ uptake and initial system clearance, followed by more general systemic removal that lasts for many days. So a typical sampling scheme (whether involving animal sacrifice and organ counting/autoradiography or in vivo imaging using small animal imaging techniques) is to collect several samples in the first hours after administration (for example at 1, 4, 10, and 24 hours), then about once or twice a day for a few days to two weeks. In human studies, similar approaches are used, but the balancing of logistic and cost issues against the desire for more data often require some compromises.

Image Quantification Techniques—Planar, Single Photon Emission Computed Tomography

In human studies, all data are obtained from quantitative imaging. Specific quantification techniques have been summarized by many authors, and were discussed in overview in a document published by the MIRD Committee in 1999 (23). As noted in the previous section, the timing of these studies must be carefully planned to observe all phases of uptake and clearance. An absolute minimum of two data points per phase of uptake or clearance is needed to characterize the kinetics of this phase; more data points are naturally always desirable, given logistic and cost constraints.

With the use of planar data, the most accepted technique is to obtain images from the posterior and anterior projections, then correct the projected data in each region of interest for attenuation and scatter. A number of approaches have been used to address both issues. The most popular technique for attenuation correction involves the use of a Co-57 (or other) projection source imaged with and without the patient in the view, with the attenuation coefficient for the system having been characterized in advance (23). For scatter correction, the two- or three-energy window method proposed by Ogawa et al. (24) is widely accepted, and applied where gamma camera software permits simultaneous acquisition in multiple energy windows.

Quantitative imaging using single photon emission computed tomography (SPECT) methods is considerably more complex, and is not widely practiced for the purposes of calculating internal doses. Quantitative imaging is used widely for cardiac imaging and evaluation and, similarly, for positron emission tomography

(PET) evaluations of cardiac (25) and functional neuroimaging (26), among other applications. An excellent overview of the applications and limitations of this technology was given recently by King (27).

Treatment of Kinetic Data

Once a satisfactory set of kinetic data is obtained and quantified, the integral of the time-activity curve for each source organ may be obtained by:

1. *Direct integration*: directly integrating under the actual measured values by a number of methods. This does not give very much information about your system, but it does allow you to calculate τ rather easily. The most common method used is the Trapezoidal Method, simply approximating the area by a series of trapezoids.

2. *Use of a least squares analysis*: fit curves of a given shape to the data, which can be analytically integrated. The most common approach is to attempt to characterize a set of data by a series of exponential terms, as many systems are well represented by this form, and exponential terms are easy to integrate. In general, the approach is to minimize the sum of the squared distance of the data points from the fitted curve. The curve will have the form:

$$A(t) = a_1 e^{-b_1 t} + a_2 e^{-b_2 t} + \cdots$$

The method looks at the squared difference between each point and the solution of the fitted curve at that point, and minimizes this quantity by taking the partial derivative of this expression with respect to each of the unknowns a_i and b_i and setting it equal to zero. Once the ideal estimates of a_i and b_i are obtained, the integral of $A(t)$ from zero to infinity is simply:

$$\int_0^\infty A(t)\,dt = \frac{a_1}{b_1} + \frac{a_2}{b_2} + \ldots$$

If the coefficients a_i are in units of activity, this integral represents cumulated activity (the units of the b_i are time^{-1}).

3. *Use of compartmental models*: if one either knows quite a bit about the biological system under investigation or you would like to know in greater detail how this system is working, one can describe the system as a group of compartments linked through transfer rate coefficients. Solving for $\tilde{A}$ of the various compartments involves solving a system of coupled differential equations describing transfer of the tracer between compartments and elimination from the system. The solution to the time activity curve for each compartment will usually be a sum of

exponentials, but not obtained by least squares fitting each compartment separately, but by varying the transfer rate coefficients between compartments until the data are well fit by the model. The Simulation Analysis and Modeling (SAAM) code is widely applied for this purpose (28).

Dose Calculations

Once suitable time-integrals are available, and DFs from a reasonably representative standardized model are selected, the process of calculating the absorbed doses to the various organs in the body is a very straightforward although quite tedious task, involving the repetitive application of equation 1 above, for each source and target region in the system. A correction is needed, if activity in the remainder of the body is calculated, for use with (the available) DFs for "total body," as described by Cloutier et al. (29). These calculations can be done by hand (taking perhaps hours); of course, most prefer a computerized approach, using individually tailored mathematical spreadsheets or computer programs, as are discussed below.

Patient-Specific Modifications

Some patient-specific modifications to dose calculations made with standardized anthropomorphic phantoms are possible, and are certainly indicated in therapy applications. One *can* make the dose estimates calculated with standardized anthropomorphic phantoms more patient-specific through mass-based adjustments to the organ self doses (30):

1. Specific AFs for electrons and alphas scale linearly with mass $[\Phi' = \Phi (m'/m)]$.
2. AFs for photons scale with mass to the 1/3 power $[\phi' = \phi (m'/m)^{1/3}]$.

Cross-irradiation AFs do not change appreciably with changes in organ mass, in most cases, so the adjustments to organ self-dose are usually all that are needed. One generally *cannot* adequately account for patient-specific differences in organ geometry, account for patient-specific marrow characteristics, or calculate dose distributions within organs. Patient-specific considerations should be made as much as is possible. Use of a uniform activity or activity per kg or m^2 approach to radiation therapy with internal emitter treatments is not likely to be adequate (due to the narrow range between tumor ablation and bone marrow toxicity). Individual patients not only have significantly different uptake and retention half-times of activity of the radioactive agent, but also have significantly different physical characteristics and radiosensitivities. Many cancer patients have failed other treatments, and may enter radiotherapy with compromised marrow due to their previous treatments. Thus, their therapies should be optimized, taking into account effects of previous therapy as well as the other measured parameters as much as is possible.

RESOURCES FOR PERFORMING CALCULATIONS

Literature Resources

MIRD Literature—The MIRD Pamphlets

A MIRD Pamphlet is a document which generally contains material needed to implement the MIRD schema for internal dose calculations, including equations, data, methods, etc. Several of the MIRD Pamphlets were issued and then revised and reissued; therefore, some of the MIRD Pamphlet titles contain the word 'revised'. Most of the important MIRD Pamphlets are shown below (Table 1). MIRD 1, revised has been superceded by the MIRD Primer (see books, below). MIRD 5 and 5, revised are not much in use, as the Cristy/Eckerman (20) phantom series is widely used. MIRD Pamphlets 3 and 8 are also not much in use, as new AFs for spheres were calculated (31), and problems with the MIRD values were pointed out.

MIRD Literature—The MIRD Dose Estimate Reports

The MIRD Dose Estimate Reports contain radiation dosimetry for particular radiopharmaceuticals, along with the kinetic model employed. They were published as separate articles in the Journal of Nuclear Medicine (as are the reports after number 12) and are mostly quite similar. The first table in the article is usually a summary of the dose estimates for all significant organs for unit administrations of the pharmaceutical. Later tables and figures show some of the developmental material used to calculate the dose estimates. All of these estimates contain some useful information, except perhaps in cases in which the pharmaceutical is no longer in use. The kinetic models are presented in various ways which must be studied individually (Table 2).

The MIRD Literature—MIRD Books

The MIRD Committee has published a number of books as well:

1. The MIRD Primer (15), described above
2. A set of decay data was published in 1989 (32), which replaced old MIRD compendia of decay data (MIRD pamphlets 4, 6, and 10). These data are, however, also now somewhat dated
3. In 1998, a tabulation of S values was published for cellular sources and targets, with activity being on the surface of a cell (of various dimensions), in the cytoplasm, or uniformly throughout the entire cell, with the target being the whole cell or the nucleus (33).

Table 1 Selected Medical Internal Radiation Dose Pamphlets

Pamphlet	Publication and date	Main information	Comments
1, 1 revised	1968, 1976	Discussion of MIRD internal dose technique	Superceded by the MIRD primer (1988)
3	1968	Photon absorbed fractions for small objects	Superceded by J Nucl Med 41:149–160, 2000
5, 5 revised	1969, 1978	Description of anthropomorphic phantom representing reference man, photon absorbed fractions for many organs	Superceded by availability of Cristy/ Eckerman phantom series (1987)
7	1971	Dose distribution around point sources, electron, beta emitters	Good data, difficult to use; use of Monte Carlo codes like MCNP, EGS is generally preferred
8	1971	Photon absorbed fractions for small objects	Same as Pamphlet 3, smaller objects, also superceded by J Nucl Med 41:149–160, 2000
11	1975	S-values for many nuclides	Newer S values available, see *RADAR dose factor page*
12	1977	Discussion of kinetic models for internal dosimetry	
13	1981	Description of model of the heart, photon absorbed fractions	
14, 14 revised	1992, 1999	Dynamic urinary bladder for absorbed dose calculations	Software to be made available, see *RADAR software page*
15	1996	Description of model for the brain, photon absorbed fractions	
16	1999	Outline of best practices and methods for collecting and analyzing kinetic data	Widely cited, useful document
17	1999	S values for voxel sources	
18	2001	Administered activity for xenon studies	
19	2003	Multipart kidney model with absorbed fractions	

Abbreviations: MIRD, medical internal radiation dose; RADAR, radiation dose assessment resource.

Table 2 Selected Medical Internal Radiation Dose Estimate Reports

Dose estimate report number	Publication reference	Compound or pharmaceutical studied
1	J Nucl Med 14:49–50,1973	Se-75-L-selenomethionine
2	J Nucl Med 14:755–756,1973	Ga-66-, Ga-67-, Ga-68-, and Ga-72-Citrate
3	J Nucl Med 16:108A–108B,1975	Tc-99m-sulfur colloid in various liver conditions
4	J Nucl Med 16:173–174, 1975	Au-198-colloidal gold in various liver conditions
5	J Nucl Med 16:857–860,1975	I-123, I-124, I-125, I-126, I-130,I-131, and I-132 as sodium iodide
6	J Nucl Med 16:1095–1098,1975	Hg-197- and Hg-203-labeled chlormerodrin
7	J Nucl Med 16:1214–1217,1975	I-123, I-124, I-126, I-130, and I-131 as sodium rose bengal
8	J Nucl Med 17:74–77,1976	Tc-99m as sodium pertechnetate
9	J Nucl Med 21:459–465, 1980	Radioxenons in lung imaging
10	J Nucl Med 23:915–917,1982	Albumin microspheres labeled with tc-99m
11	J Nucl Med 24:339–348,1983	Fe-52, Fe-55, and Fe-59 used to study ferrokinetics
12	J Nucl Med 25:503–505,1984	Tc-99m Diethylenetriamine pentaacetic acid
13	J Nucl Med 30:1117–1122, 1989	Tc-99m labeled bone imaging agents
14	J Nucl Med 31:378–380, 1990	Tc-99m labeled red blood cells
15	J Nucl Med 33:777–780, 1992	Radioindium-lableled autologous platelets
16	J Nucl Med 33:1717–1719, 1992	Tc-99m diethylenetriamine pentaacetic acid aerosol
17	J Nucl Med 34:1382–1384, 1993	Inhaled Kr-81m Gas in lung imaging
18	J Nucl Med 39:671–676, 1998	Indium 111 B72.3 (IgG antibody to ovarian and colorectal cancer)

Software and Internet Resources

The MIRDOSE and Organ Level Internal Dose Assessment Software

The MIRDOSE code series began with a Tektronix PC-based MIRDOSE 1 code (34), then migrated to the MIRDOSE 2 code in the PC-DOS environment, and

MIRDOSE 3 and 3.1 in the PC-Windows environment (21). MIRDOSE has been widely used in the nuclear medicine community and cited in the literature and in presentations at scientific meetings as the basis for presented internal dose estimates. The MIRDOSE 2 and 3 codes implemented the use of whole body MIRD stylized mathematical phantoms representing adult males and females, children, and pregnant women. The codes automated the calculation of internal dose for a large number (>200) radiopharmaceuticals in these phantoms, the rapid comparison of calculations for different cases, examination of dose contributions to different organs, and regional marrow dose calculations. The code was also widely used as a tool for teaching internal dosimetry in universities and professional training centers. Sample input and output screens from the code are shown in Figure 1. The top panel in Figure 1 illustrates a user interface where information such as the type of radionuclide and element, age, sex, and physiological parameters are specified. The bottom panel in Figure 1 illustrates the output of the total dose for a reference adult male who is injected with Y-90. The output also include information on doses for various organs that are clinically important. MIRDOSE is being updated to a new generation code, named OLINDA (Organ Level INternal Dose Assessment) (35), employing the Java programming language and the Java Development Kit environment. The entire code was rewritten, but all of the basic functions of the MIRDOSE code were retained, and others were extended. More individual organ phantoms were included, the number of radionuclides was significantly increased (to over 800, including many alpha emitters), and the ability to perform minor patient-specific adjustments to doses reported for the standard phantoms was made available. A sample output screen from the OLINDA code, and a screen involving the implementation of patient-specific organ mass adjustments are shown in Figure 2.

The Radiation Dose Assessment Resource System

In an effort to provide data needed for dose calculations to the user community rapidly and in electronic form, the RAdiation Dose Assessment Resource (RADAR) group was formed (36). The group maintains an internet web site (current address www.doseinfo-radar.com) where information on internal and external dose assessment is provided; most data are available directly from the site for immediate download. The last publication of dose factors for radionuclides of interest in nuclear medicine in this format from the MIRD Committee was provided in 1975 (19). Tables of S values (rem/μCi-day) were also published as an ORNL document (37), and selected SEE values were presented in ICRP Publication 30 (38). Dose factors, principally for nuclides of interest in nuclear medicine, were made available with the distribution of the MIRDOSE software (21), but the factors themselves were never published.

Publication of the technical basis for these factors is important to users. With the advent of "electronic publishing" approaches, it is possible for the

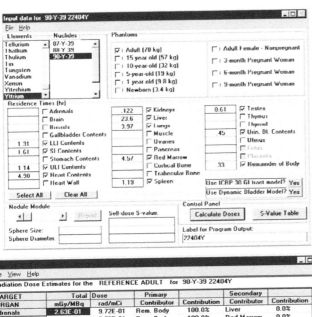

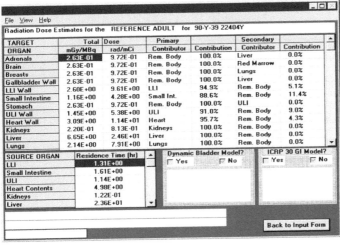

Figure 1 Sample input (*top*) and output (*bottom*) screens from the MIRDOSE 3.1 software.

voluminous data tables to be distributed through peer reviewed journals, with the technical basis for the data being published in a few pages of journal text. RADAR has employed this method in a number of publications (39,14), to document the basis for these dose factors and facilitate their distribution to users through an electronic format.

PROGRESS IN 3D DOSIMETRY AND TREATMENT PLANNING

Several of the efforts to use image data to perform dose calculations, as described above, include the 3D-ID code from the Memorial Sloan-Kettering Cancer

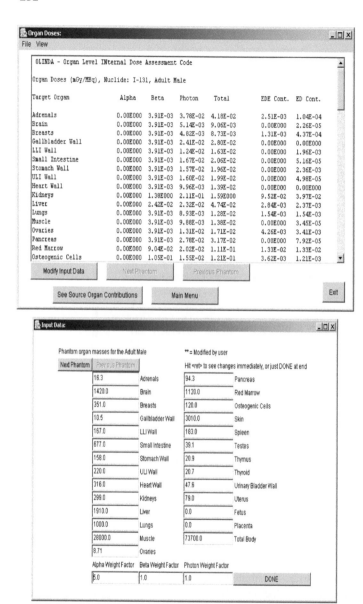

Figure 2   Sample output screens from the OLINDA software.

Center (40), the SIMDOS code from the University of Lund (41), the RTDS code
at the City of Hope Medical Center (42), the MABDose computer code (43), and
the DOSE3D code (44). The code with the most clinical experience to date is the
3D-ID code. These codes either rely on the standard geometrical phantoms

(MABDose and DOSE3D) or patient-specific voxel phantom data (3DID and SIMDOS) and usually employ in-house written routines to perform photon transport. Neither has a particularly robust and well supported electron transport code, such as is available in EGS or MCNP. The PENELOPE code (PENetration and Energy Loss of Positrons and Electrons) (45) performs Monte Carlo simulation of electron-photon showers in any kind of material, treats radiation transport across a broad energy range, and generates electron-photon showers in complex material structures consisting of any number of distinct homogeneous regions (bodies) with different compositions.

A common approach used in modeling is to assume that electron energy is absorbed wherever the electron is first produced. The development and support of electron transport methods is quite complex, as evidenced by ongoing intensive efforts by both the EGS4 (46) and MCNP (47) computer code working groups. It is not reasonable to expect in-house written codes to deal effectively with electron transport. In areas of highly nonuniform activity distribution, such as an organ with multiple tumors evidencing enhanced uptake of an antibody, explicit transport of both photons and electrons is needed to characterize dose distributions adequately.

Investigators at Vanderbilt University have already demonstrated the capability for performing radiation transport in voxel phantoms with the MCNP Monte Carlo radiation transport code for internal sources (48,49) in the voxel phantom provided by the group at Yale (50), and Investigators at Rensselaer Polytechnic Institute have demonstrated the capability using the EGS code for external sources (51) in the VIP man voxel phantom (52). Jones reported work performed at the NRPB, U.K. on an adult male model called NORMAN using MR images of 2-mm$\times$2-mm resolution and 10-mm slice thickness (53). Their model was used to estimate organ doses from external photon sources over a range of energies and irradiation geometries. When comparing their calculations to those which used a MIRD-type stylized model, differences in organ doses were found to range from a few percent to over 100% at photon energies between 10 and 100 keV. Petoussie-Henss et al. reported a family of tomographic models developed from CT images of 2-mm$\times$2-mm resolution and 8-mm slice thickness (54). Dose coefficients from external irradiation with these phantoms were substantially different than values derived using the MIRD phantom, suggesting to these authors that the MIRD models do not represent well a large proportion of the population.

RELATING OBSERVED DOSES TO BIOLOGICAL EFFECTS

Knowledge Gained from External Therapy

The goal of all forms of radiation therapy against cancer is to give lethal doses of ionizing radiation to malignant cells while not exceeding the radiation tolerance of involved normal tissues. Knowledge of the tolerance of normal tissues to radiation is thus essential to the successful design of therapy. Understanding of these tolerances has grown over the years since radiation therapy has become routine, from experience with many patients and sharing of data. A number of standard toxicity scoring systems have been developed, including those of the National Cancer Institute (NCI), Southwestern Oncology Group, Radiation Therapy Oncology Group (RTOG), and World Health Organization (55). In these systems, severity of effects is separated into categories, or "grades," with scores ranging from 0 to 4 or 5, with higher grades implying more severe toxicity, even to the point of mortality. For hematological parameters, grades are generally associated with numerical values of the levels of various elements in peripheral blood (platelets, lymphocytes, etc.), whereas for organs the grades are established by less objective, phenomenological observations (inflammation, degradation of function, ulceration, etc.). It is important to remember that criteria for grading may be quite circumstance-dependent, e.g., the definition of "normal" blood levels in cancer patients (and thus the changes that suggest that a particular grade of toxicity is indicated) may vary from that for normal healthy adults. Some scales, e.g., the RTOG, use different criteria for acute (defined as up to 90 days post-treatment) versus late toxicity. Quality of Life indicators may also be employed in clinical trials and other evaluations, including measures such as pain, use of analgesics, constipation, mood, fatigue, and other measures of performance status, e.g., physical activity.

New radiolabeled agents under investigation for possible use in treatment of cancer are evaluated in clinical trials in which safety and efficacy are studied carefully. Safety concerns include possible toxicity associated with radiation exposure of healthy tissues in the body. Generally, dosages thought to be useful against the disease are given in graded steps, with careful observation of deleterious side effects. If a drug can be shown to have good efficacy while resulting in low, manageable rates of occurrence of normal tissue toxicity, it is likely to be approved for more widespread use. Patient cohort size varies, as do the definitions of maximum tolerable doses (MTDs), but generally at least five patients must be studied in Phase I trials, and the MTD is generally defined as the dose that results in moderate to severe toxicity in the majority of this cohort. Escalation of administered dosages (and thus radiation doses) is generally accomplished in fixed steps of 20-25%, while maintaining vigilance over undesired side effects of the treatment. In Phase II and III trials, more patients are evaluated and doses lower than MTDs are given, with an eye on efficacy and clinical feasibility. The use of MTD as the target dose is open to some debate as there are circumstances in which different effects are induced at high doses that may block the beneficial effects observed at lower doses.

Organ tolerance data for external beam irradiation has been derived generally using treatment plans which deliver doses at high dose rates (HDR), perhaps 2 Gy in a single fraction at dose rates of around 1 Gy/min, with five fractions received per week for up to eight weeks. Thus the actual dose rates for a single treatment are high, but 24 hours elapse between most fractions, with

72 hours between some. When radiation is delivered using radionuclides, the dose is delivered in a continuous but constantly decaying fashion over periods of days to weeks, depending on the effective half-life of the radiopharmaceutical in the tumor or organ. The dose rates experienced will be generally lower, but there are no time periods when radiation dose is not being received. Thus the relationship to be expected between known organ tolerances for fractionated HDR external beam therapy and dose from continuous, LDR internal sources is not well established. In addition, profound differences may exist among radionuclides with respect to their radiotoxicity.

From both several decades of widely published data and from the multi-year focused effort funded by the NCI in the late 1980's, tolerances to external beam fractionated radiation for a number of normal tissues in the human have been well documented. Data are expressed in terms of NTCPs of 5/5 and 50/5 (i.e., a 5% or 50% complication probability in five years following exposure) for 1/3, 2/3, or 3/3 of an organ or tissue being irradiated (56). By contrast, tolerance doses for radionuclides are only available from a relatively small number of patients. A recent overview article by Meredith (57), summarizes current knowledge in this area.

Relation of External Dose to Internal Dose

In her paper, Dr. Meredith points out several problems with the interpretation of these data, namely that (1) the internal dose data are generally not as accurate as external dose data, as they do not as carefully account for lack of radionuclide homogeneity within the tissues, tissue density changes which may have affected the image quantification, and other factors, (2) tracer studies used to establish the biokinetics (and thus the dosimetry) may have different biokinetic patterns than when the full therapeutic dose is given, as has been documented in several studies, and (3) lack of uniformity of reporting of internal dose results, depending on which image quantification methods, computer programs, dose conversion factors, etc. were used. Interpretation of the findings is difficult due to the complexities in the format of the reported results as well. Nonetheless, the data may suggest that a higher tolerance has been observed for internally administered radionuclides, implying that the low dose rate effects cause a lower tissue response given the same level of absorbed dose (Gy). It is also, however, reasonable to expect that this effect will vary considerably with differences in radiopharmaceutical effective half-time in the tissue. Short-lived agents will deliver their dose in a shorter time, thus more approximating the dose rates of external beam radiation, while longer-lived agents, whose dose is delivered over many days to weeks, will deliver the dose to the tissues at a considerably lower dose rate especially at later times.

Bone marrow toxicity is the major dose-limiting factor in RIT, but there is no consensus on how to calculate that dose accurately, or of individual patients' ability to tolerate the planned therapy (58–65). Experience with external beam therapy has shown that there is a narrow margin between the delivered dose that kills a tumor and that which causes serious injury to the patient. Given that with modern methods the dose from external beam treatments is accurately known, the remaining major issues are tumor sensitivity and patient tolerance. In nuclear medicine, in contrast to beam radiotherapy, marrow-absorbed dose is not accurately evaluated, even when a treatment planning dosimetry study is performed (66). Both external beam and internal emitter therapy share the same uncertainty regarding predicted patient tolerance. Another problem is that nuclear medicine physicians, in general, have less experience in the therapy regime and typically undertreat patients in order to minimize the risk of even low-grade toxicity. If treatment of bone cancer with radioisotopes and RIT are to become a primary means of treating cancer patients, we need better ways of determining the amount of activity to be administered to individual patients, which is based on dose needed to treat the tumor and patient tolerance (67).

Hepatotoxicity with labeled ^{90}Y labeled microspheres was suggested to be lower than would have been expected from knowledge of dose-related toxicity from external sources of radiation (68). Behr et al. have extensively studied radiation nephrotoxicity following therapy with radiopeptides and antibody fragments, including the development of methods to prevent these side effects in pre-clinical as well as clinical settings (69–71). In a recent editorial (70) they point out that "…no maximum tolerated renal dose (MTD) is known for internal emitters. The assumption of similarity between external beam irradiation (doses ~20–25 Gy may cause nephrotoxicity in 1–5% of patients) …and internal emitter tissue tolerance doses may be a conservative and thus a safe one, but it is not supported by any experimental or clinical evidence" and that "…dose rate, penetration range and heterogeneity of microdosimetry differences suggest higher MTDs for internal emitters than for external beam radiation." Behr et al. (72) have suggested that the nephrotoxic potential of Auger electron emitters (such as ^{111}In, ^{67}Ga, or ^{140}Nd) is much lower than that of of ^{177}Lu labeled peptides. They suggest that perhaps as a consequence of their short path length, they selectively irradiate the tubular cells, thereby sparing the much more radiosensitive glomeruli. Auger electron radiation has demonstrated in some preclinical trials higher anti-tumor effects when the radionuclide is internalized into the tumor cells, as is the case for most peptide type radiopharmaceuticals. Auger electron emitters such as ^{195m}Pt may prove to be more effective than traditional beta emitters in therapy (73,74).

REFERENCES

1. Larson SM, Carrasquillo JA, McGuffin RW, et al. Preliminary clinical experience using an I-131 labeled, murine fab against a high molecular weight antigen of human melanoma. Radiology 1985; 155:487–492.

2. Kaminski MS, Zasadny KR, Francis IR, et al. Radioimmunotherapy of B-cell lymphoma with [131I]anti-B1 (anti-CD20) antibody. N Engl J Med 1993; 329:459–465.

3. Press OW, Eary JF, Applebaum FR, Bernstein ID. Radiolabeled antibody therapy of lymphomas. In: DeVita VT, Hellmam S, Rosenberg SA eds. Biologic Therapy of Cancer. Philadelphia, PA: J.B. Lippincott, 1994:1–13.

4. Siegel JA, Wessels BW, Watson EE, et al. Bone marrow dosimetry and toxicity for radioimmunotherapy. Antibody Immunoconjugates Radiopharm 1990; 3:213–233.

5. Sisson JC, Shulkin BL, Lawson S. Increasing efficacy and safety of treatments of patients with well-differentiated thyroid carcinoma by measuring body retentions of 131I. J Nucl Med 2003; 44:898–903.

6. Jonsson H, Mattsson S. Excess radiation absorbed doses from non-optimised radioiodine treatment of hyperthyroidism. Radiat Prot Dosimetry 2004; 108:107–114.

7. Traino AC, Di Martino F, Lazzeri M, Stabin MG. Study of the correlation between administered activity and radiation committed dose to the thyroid in 131I therapy of Graves' disease. Radiat Prot Dosimetry 2001; 95:117–124.

8. DeNardo SJ. Tumor-targeted radionuclide therapy: trial design driven by patient dosimetry. J Nucl Med 2000; 41:104–106.

9. International Commission of Radiation Units and Measurements, ICRU Report 33, Radiation Quantities, and Units, ICRU 33. Washington, DC: International Commission on Radiation Units and Measurements 1980.

10. International Commission on Radiological Protection. 1990 Recommendations of the International Commission on Radiological Protection. ICRP Publication 60. New York: Pergamon Press, 1991.

11. Hall EJ. Radiobiology for the Radiologist. 5th ed. Philadephia, PA: Lippincott Williams & Wilkins, 2000.

12. Shen S, Meredith RF, Duan J, et al. Improved prediction of myelotoxicity using a patient-specific imaging dose estimate for non-marrow-targeting 90Y-antibody therapy. J Nucl Med 2002; 43:1245–1253.

13. Siegel JA, Yeldell D, Goldenberg DM, et al. Red marrow radiation dose adjustment using plasma FLT3-1 cytokine levels: improved correlations between hematologic toxicity and bone marrow dose for radioimmunotherapy patients. J Nucl Med 2003; 44:67–76.

14. Stabin MG, Siegel JA. Physical models and dose factors for use in internal dose assessment. Health Phys 2003; 85:294–310.

15. Loevinger R, Budinger T, Watson E. MIRD primer for absorbed dose calculations. Soc Nucl Med 1988.

16. Snyder W, Ford M, Warner G, Watson, S. A tabulation of dose equivalent per microcurie-day for source and target organs of an adult for various radionuclides. ORNL-5000. Oak Ridge, TN: Oak Ridge National Laboratory, 1975.

17. International Commission on Radiological Protection: Report of the Task Group on Reference Man. ICRP Publication 23 New York: Pergamon Press, 1975.

18. Snyder W, Ford M, Warner G. MIRD Pamphlet No 5, revised—estimates of specific absorbed fractions for photon sources uniformly distributed in various organs of a heterogeneous phantom. New York: Society of Nuclear Medicine, 1978.

19. Snyder WS, Ford MR, Warner GG, Warner SB. MIRD Pamphlet No. 11—"S" absorbed dose per unit cumulated activity for selected radionuclides and organs. New York: Society of Nuclear Medicine, 1975.

20. Cristy M, Eckerman KF, Specific Absorbed Fractions of Energy at Various Ages from Internal Photon Sources. ORNL/TM-8381. Oak Ridge, TN: Oak Ridge National Laboratory, 1987.

21. Stabin MG. MIRDOSE: personal computer software for internal dose assessment in nuclear medicine. J Nucl Med 1996; 37:538–546.

22. Stabin M, Watson E, Cristy M, et al. Mathematical models and specific absorbed fractions of photon energy in the nonpregnant adult female and at the end of each trimester of pregnancy. ORNL Report ORNL/TM-12907. Oak Ridge, TN: Oak Ridge National Laboratory, 1995.

23. Siegel J, Thomas S, Stubbs J, et al. MIRD pamphlet no 16—techniques for quantitative radiopharmaceutical biodistribution data acquisition and analysis for use in human radiation dose estimates. J Nucl Med 1999; 40:S37–S61.

24. Ogawa K, Harata Y, Ichihara T, Kubo A, Hashimoto A. A practical method for position-dependent compton-scatter correction in single photon emission CT. IEEE Trans Med Imag 1991; 10:408.

25. Keng FY. Clinical applications of positron emission tomography in cardiology: a review. Ann Acad Med Singapore 2004; 33:175–182.

26. Sadek JR, Hammeke TA. Functional neuroimaging in neurology and psychiatry. CNS Spectr 2002; 7:286–290.

27. King MA, Glick SJ, Pretorius PH, et al. Attenuation, scatter, and spatial resolution compensation in SPECT. In: Wernick MN, Aarsvold JN, eds. Emission Tomography: The Fundamentals of PET and SPECT. New York: Academic Press, 2003.

28. Foster D, Barrett P. Developing and testing integrated multicompartment models to describe a single-input multiple-output study using the SAAM II software system. In: Proc. Sixth International Radiopharmaceutical Dosimetry Symposium. Oak Ridge, TN: Oak Ridge Institute for Science and Education, 1999; 577–599.

29. Cloutier R, Watson E, Rohrer R, Smith E. Calculating the radiation dose to an organ. J Nucl Med 1973; 14:53–55.

30. Snyder W. Estimates of absorbed fraction of energy from photon sources in body organs. In: Medical Radionuclides: Radiation Dose and Effects. Springfield, VA: US Atomic Energy Commission, 1970:33–50.

31. Stabin MG, Konijnenberg M. Re-evaluation of absorbed fractions for photons and electrons in small spheres. J Nucl Med 2000; 41:149–160.

32. Weber D, Eckerman K, Dillman L, Ryman J. MIRD: Radionuclide Data and Decay Schemes. New York: Society of Nuclear Medicine, 1989.

33. Howell RH, Rao DV, Bouchet LG, Bolch WE, Goddu SM. MIRD Cellular S Values. New York: Society of Nuclear Medicine, 1997.

34. Watson EW, Stabin MG. BASIC alternative software package for internal dose calculations. In: Computer Applications in Health Physics, Proceedings of the 17th Midyear Topical Symposium of the Health Physics Society, Pasco, WA, 1984; 7.79–7.86.

35. Stabin MG, Sparks RB, Crowe E. OLINDA/EXM: the second-generation personal computer software for internal dose assessment in nuclear medicine. J Nucl Med 2005; 46:1023–1027.

36. Stabin M, Siegel J, Hunt J, Sparks R, Lipsztein J, Eckerman K. RADAR—the radiation dose assessment resource. An online source of dose information for nuclear medicine and occupational radiation safety. J Nucl Med 2001; 42:243. Abstract.

37. Snyder W, Ford M, Warner G, Watson S. A tabulation of dose equivalent per microcurie-day for source and target organs of an adult for various radionuclides. ORNL-5000. Oak Ridge, TN: Oak Ridge National Laboratory, 1975.

38. International Commission on Radiological Protection. Limits for Intakes of Radionuclides by Workers. ICRP Publication 30. New York: Pergamon Press, 1979.

39. Stabin MG, da Luz CQPL. New decay data for internal and external dose assessment. Health Phys 2002; 83:471–475.

40. Sgouros G. Treatment planning for internal emitter therapy: methods, applications, and clinical implications. Presented at the Sixth International Radiopharmaceutical Dosimetry Symposium, Stelson A, Stabin M, Sparks R eds., held May 7–10, 1996 in Gatlinburg, TN. Oak Ridge, TN: Oak Ridge Associated Unversities, 1999: 13–25.

41. Tagesson M, Ljungberg M, Strand S-E. The SIMDOS Monte Carlo code for conversion of activity distributions to absorbed dose and dose-rate distributions. Presented at the Sixth International Radiopharmaceutical Dosimetry Symposium, Stelson A, Stabin M, Sparks R eds., held May 7–10, 1996 in Gatlinburg, TN. Oak Ridge, TN: Oak Ridge Associated Unversities, 1999: 416–424.

42. Liu A, Williams L, Lopatin G, Yamauchi D, Wong J, Raubitschek A. A radionuclide therapy treatment planning and dose estimation system. J Nucl Med 1999; 40:1151–1153.

43. Johnson T, McClure D, McCourt S. MABDOSE I: characterization of a general purpose dose estimation code. Med Phys 1999; 26:1389–1395.

44. Clairand I, Ricard M, Gouriou J, DiPaola M, Aubert B. DOSE3D: EGS4 Monte Carlo code-based software for internal radionuclide dosimetry. J Nucl Med 1999; 40:1517–1523.

45. Salvat F, Fernandez-Varea JM, Costa E, Sempau J. PENELOPE—A Code System for Monte Carlo Simulation of Electron and Photon Transport. Workshop Proceedings, Issy-les-Moulineaux, France. ISBN 2001 92-64-18475-9.

46. Bielajew A, Rogers D. PRESTA: the parameter reduced electron-step transport algorithm for electron monte carlo transport. Nucl Instrum Methods 1987; B18:165–181.

47. Briesmeister J. MCNP—a general Monte Carlo n-particle transport code, version 4B. Los Alamos National Laboratory, report LA-12625-M, 1997.

48. Yoriyaz H, Stabin MG, dos Santos A. Monte Carlo MCNP-4B-based absorbed dose distribution estimates for patient-specific dosimetry. J Nucl Med 2001; 42:662–669.

49. Stabin M, Yoriyaz H. Photon specific absorbed fractions calculated in the trunk of an adult male voxel-based phantom. Health Phys 2002; 82:21–44.

50. Zubal IG, Harrell CR, Smith EO, Rattner Z, Gindi G, Hoffer PB. Computerized 3-dimensional segmented human anatomy. Med Phys 1994; 21:299–302.

51. Chao TC, Bozkurt A, Xu XG. Conversion coefficients based on the VIP-man anatomical model and EGS4-VLSI code for external monoenergetic photons from 10 keV TO 10 MeV. Health Phys 2001; 81:163–183.

52. Xu XG, Chao TC, Bozkurt A. VIP-man: an image-based whole-body adult male model constructed from color photographs of the visible human project for multi-particle Monte Carlo calculations. Health Phys 2000; 78:476–486.

53. Jones DG. A realistic anthropomorphic phantom for calculating specific absorbed fractions of energy deposited from internal gamma emitters. Radiat Prot Dosim 1998; 79:411–414.

54. Petoussi-Henss N, Zankl M, Fill U, Regulla D. The GSF family of voxel phantoms. Phys Med Biol 2002; 47:89–106.

55. Trotti A, Byhardt R, Stetz J, et al. Common toxicity criteria: version 2.0 an improved reference for grading the acute effects of cancer treatment: impact on radiotherapy. Int J Radiat Oncol Biol Phys 2000; 47:13–47.

56. Emami B, Lyman J, Brown A, et al. Tolerance of normal tissues to therapeutic irradiation. Int J Rad Oncol Biol Phys 1991; 21:109–122.

57. Meredith R. Clinical trial design and scoring of radionuclide therapy endpoints: 83 normal organ toxicity and tumor response. Cancer Biother Radiopharm 2002; 17:83–100.

58. DeNardo DA, DeNardo GL, O'Donnell RT, et al. Imaging for improved prediction of myelotoxicity after radioimmunotherapy. Cancer 1997; 80:2558–2566.

59. Siegel JA, Lee RE, Pawlyk DA, Horowitz JA, Sharkey RM, Goldenberg DM. Sacral scintigraphy for bone marrow dosimetry in radioimmunotherapy. Int J Radiat Appl Instrum B 1989; 16:553–559.

60. Siegel JA, Wessels BW, Watson EE, et al. Bone marrow dosimetry and toxicity for radioimmunotherapy. Antibody Immunoconj Radiopharmacol 1990; 3:213–233.

61. Lim S-M, DeNardo GL, DeNardo DA, et al. Prediction of myelotoxicity using radiation doses to marrow from body, blood, and marrow sources. J Nucl Med 1997; 38:1378–1474.

62. Breitz H, Fisher D, Wessels B. Marrow toxicity and radiation absorbed dose estimates from rhenium-186-labeled monocolonal antibody. J Nucl Med 1998; 39:1746–1751.

63. Eary JF, Krohn KA, Press OW, Durack L, Bernstein ID. Importance of pre-treatment radiation absorbed dose estimation for radioimmunotherapy of non Hodgkin's lymphoma. Nucl Med Biol 1997; 24:635–638.

64. Behr TM, Sharkey RM, Juweid ME, et al. Hematological toxicity in the radioimmunotherapy of solid cancers with 131I-labeled anti-CEA NP-4 IgG1: dependence on red marrow dosimetry and pretreatment. In Proceedings of Sixth International Radiopharmaceutical Dosimetry Symposium, Stelson A, Stabin M, Sparks R eds., May 7–10, 1996, Gatlinburg, TN. Oak Ridge, TN: Oak Ridge Associated Universities, 1999; 113–125.

65. Juweid ME, Zhang C-H, Blumenthal RD, Hajjar G, Sharkey RM, Goldenberg DM. Prediction of hematologic toxicity after radioimmunotherapy with 131I-labeled anticarcinoembryoinic antigen monoclonal antibodies. J Nucl Med 1999; 10:1609–1616.

66. Erdi AK, Erdi YE, Yorke ED, Wessels BW. Treatment planning for radio-immunotherapy. Phys Med Biol 1996; 41:2009–2026.

67. DeNardo GL, DeNardo SJ, Macey DJ, Shen S, Kroger LA. Overview of radiation myelotoxicity secondary to radioimmunotherapy using 131I-lym-1 as a model. Cancer Supp 1994; 73:1038–1048.

68. Gray BN, Burton MA, Kelleher D, Klemp P, Matz L. Tolerance of the liver to the effects of Yttrium-90 radiation. Int J Radiat Oncol Biol Phys 1990; 18:619–623.

69. Behr TM, Sharkey RM, Sgouros G, et al. Overcoming the nephrotoxicity of radiometal-labeled immunoconjugates: improved cancer therapy administered to a nude mouse model in relation to the internal radiation dosimetry. Cancer 1997; 80:2591–2610.

70. Behr TM, Béhé M, Kluge G, et al. Nephrotoxicity versus anti-tumor efficacy in radiopeptide therapy: facts and myths about the Scylla and Charybdis. Eur J Nucl Med 2002; 29:277–279.

71. Behr TM, Goldenberg DM, Becker W. Reducing the renal uptake of radiolabeled antibody fragments and peptides for diagnosis and therapy: present status, future prospects and limitations. Eur J Nucl Med 1998; 25:201–212.

72. Behr TM, Béhé M, Angerstein C, Rosch F, Becker W. Radiopeptide therapy with cholecystokinin (CCK)-B/gastrin receptor ligands:toxicity and therapeutic efficacy of Auger e- versus α or β emitters. J Nucl Med 2001; 42:68P.

73. Willins JD, Sgouros G. Modeling analysis of platinum-195m for targeting individual blood-borne cells in adjuvant radioimmunotherapy. J Nucl Med 1995; 36:315–319.

74. Howell RW, Kassis AI, Adelstein SJ, et al. Radiotoxicity of platinum-195m-labeled trans-platinum (II) in mammalian cells. Radiat Res 1994; 140:55–62.

14

Dosimetry Applied to Peptide Radionuclide Receptor Therapy

Marta Cremonesi

Medical Physics Department, European Institute of Oncology, Milan, Italy

INTRODUCTION

The interrelated aspects of molecular biology, radiochemistry, nuclear medicine, and radiobiology have played an essential role in the evolution of new radiolabeled molecules for the diagnosis and therapy of positive somatostatin receptor tumors. The experience acquired in the diagnosis of neuroendocrine tumors represented the basis for the development of peptide radionuclide receptor therapy (PRRT), with a constantly increasing spectrum of applications. The clinical trials carried out over the last few years represented not only a promising new option in the management of patients with inoperable or metastasized neuroendocrine tumors but also a source of essential data for further PRRT developments. In such challenging perspectives, the efforts of dosimetrists have been focused on providing useful information for treatment planning and toxicity prevention. Many important results have been obtained, but many new or unsolved problems still require solution, with the final aim of finding a dose–effect relationship.

In this section, the dosimetry experience of several investigators is reviewed in the light of the literature. Methodological aspects and practical approaches are summarized, including the suitable characteristics of the radiopharmaceuticals, the data acquisition and processing for dosimetry, the overview of the results, and the principal methods to reduce radiation doses to critical organs. The recent models specifically studied to improve the accuracy of the dosimetric evaluations as well as a dose–effect relationship are finally reported.

RADIONUCLIDES AND RADIOCOMPOUNDS

The realization of new radiolabeled somatostatin analogs for imaging and therapy is, at present, a field of active research (1–4). Several compounds and radionuclides have been proposed based on their affinity for somatostatin receptor subtypes, labeling stability, chemical, and physical characteristics. In the perspective of dosimetry, the radiopharmaceuticals mostly used in this field can be grouped by the radionuclide, which physical properties are summarized hereafter (Table 1):

^{111}In

The γ-ray emission (173 and 247 keV) and the relatively long physical half-life (2.83 days) of ^{111}In allow to collect pharmacokinetics and biodistribution data up to at least three days. This makes this radionuclide suitable for diagnosis and staging of somatostatin-receptor-positive tumors, and for dosimetry as well. The experience in the diagnostic applications suggested the idea of using ^{111}In-coupled peptides also for therapeutic applications, supported by the possible benefit related to the Auger emission of this radionuclide. Auger electrons are high LET (Linear Energy Transfer) particles, able to deliver high doses within a very short penetration range in tissue (<10 µm). To be effective as a cytotoxic agent, the targeting ^{111}In-labeled molecule must be internalized within the nucleus of the target cell, preferably intercalating with DNA (5,6). A negligible effect is produced on adjacent cells, whether normal or neoplastic. A non-homogeneous distribution of the receptors throughout the target results in a non-uniform dose distribution and in a high probability of failing the therapeutic effect. Therefore, only studies in patients could eventually establish the efficacy in PRRT of a compound labeled with a high LET particle emitter, as ^{111}In is. ^{111}In-DOTATOC and ^{111}In-DTPA-octreotide (Octreoscan®) are the ^{111}In-labeled radiopharmaceuticals principally used.

^{90}Y

^{90}Y is a pure β^- emitter ($E_{max} = 2.3$ MeV). The long penetration range of its β^- particles (the average range in tissue is of several millimetres in tissue, equivalent to ~ 500 cell diameters) generates the possible benefit related to the cross-fire effect. ^{90}Y is particularly suitable for therapy. The resulting quite homogeneous dose distribution enhances the probability of killing all neoplastic cells, but at the cost of high radiation exposure of normal tissues. ^{90}Y-DOTATOC, ^{90}Y-DOTATATE, and ^{90}Y-lanreotide are the principal ^{90}Y-labeled radiopharmaceuticals used for therapy.

Table 1 Radionuclides and Radiopharmaceuticals for Diagnostics and Therapy

Radionuclide and $T_{1/2}$	Useful particle emission	Energy	Particle range in tissue[a]	Radiolabeled peptides	Clinical application
^{111}In 67.4 hours	γ e^- Auger e^- Internal conversion	Eγ: 173 (87%), 247 (94%) keV E: 0.5–25 keV E: 144–245 keV	R_{max}: 0.02–10 μm R_{max}: 200–550 μm	^{111}In-DTPA ^{111}In-DOTATOC	Patient recruitment, follow-up; pre-therapeutic dosimetry; therapy
^{90}Y 64.1 hours	$β^-$	$E_{max, β}$: 2.28 MeV $E_{ave, β}$: 0.935 MeV	R_{max}: 11.3 mm R_{ave}: 4.1 mm	^{90}Y-DOTATOC ^{90}Y-DOTATATE ^{90}Y-Lanreotide	Therapy
^{177}Lu 6.73 d	$β^-$ γ	$E_{max, β}$: 0.497 MeV $E_{ave, β}$: 0.149 MeV Eγ: 113 (6%), 208 (11%) keV	R_{max}: 2 mm R_{ave}: 0.5 mm	^{177}Lu-DOTATATE	Pre-therapeutic dosimetry; therapy
^{86}Y 14.7 hours	$β^-$	Eγ: 511 keV (33%)		^{86}Y-DOTATOC	Patient recruitment, follow-up; pre-therapeutic dosimetry

[a] R_{max}, R_{ave}: maximum and average range in tissue of β particles, internal conversion electrons, Auger electrons.

^{177}Lu

The physical properties of ^{177}Lu offer suitable characteristics for PRRT, with intermediate advantages between ^{90}Y and ^{111}In. ^{177}Lu is a β^--particle emitter ($E_{max} = 0.50$ MeV), with quite long half-life (6.7 days), and an average penetration range in tissue of approximately 1 mm ($\sim$ 100 cell diameters). It is also a γ emitter (113 and 208 keV) of low emission abundance. Therefore, imaging, dosimetry, and radionuclide therapy are enabled with the same complex. Comparison of its physical parameters with those for ^{90}Y indicates a lower "cross-fire" induced damage, partially compensated by a higher percentage of radiation energy absorbed in very small volumes. This suggests ^{177}Lu as an appropriate radionuclide especially for the treatment of small tumors (optimal diameter $\sim$ 2 cm) and micrometastases, while ^{90}Y seems to be more advantageous for larger tumors (optimal diameter $\sim$ 3.4 cm). ^{177}Lu-DOTATATE is considered, at present, a promising radiopharmaceutical for PRRT.

PET Radionuclides

The interest for new PET imageable peptides has greatly raised in the last years. Positron emitters allow increased quantitative accuracy and spatial resolution, and the possibility of analyzing non-uniform distributions in normal organs. These advantages reflect into improved dosimetry.

^{86}Y is a 14.7 hour half-life β^+-emitter that has been proposed to image surrogates chemically identical to ^{90}Y-labeled compounds and to determine their biokinetics. However, its physical half-life and its relatively low emission abundance (33%) enable delayed acquisitions. ^{86}Y also emits multiple high energy γ-rays in cascade. ^{86}Y-DOTATOC and ^{86}Y-DOTATATE have been used to predict the in vivo behavior of the corresponding ^{90}Y-labeled therapeutical pharmaceuticals.

Besides ^{86}Y applications, important results have also already been obtained with ^{68}Ga (7–9) and ^{110m}In (10) labeled peptides. ^{68}Ga is a particularly interesting positron emitter ($T_{1/2} = 68$ minutes) that can be produced by a ^{68}Ge/^{68}Ga generator. This represents a practical advantage in centers with PET facility without a cyclotron. ^{110m}In can act as a radiotracer for ^{90}Y or ^{111}In therapeutic agents.

METHODS FOR PRETHERAPY DOSIMETRY

Dosimetry of normal organs, critical organs, and tumor tissues can be of help in patient selection and therapy planning for PRRT.

Dose estimates to target organs are generally performed using the MIRD scheme previously described in this book by M.G. Stabin. Once the integral activities in organs of interest are determined by numerical or compartmental models (11,12), absorbed dose calculations are generally performed using dedicated software [MIRDOSE3 (13), OLINDA/EXM (14–16)]. These programs offer different kinetic models and phantoms with reference parameters for the anatomy of different age and sex patients, and the possibility of including also some patient-specific adjustments to the standard models. For a more accurate dosimetry, new sophisticated models can be applied, taking into account patient-specific differences in organ shape or size or inhomogeneous activity distributions. Some methods proposed include 3D absorbed dose evaluations, fused CT, and SPECT, and Monte Carlo codes (17).

For PRRT applications, dosimetry needs to predict accurate absorbed doses for compounds labeled with radionuclides (such as ^{111}In, ^{90}Y, ^{86}Y, ^{177}Lu) that present very different characteristics and drawbacks for data acquisition and computation. Many methods can be selected for dosimetry. Most sophisticated evaluations are usually time-consuming and require expensive facilities not commonly available. Practical methods are desirable also for clinical reasons related to patient compliance, but their reliability has to be ensured. The existence of widely accepted protocols to be used in different centers for image acquisition and analysis is certainly appealing, but still arduous.

Nevertheless, common aspects subsist in the assessment of the absorbed doses, despite differences in the generation of the time–activity curves. Radionuclides and molecules may influence differently the in vivo behavior of a radiocompound, but the biokinetics of the somatostatin analogs share some characteristics which are similar for the approaches of dosimetry.

In fact, all the radiolabeled peptides show typically a very fast blood clearance, a very fast activity elimination through the urine, and a biodistribution with spleen, kidneys, and liver as main source organs. These characteristics establish the essential data set required for a dosimetric study, which includes *blood samples* and complete *urine* collection within pre-selected time intervals, and *scintigraphic images* (anterior and posterior whole body (WB) and SPECT acquisitions). Although, in principle, planar views are not ideal for dosimetry, the availability of 5–7 WB serial images (2–3 hours p.i. up to almost 3 days p.i.) might offer complete and satisfactory information on biodistribution and its variation in time. This represents a good alternative to the time-consuming SPECT technique alone, whose limited field of view requires almost two acquisitions for each time point. SPECT acquisitions are frequently focused on certain areas of the body (tumor site, critical organs) and limited at a few time points (18). Once these rough data are analyzed, the activity in normal and tumor tissues has to be converted into time–activity curves, and the absorbed doses finally estimated.

Briefly reported hereafter is an overview of the dosimetric approaches currently applied for the therapeutical radiocompounds.

Therapy Trials with ^{111}In-Peptides

The use of ^{111}In-peptides is limited to therapeutical trials with Octreoscan (19), due to its commercial availability. The dosimetric methods to apply are those commonly required by ^{111}In-labeled compounds. The physical half-life of ^{111}In is adequate to follow the biological half-life of the labeled peptide, long enough to allow the acquisition of a suitable number of scintigraphic images. A tracer amount of Octreoscan has to be administered for dosimetry in a pre-therapeutical setting. Conversely, the high activities injected for therapy produce a very intense γ-emission, precluding early acquisitions (20,21).

Therapy Trials with ^{90}Y-Peptides

The major practical difficulty in the therapy with ^{90}Y labeled peptides—^{90}Y-DOTATOC (22,23) and ^{90}Y-Lanreotide (24,25)—is due to the lack of γ-emission of this radionuclide. The Bremsstrahlung of ^{90}Y does not allow the direct estimate of biokinetics of the radiopharmaceutical. For adequate pre-treatment dosimetry, alternative methods mimicking the therapeutic radionuclide had to be envisioned. Options include imaging with similar analogs labeled with ^{111}In or with the same analogue labeled with a positron emitter (e.g., ^{86}Y) (26,27).

^{111}In-Based Methods

The first approach used in some centers consisted of simulating therapy with ^{90}Y-compunds by the administration of diagnostic activities of Octreoscan (18,28–30). However, Octreoscan is composed not only by a different radionuclide but also by a different targeting molecule than any ^{90}Y-compound used for therapy. Therefore, its use should be limited to patient enrollment and follow-up, while it is not appropriate for dosimetric purposes of peptides with intrinsic different affinity, and, consequently, kinetics. As a more suitable alternative, the same analogue of the therapeutic agent labeled with ^{111}In has been considered as radiotracer to depict the trend of ^{90}Y-peptides (e.g., ^{111}In-DOTATOC for ^{90}Y-DOTATOC). Based on the hypothesis of a similar chemical behavior in-vivo of ^{111}In and ^{90}Y, this represented the natural step for dosimetry in therapeutical applications (31–36). Images derived from ^{111}In-DOTATOC visibly reflect the higher in vivo affinity and specific uptake in somatostatin receptor-expressing tissues, and especially in the tumor compared with Octreoscan. This was demonstrated in a study comparing the two radiotracers (28). In a therapeutic planning perspective, ^{111}In-DOTATOC has been preferably used by several authors to mimic the behavior of ^{90}Y-DOTATOC for dosimetric purposes, given to the presence of the identical molecule in these two radiocompounds (37).

To date, planar and SPECT imaging and kinetics analysis with ^{111}In labeled peptides remains a standard and feasible procedure, not requiring PET technology (18,31,34). A further and most relevant advantage of this approach is in the possibility of collecting data for a proper period of time, enabling depiction of the descending trend of time–activity curves.

^{86}Y-Based Methods

It is unquestionable that, although the chemical behavior of ^{111}In-DOTATOC is similar to that of the analogue labeled with ^{90}Y, the chemical nature of the radionuclide possibly affects the binding affinity for somatostatin receptors (38–40). In this case, the behavior of ^{111}In-derivatives could not be supposed identical to that of the correspondent ^{90}Y-derivatives. To totally preserve the chemical structure of the therapeutical radiocompound, the labeling of the same compound with a positron emitter of the same element ([86]Y) has been introduced. In particular, the biokinetics of [86]Y-DOTATOC was investigated, and the use of [86]Y-DOTATOC has often been considered as the gold standard method for mimicking therapy with ^{90}Y-DOTATOC. Actually, the influence of the radionuclide and the variations produced to the in vivo biodistribution and in dosimetric estimates—were they significant or negligible—have not been specifically explored. A direct comparison of ^{111}In-DOTATOC versus [86]Y-DOTATOC in the same patients should be of major interest. This would solve doubts and definitively establish the reliability of the ^{111}In-based dosimetric methods. Unfortunately such a study lacks in the literature. The biokinetics of Octreoscan versus [86]Y-DOTATOC has been compared instead. The results indicated that Octreoscan can be considered not really predictive of ^{90}Y-DOTATOC therapy but a conservative evaluation, offering preliminary information for patient recruitment and prospective radiation burden to the kidneys. This study evidenced different affinities for tumors and tissues expressing somatostatin receptors, with general Octreoscan overestimates in kidney dose and underestimates in tumor dose. This was not surprising, differences being comprehensibly explained by the different spatial resolution of PET versus SPECT, by the influence of the molecule affinity, and by a possible, but unsolved, influence of the radionuclide (18,27,30).

The use of PET imaging has the great advantage of identifying smaller lesions and to provide more accurate evaluation of tumor uptake (18,41). However, once considering [86]Y for dosimetry, some considerations should alert on the drawbacks which preclude its routine clinical use. The first practical difficulty is in the availability of PET scanners, as well as of the necessary facilities and expertise to produce [86]Y, which are still limited to privileged centers. Moreover, biokinetics evaluations with [86]Y-peptides need a relatively large number of time-consuming acquisitions and biological samples, which have to compete with the short physical half-life of the isotope and its relatively low branching. This results in the possibility of collecting data only within $\sim$ 40 hours after injection. High patient compliance and ample availability of the equipment to collect 5 to 6 PET acquisitions within this time is required. The late activity uptake in organs and blood, not experimentally obtainable, must be estimated by extrapolation methods (18). The reliability of the integrated activities is consequently affected, especially for tissues with a delayed metabolic uptake, for which the trend of the descending part of the time–activity curves can be determinant.

A further problem is represented by the decay characteristics of [86]Y, which include the emission of a high number of prompt γ-rays of high energy. These photons, attenuated by the patient, the scanner septa, and the detectors, can result in spurious—but accepted as valid—true coincidences. This produces consistent over-estimations in background regions and anomalous apparent activity in inactive high density regions. Some authors (42–44) examined the accuracy of [86]Y-PET by measurements with tissue-equivalent phantoms. When standard reconstruction and corrections were applied, they observed a considerably increased activity especially in regions of high physical density (up to ~70% and ~150% in soft tissue and bone, respectively). To compensate, background subtraction or sinogram tail subtraction methods (43,44) have been proposed, but the algorithms need to be specifically determined with respect to scanner design, acquisition mode, and, eventually, patient characteristics. In conclusion, corrections are not easy to apply, and if they are not adequate, implications to dosimetry estimates of ^{90}Y-labeled compounds may be important, with particularly over-estimations of the activity in bone and bone marrow.

All the methods described above evidenced inherent advantages and drawbacks in the prediction of radiation doses of ^{90}Y-conjugates. Several authors compared the biokinetics behavior of the available radiotracers used to predict therapy and to discuss the reliability of [111]In- versus [86]Y- based results(26,45,46). As a conclusion, it can be said that although [86]Y-techiniques provide more accurate diagnostics and tumor activity estimates, they do not totally replace ^{111}In-labeled surrogates, which remain the most attractive options for pre-treatment dosimetry. ^{111}In-based methods can be considered simple and satisfactory alternatives, easy to apply and less expensive.

Therapy Trials with ^{177}Lu-Peptides

[177]Lu-peptides (e.g., ^{177}Lu-DOTATATE), with the special characteristics of its radionuclide, represent the most recent interest of PRRT (47). Besides the therapeutical potential of the β radiation, ^{177}Lu has the practical advantage of emitting γ-rays useful for scintigraphy. The low γ abundance of ^{177}Lu allows to study the actual biokinetics of the radiopharmaceutical also during therapy, without saturation problems. As a slight effect of Bremsstrahlung contribution from β-emission, [177]Lu- images may appear slightly blurred, but image analysis is not affected.

The long physical half life of ^{177}Lu and the enhanced uptake in receptor-positive tissues of ^{177}Lu-DOTATATE provide good information of tumor kinetics and improves the experimental estimates of the last part of the time–activity curves in normal organs.

For a pre-treatment study, activities higher than in case of ^{111}In-peptides need to be administered, but methods for data collection and time schedule similar to those considered for ^{111}In-peptides result to be adequate also for the dosimetry of ^{177}Lu-peptides. This has been demonstrated in a study comparing the biokinetics of ^{177}Lu-DOTATATE to that of Octreoscan (48). In fact, similar biological half-lives and principle source organ involvement were observed in the two radiocompounds, of course with different uptake in organs, and lesions with high somatostatin receptor expression due to different affinity.

Critical Organ and Tumor Dosimetry

Red Marrow Dosimetry

Red marrow toxicity represents the limiting factor in the majority of radionuclide therapies. For this reason, great efforts have been made to study proper models for red marrow dosimetry and tolerance.

Red marrow is a very radiosensitive tissue, with complex and non-homogeneous structure, including trabecular bone, cortical bone, active, and inactive red marrow. This microstructure was taken into account within the MIRD scheme. The computation of the S factors was revised (13,15,49–51) and included in MIRDOSE 3.1 and OLINDA codes. Nevertheless, the mechanisms have not yet been completely explained. They depend on the radiolabeled molecules used, on the specific binding to the components of marrow, on the transchelation of the metal label to transferrin, or simply on the presence of the radiocompound in the bloodstream. Difficulties in modeling the dose estimate of active marrow are therefore comprehensive. Reviews published on this topic (16,52–54) may clarify this issue.

The principal approaches used to evaluate the red marrow dose can be distinguished in "blood-based methods" and "imaging-based methods."

The *blood-based method* was expressly investigated in the study of intact radiolabeled antibodies, to apply in case of no specific uptake of the MoAbs in the red marrow (55). The activity concentration in the red marrow $[A]_{RM}$ was linearly related to the activity concentration in the blood $[A]_{blood}$ or in the plasma $[A]_p$ by an appropriate factor, likely related to the molecular weight of MoAbs. This factor was experimentally determined to be 0.2–0.4.

The possibility of implementing this method also in PRRT was first supported by animal studies (45,56). Moreover, the results obtained in bone marrow samples taken in patients administered with Octreoscan showed a red marrow activity concentration equal to that in plasma at the same time points (57). However, being the molecular weight of peptides is much lower than those of MoAbs, it was observed that the peptide-bound activity in the red marrow probably distributes in a volume larger than the extracellular space. Conse-quently, a factor for the red marrow-to-blood concentration ratio close to 1 has been accepted, conservatively, in place of the 0.2–0.4 for MoAbs (54,58). This hypothesis states that the concentration in the blood can be considered repre-sentative of that in the red marrow ($[A]_{RM} \cong [A]_{blood}$).

The *image-based method* applies in case of specific uptake in bone or bone marrow. The activity in selected areas of known red marrow volume (such as sacrum, lumbar vertebrae, femur) is quantified from images, and scaled for the whole red marrow mass. This method applies when images clearly demonstrate uptake in the marrow—as typically occurs in many therapies with radiolabeled MoAbs.

In PRRT, uncertainties still remain on the optimal procedure for the assessment of bone marrow doses. Images of [111]In- or [177]Lu- labeled somatostatin analogs usually do not evidence any specific uptake in red marrow nor in bone. Consequently, many authors prefer to extrapolate the red marrow dose from the time–activity curve in the blood, the plasma, or even the remainder of the body (27,33). However, controversial results have been shown by PET images studies with [86]Y-DOTATOC. Some authors reported a non-evident specific peptide uptake in the marrow, while others claimed an uptake in the red marrow, suggesting the need of a image-derived method (18,59). It has been demonstrated that [86]Y-based dosimetry for bone and red marrow must be regarded with caution as artifacts typically cause consistent overestimates and the reliability of activity determination is doubtful in these regions (44). Conversely, the blood-derived method generally provides very low doses, which do not satisfactorily predict haematological toxicity. Marrow toxicities—even if mild and reversible—are not uncommon, especially in PRRT with ^{90}Y-DOTATOC. Some authors considered the possibility that the red marrow to blood activity concentration ratio was also time dependent (60). Finally, it has been suggested that the relationship between dose and myelotoxicity could be better predicted including patient-specific parameters to dose evaluation (61) and examining the individual red marrow sensitivity. Patients undergoing radionuclide therapies are frequently exposed to previous aggressive chemotherapies which can provoke major alterations of the marrow reserve. In this regard, results have been published (54,56,61–63).

Kidney Dosimetry

The radiopharmaceuticals used for PRRT have in common a high renal activity concentration, yielding to shift—or to expand—the general concern of toxicity from red marrow to kidneys. In fact, kidneys have been identified as dose–limiting organs for PRRT, in particular during therapy with ^{90}Y-DOTATOC (18,19,64–67). Accurate kidney dosimetry plays a key role for the assessment of radiation nephropathy. Nonetheless, the radiation dose that can be safely delivered to the kidneys during PRRT remains to be established. Methods usually proposed to estimate absorbed doses to normal organs are based on the MIRD scheme and with the assumption of homogeneous activity distribution in the source organs of standard man/woman masses. The preliminary dosimetric evaluations were usually obtained by this method, proven to be a robust and standard approach for clinical use. However, a more careful analysis of the data, with extremely wide inter-patient variability of kidney absorbed doses, strongly oriented towards direct individual measurements, and suggested the need of more accurate dosimetry in this context.

A first crucial improvement was represented by the inclusion in the dosimetric estimates of the actual renal volumes (assessed by CT). A high inter-individual variability was observed in the kidney volumes of patients [range: 231–503 ml, in 25 patients (18)], some of which resulting very far from the reference values of 288 ml (male) and 264 ml (female). Consequently, kidney-absorbed doses rescaled by the true renal masses provided values differing up to 100%. The relevance of this simple correction was recently confirmed in a clinical study, in which the unexpected renal toxicity experienced by few patients could be retrospectively explained by the significantly smaller kidney mass (18).

A further contribution to accuracy can be derived considering that radioactivity remains confined to certain areas of the kidney. Actually, a different uptake between cortex and medulla was promptly suggested by SPECT and planar images—visually showing much higher and persisting activity concentration in the cortex. Unfortunately, the spatial resolution of the SPECT scanners (>1 cm) is not adequate for an accurate measurement of the subregional distribution. The CT-PET facility is of help in investigating this difference, but the examination still presents difficulties. The non-uniform distribution of radiolabeled peptides in the kidneys has been recently demonstrated by ex vivo autoradiography in patients injected with Octreoscan (68). These experimental findings are very important and may guide to the choice of appropriate parameters and dosimetric models. With acceptable approximation, for example, these autoradiographic results might suggest an uptake ratio between cortex and medulla to be included in a multiregional kidney model, and provide improved dose estimates (69).

Despite the possible methods and corrections, the absorbed doses in the kidneys remain high. Given the vital metabolism and the radiosensitivity of the parenchyma, radiation injury of the kidneys, which typically reveals late, severe, and irreversible, is at present under the greatest investigation (70). Special attention is paid on the kidney irradiation processes and on the possible methods to reduce renal uptake.

The study of the mechanisms causing the high radioactivity accumulation in the renal tissues has resulted in a source of precious information and suggestions for renal protection. It was observed that renal uptake is not somatostatin receptor-driven (39,71), mostly related instead to the very rapid clearance from the circulation of the small peptides (molecular weight ~60 kDa (40) compared to ~150 kDa (54) of intact MoAbs). Radiopeptides are filtered through the glomerular capillaries and subsequently reabsorbed in the proximal tubular cells (18,54). Dishomogeneity of their distribution is a natural consequence. On the other hand, the absence of specific binding does not preclude the possibility of interfering with peptide reabsorption by appropriate molecules, for instance. These observations opened the way to the research on possible renal protector agents. In this case, the receptor specificity loses relevance compared to the fast elimination process (which is a characteristic of the peptide), thus allowing lower restrictions in the choice of a surrogate to mimic a therapeutical radiocompound.

Methods Investigating Kidney Dose Reduction

Preclinical and clinical studies have shown that the infusion of basic positive charged amino acids (e.g., lysine, arginine)—before, during, and after the injection of the radioligand—provide a sort of tubular saturation that blocks the tubular peptide reabsorption process (7,39,72–75). Based on these findings, the efficacy and side-effects of several renal protector regimens have been tested by different groups, principally in view of therapies with Octreoscan and ^{90}Y-DOTATOC. Different amounts of amino acid solutions and combinations with other positive charged molecules have been studied. Moreover, the influence of timing, duration of the infusion and possible amino acid toxicity (58,76–79) have been analysed.

Dosimetry had the important task to evaluate the protective efficacy of different molecules and administration schemes, and to determine the possible increment of the cumulative activity to be administered in case of protection. Due to the high individual variability, more reliable methods required direct intra-patient comparison of the radiopharmaceutical biokinetics with and without the infusion of a renal protector. These studies have been carried out differently. Some authors predicted ^{90}Y-DOTATOC therapy by ^{86}Y-DOTATOC (39,46), other authors used ^{111}In-DOTATOC or Octreoscan. All the methods have provided evidence to be reliable, especially considering that the retention in the kidneys is affected by the nature of the peptides, and not by the radionuclide (39). In any case, as opposed to absolute dosimetry calculation, the aim being to assess the variation on biodistribution due to renal protection, the use of ^{111}In-derivatives allowed to overcome the limiting factor represented by the quite short half-life of ^{86}Y, and offered the possibility to acquire late images after 48 hours. This represents a most important advantage when comparing the area under the time–activity curves of the kidneys, the trend of the delayed part of which is known to possibly give an important contribute to the dose.

The results obtained by the wide number studies are reported in Table 2 with special emphasis to dose sparing and toxicity. Although the absolute absorbed dose was very patient-dependent, findings were in substantial agreement among the different groups and can be summarized by the following considerations:

- blood clearance is not substantially modified by the renal protectors;
- urine elimination curves do not differ greatly (difference up to 10% in the cumulative activity eliminated in the first 60 hours);
- tumor uptake is not altered when an agent protector is administered;
- time–activity curves in kidneys typically show a bi-exponential trend, with high uptake values in the first few hours, decreasing within 3–4 hours, and with a low gradient in the second part of the curve.
- protector agents maintain the curve trend but reduce the kidney uptake at all time points;
- integral activities of the time–activity curves for kidneys and absorbed doses are consistently lowered (approximately by 30%, with a maximum of 40%, for amino acids, and up to 55% for other positive charged molecule combinations);
- besides the amount of molecules, the duration of the infusion has an important role in the reduction of kidney uptake, lowering the second part

Table 2 Renal Protection Schemes Studied in Different Centers: Efficacy, Dosage, and Side Effects

Center	Radiopharmaceutical	Renal protection scheme[a]	Mean dose sparing (%)	Notes on toxicity[b]
Milan (78)	^{111}In-DOTATOC	Lys 20 g + arg 40 g, over 3–4 hours before T	20%	Grade I/II GI in 69% of pts
	^{90}Y-DOTATOC (6 pts)	Lys 10 g + arg 20 g over 1–2 hours before T; lys 10 g over 2–3 hours after T	25%	Grade I/II GI in 50% of pts
		Lys 10 g over 1 hour before T; lys 15 g over 2 hours after T	24%	Grade I/II GI in 10% of pts
Milan (79)	^{111}In-DOTATOC	Lys 15 g + arg 20 g before T; 10 g of each after T	37%	Grade I/II GI
	^{90}Y-DOTATOC (16+°2 pts)	Lys 10 g + avidin 2 mg/kg before T	50%	Allergic reactions to avidin
		Lysinated dextran 2–8 mg/kg + lys 10 g before T	55%	
		°Same as previous one + lys 10 g after T + lys 10 g ×2 up to 2 days after T	60%	
Rotterdam – Brussels (46)	^{86}Y-DOTATOC	Mixed AA (lys + arg 26.4 g), over 4 hours	21%	Nausea, vomiting, hypophosphatemia Transient hyperkalemia
	^{90}Y-DOTATOC (24 pts)	Lys 50 g over 4 hours	Similar to mixed AA	
		Mixed AA (lys + arg 52.8 g), over 10 hours	+ 18% versus 4-hours infusion	Nausea, vomiting, hypophosphatemia Transient hyperkalemia
		25 g lys + 25 g arg, over 4 hours	+ 13% versus 4-hours infusion	

(Continued)

Table 2 Renal Protection Schemes Studied in Different Centers: Efficacy, Dosage, and Side Effects (*Continued*)

Center	Radiopharmaceutical	Renal protection scheme[a]	Mean dose sparing (%)	Notes on toxicity[b]
Rotterdam (77)	Octreoscan (26 pts)	Mixed AA (lys 10.3 g + arg 16.1 g) over 4 hours	21%	Vomiting (50% of pts)
		Lys 25 g over 4 hours	17%	
		Lys 50 g over 4 hours	15%	
		Lys 75 g over 4 hours	44%	Severe hyperkalemia
		Lys 25 g + arg 25 g over 4 hours	33%	Vomiting (9%), hyperkalemia

[a] Lys, lysine; Arg, arginine.
[b] GI, nausea and vomiting (grade I/II-NCI, National Cancer Institute Common Toxicity Criteria).
Abbreviations: D, diagnostic; T, therapy.

the time–activity curve (up to 65% with a combination of positive charged molecules + lysine over two days after therapy);
- biodistribution in the other source organs may show minor or unrelevant variations, particularly in the spleen, and in the total body.

All the results confirmed that renal protectors are essential in optimizing the therapeutical setting. Higher tumor to kidney ratios can be achieved, and consequently, higher activities can be injected in relation to the efficacy of the regimen applied.

Tumor Dosimetry

The high variability of intra-patient and intra-lesion tumor uptake has been remarked in all PRRT studies. The wide range of tumor doses was not surprising, likely related to biological and pathological factors—differences in tumor volume, hypoxia, necrosis, viability, interstitial pressure, heterogeneity in binding affinity, receptor density, etc (80). It is well known that receptor densities can vary markedly not only among patients but also among lesions. In any case, several encouraging results have testified the efficacy of PRRT. In particular, tumor size reductions have been obtained for neuroendocrine tumors with relatively low rate of (~25%; range: 10–30%), despite their usually radioresistance and the limited amount of safely administered activities due to toxicity.

Aiming to help patient recruitment and therapy planning, some authors investigated several predictive parameters to possibly trace a dose–efficacy relationship. Very interestingly, a significant correlation has been found between radiation dose to the tumor and tumor mass reduction. In a study, responding tumors could be identified as tumors receiving much higher mean absorbed doses up to 6-fold (232 Gy) compared to non-responding tumors (37 Gy) (18). This emphasised the challenge to deliver the highest activity to the tumor while sparing normal tissues. Accurate pre-therapeutic tumor dosimetry with CT-derived tumor volumes and, whenever possible, quantitative PET tumor uptake, can profitably improve the patient management.

The selection of the radiopharmaceutical is crucial to improve the tumor radiation dose and hence the success of therapy. The most suitable choice may be performed once the characteristics of tumor volume, localization, adjacent tissues, and affinity for the targeting compound are well known. Peptides show the important ability to penetrate into the cell, which is one of the major advantages of PRRT. In the hypothesis of comparable tumor uptake, the physical characteristics of the radionuclide may be therefore fully exploited. Among the radionuclides mostly used in PRRT, it seems reasonable to expect that the lower tissue penetration range of ^{177}Lu may exert a more favourable effect on small tumors as compared with ^{90}Y. With small dimensions, part of the ^{90}Y radiation could be delivered in the surrounding tissues. Conversely, the radiation burden induced by ^{90}Y-labeled radiocompounds should be superior in larger lesions, successfully applying the cross-fire effect of ^{90}Y. Preliminary data seem to confirm these indications (81–83).

Biodistribution of ^{90}Y, ^{111}In, ^{177}Lu as Free Radionuclides

The natural tropism of the radionuclides selected for labeling the therapeutical compounds can be of minor relevance but cannot be neglected. It is always essential to carefully evaluate the chemical quality of the radiopharmaceutical before its administration, and to be aware of the biodistribution of the free radionuclide in case of deconjugation (33,84). In the perspective of myelotoxicity concern, this can be particularly important for bone seeker radionuclides. Considering ^{90}Y, for example, knowledge on the amount of activity in bone is necessary, because the energetic beta rays may irradiate the adjacent marrow. The literature reports bone localization also for free ^{177}Lu, while free ^{111}In is captured by the transferrin in the bloodstream and trapped into the liver. Thus, additional absorbed doses (85–87) have to be taken into account, depending on the percent of labeling and the in vivo stability of the radiocompound (Table 3).

DOSIMETRIC RESULTS IN PRRT TRIALS

Critical Organs and Decision Making on Administered Activity

In an ideal scenario, a pre-therapeutical, individual dosimetry could establish the activity that would deliver a prescribed tumor dose in every patient. In clinical

Table 3 Biodistribution and Absorbed Doses of Free Radionuclides

Free radionuclide	Biodistribution (%) in the body (85–87)	$T_{\frac{1}{2}\ eff}$	Absorbed doses (mGy/MBq)
^{111}In	Liver: 33% Red marrow: 33% Remainder of the body: 33%	67.4 hours In all tissues	Liver: 1.2 Red marrow: 0.76 Total body: 0.16
^{90}Y	Trabecular bone: 25% Cortical bone: 25% Liver: 15% Remainder of the body: 10% Excreted: 25%	64.1 hours In all tissues	Liver: 3.89 Red marrow: 3.26 Osteogenic cells: 3.91 Total body: 0.52
^{177}Lu	Trabecular bone: 40% Cortical bone: 40% Excreted: 20%	6.73 days In all tissues	Red marrow: 1.47 Osteogenic cells: 10.2 Total body: 0.24

practice, the potential toxicity is most frequently the limiting factor, and dosimetry represents a helpful tool to explore the maximum tolerated activity, to identify patients at risk and, possibly, to avoid unwanted outcomes.

A glance to the dosimetric data reported in the literature for the principal PRRT trials (Table 4A for Octreoscan, Table 4B for ^{90}Y-DOTATOC, Table 4C for ^{177}Lu-DOTATATE) revealed large ranges of variability. Besides the different methods used for dosimetry, inter-individual differences are attributable to differences in organ functionality, metabolism, or receptor density of parenchymatous organs. Therefore mean values of absorbed doses among patients—even if averaged on a large cohort of patients—should not be considered to plan PRRT.

Table 4A Dosimetry of Octreoscan$^{®}$

	Mean absorbed doses ± 1 SD (mGy/MBq)				
	10 pts (21)	8 pts (28)	1 pt (98)	3 pts (27)	6 pts (30)[a]
RM	0.03 ± 0.01		0.06	0.02 ± 0.00	0.015 ± 0.01
Kidneys	0.52 ± 0.25	0.47	0.91	0.24 ± 0.07	0.17 ± 0.06[a]
Liver	0.07 ± 0.02	0.07	0.24	0.08 ± 0.020	0.06 ± 0.04
Spleen	0.34 ± 0.17	0.36	0.85	0.24 ± 0.13	0.27 ± 0.09
LLI	0.08 ± 0.05		0.21	0.04 ± 0.01	
SI	0.04 ± 0.02		0.15	0.03 ± 0.01	
ULI	0.06 ± 0.03		0.19	0.04 ± 0.01	
Urinary bladder	0.35 ± 0.06	0.19	0.25	0.11 ± 0.00	
Total body	0.03 ± 0.01		0.07	0.02 ± 0.00	
Blood clearance		13% after 1 hour 4% after 12 hours			
Cumulative urine elimination	$77\% \pm 11\%$ after 24 hours	93% after 24 hours			$59\% \pm 21\%$ after 24 hours
Tumors	For tumor mass $= 10$ g, mean dose: 2.83 or 11.17 mGy/MBq (for RBE $= 1$ or 20) (35) For tumor mass $= 100$ g, mean dose: 0.42 or 1.25 mGy/MBq (for RBE $= 1$ or 20) (35) For tumor mass $= 1$ g, mean dose: 6.88 mGy/MBq (48) For tumor mass $= 10$ g, mean dose: 0.72 mGy/MBq (48) Tumor 1: $(1.7 + 17.6)$[b] mGy/MBq $= 19.3$ mGy/MBq (98) Tumor 2: $(6.7 + 23.8)$[b] mGy/MBq $= 30.5$ mGy/MBq (98)				

[a] Absorbed doses evaluated in patients co-administered with renal protective agents.
[b] Tumor absorbed doses evaluated considering contributions to the absorbed dose to the nucleus from both. ^{111}In-compound bound to cell-surface (basal) and ^{111}In-compound bound to nucleus (Auger).

Table 4B   Dosimetry of ^{90}Y-DOTATOC

Radiotracer used as surrogate	Mean absorbed doses ±1 SD (mGy/MBq)				
	^{111}In-DOTATOC			^{86}Y-DOTATOC	
	8 pts (28)	32 pts (38,76)	5 pts (91)	3 pts (27)	6 pts[a] (30)
RM		0.03±0.01	0.17±0.02	0.05±0.00	0.06±0.02
Kidneys	6.05	3.84±2.02	2.84±0.64	2.73±1.41	1.71±0.89[a]
Liver	0.27	0.75±0.65	0.92±0.35	0.66±0.15	0.72±0.40
Spleen	5.36	7.20±5.21	6.57±5.25	2.32±1.97	2.19±1.11
Urinary bladder	1.59	2.61±1.21		1.03±0.23	
Total body		0.15±0.06		0.08±0.01	
Blood clearance		9%±5% after 1 hour 0.9%±0.4% after 12 hours	15% after 1 hour 4% after 12 hours	12% after 1 hour 2% after 12 hours	
Cumulative activity eliminated in the urine		73%±11% after 24 hours	77%±12% after 24 hours	60%±10% after 24 hours	51%±20% after 24 hours
Tumor		Mean dose range: 2.4–41.7 mGy/MBq (9 lesions) (90) Mean dose range: 1.4–31.0 mGy/MBq (23 lesions, tumor mass range: 2–115 g) (33) Mean dose range: 2.1–29.5 mGy/MBq (30)			

[a] Absorbed doses evaluated in patients co-administered with renal protective agents.

Table 4C Dosimetry of ^{177}Lu-DOTATATE

	Mean absorbed doses $\pm$ 1 SD (mGy/MBq) 6 pts (48)
Red marrow	0.07 ± 0.01^a
Kidneys	1.65 ± 0.47^b
	0.88 ± 0.19^c
Liver	0.21 ± 0.08
Spleen	2.15 ± 0.39
Blood clearance	13% after 1 hour; 2% after 12 hours
Cumulative urine elimation	64% after 24 hours
Tumors	For tumor mass = 1 g: mean dose: 37.92 mGy/MBq
	For tumor mass = 10 g, mean dose: 3.86 mGy/MBq

[a] Mean absorbed dose to red marrow blood derived.
[b] With no renal protection.
[c] With renal protection.

The first dosimetric evaluations combined to the preliminary clinical results were useful to identify the critical organs. Although the spleen usually receives the highest dose, no particular side effects associated to its irradiation have been ever observed. On the contrary, the red marrow radiosensibility and the high uptake in the kidneys had enhanced major concern, for radiopeptides used in single-cycle PRRT and in repeated administrations as well. Typical toxicities are observed as reversible marrow depression (Octreoscan, ^{177}Lu-DOTATATE), kidney nephropathy or low renal function deterioration (^{90}Y-DOTATOC), and reversible sterility in men (^{177}Lu-DOTATATE) (81).

These side effects have strongly influenced the administration of therapeutical activities, indicating high activities to be administered with caution in PRRT (88). However, as a dose–response or an activity-response relationship has not been found, a standard rule to establish the optimal amount of activity to administer in patients undergoing PRRT has not been defined. Consequently, many clinical trials have been carried out with a large variety of protocols, all with a suitable rational. Some protocols plan very high activities in one single administration, other protocols use much lower activities to be repeated in several cycles. In some institutes, dosimetry is not performed and the administration of radiopeptides is based on activity- or on activity per m^2– values, empirically estimated to be safe, to be increased in escalation studies. In other centers, individual dosimetry represents the basis to identify the activity that would limit, cumulatively, the radiation dose to critical organs within values "considered at risk." As precise thresholds are still not available for radionuclide therapies, conventional and cautelative limits were derived from the external radiotherapy experience [20—25 Gy to the kidneys and 2 Gy to the red marrow (89,90)] and by the directives of the local radiation protection authorities as well [e.g., 27 Gy to the kidneys, in Germany (30)].

Histogram associated to Table 4.

(A)

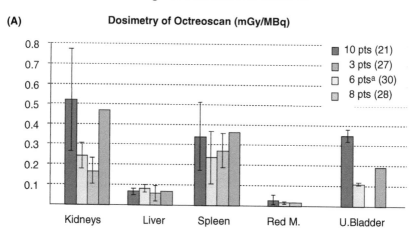

Dosimetry of Octreoscan (mGy/MBq)

(B)

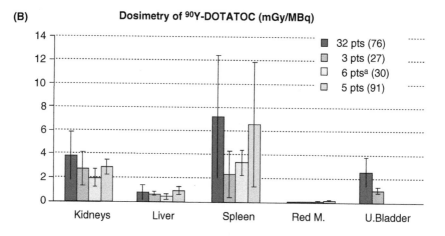

Dosimetry of ^{90}Y-DOTATOC (mGy/MBq)

(C)

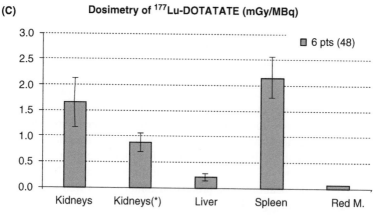

Dosimetry of ^{177}Lu-DOTATATE (mGy/MBq)

The emerging features for the main PRRT radiocompounds—Octreoscan, ^{90}Y-DOTATOC, and ^{177}Lu -DOTATATE—are summarized below.

Dosimetric Results in Therapy Trials with Octreoscan

The pharmacokinetics of Octreoscan demonstrates a very fast blood clearance and elimination, giving low irradiation of the body. Activity elimination occurs mainly through the kidneys, with low activity found in the intestine contents ($<2\%$). No specific uptake of the tracer is usually observed in bone marrow or bone, thus the blood-derived method has been mostly used for red marrow dose evaluation (0.01–0.06 mGy/MBq). Organs receiving the highest doses are the spleen (0.10–0.85 mGy/MBq), the kidneys (0.10–0.90 mGy/MBq), and the liver (0.05–0.25 mGy/MBq). The absorbed doses to tumors, evaluated as the mean energy released to the whole tumor tissue, vary in a wide range (0.7–30.5 mGy/MBq). However, being the therapeutical utility of Octreoscan in the Auger emission of ^{111}In, specific microdosimetric models should be more appropriate.

Despite some encouraging preliminary results, the clinical trials showed only rare cases of tumor regression (82). This probably relates to the too scarce release of the Auger energy close enough to the DNA. Due to the clinical outcomes, Octreoscan is no longer identified as ideal for therapy.

Dosimetric Results in Therapy Trials with ^{90}Y-DOTATOC

The need of a radiotracer to mimic the biokinetics of ^{90}Y-DOTATOC generated comprehensive controversies in the choice of proper dosimetric approaches and in some cases in the results. The data presented in Table 4B may remark differences and similarities of the radiotracers used as surrogates (^{111}In-DOTATOC and ^{86}Y-DOTATOC) and their influence on the ^{90}Y-derived dosimetry.

Pharmacokinetics data of ^{90}Y-DOTATOC show a very fast blood clearance and rapid urinary elimination from the body. The highest absorbed doses were found in the spleen (range: 1.5–19.4 mGy/MBq), the kidneys (1.06–10.3 mGy/MBq), and the liver (0.1–2.6 mGy/MBq).

As for the absorbed dose to the red marrow, the majority of the authors did not observe any significant uptake in bone or bone marrow, and provided blood-derived absorbed dose values ranging from 0.01 to 0.20 mGy/MBq when evaluated from ^{111}In-DOTATOC, and from 0.04 to 0.08 mGy/MBq if evaluated from ^{86}Y-DOTATOC. Other authors reported instead some marrow uptake resulting from ^{86}Y-DOTATOC images (59), deriving red marrow doses of 0.11–0.23 mGy/MBq, although uncertainties remain on the information obtained by ^{86}Y-images in these regions. In conclusion, red marrow-absorbed dose for ^{90}Y-DOTATOC is still difficult to assess.

Highly variable absorbed doses were found in tumors derived from ^{111}In-DOTATOC (33) (1.4–31.0) mGy/MBq and from ^{86}Y-DOTATOC (30,91) (2.1–41.7 mGy/MBq). The efficacy of PRRT with ^{90}Y-DOTATOC has been confirmed by several clinical results. The cross-fire effect of ^{90}Y together with the peptide ability of internalizing the tumor cells allow the release of doses quite uniformly distributed. The major drawback is that the activity administered has to deal with the high kidney irradiation, which can preclude the achievement of a prescribed tumor dose.

Dosimetric Results in Therapy Trials with ^{177}Lu -DOTATATE

^{177}Lu -DOTATATE is the most recent radiopharmaceutical applied for PRRT. The inherent dosimetric studies are therefore quite limited. The blood clearance and urinary excretion resulted quite fast, similar to those of the radiopharmaceutical previously described. The absorbed doses for ^{177}Lu-DOTATATE provided lower values to normal organs compared to ^{90}Y-DOTATOC, with ranges of 1.8–2.7 mGy/MBq to the spleen, 1.0–2.2 mGy/MBq to the kidneys (lowered to 0.7–1.1 mGy/MBq with protection), 0.1–0.3 to the liver, and 0.05–0.08 mGy/MBq to the red marrow—derived with the blood approach (48).

As an interesting issue, the possible sterility was also investigated by the authors, although the absorbed dose to the gonads was not specifically evaluated. This is important, especially for molecules labeled with a γ-emitter, rapidly eliminated from the body. In this case, the intense activity received in the urinary bladder within the first hours may contribute to gonad radiation dose, especially in men. In fact, a significant decrease in serum testosterone concentrations was found in patients treated with ^{177}Lu-DOTATOC, with a period of 18—24 months for reversibility (81,83). This result suggested the need to deepen this topic in future trials.

Recent publications indicated advantageous qualities of ^{77}Lu-DOTATATE compared to ^{90}Y for small lesions. Accurate comparison of dosimetry with ^{90}Y- and ^{177}Lu- derivatives is certainly interesting, almost theoretically. In the hypothesis of identical tumor uptake, of course the longer half-life of ^{177}Lu plays favorably compared to ^{90}Y, increasing the integral activity for the tumor. However, in the absorbed dose calculation, the corresponding dose factors (15) [or S values (13)], accounting for the energy emission of the radionuclide, are higher for ^{90}Y than for ^{177}Lu in most tumors. Actually, the tumor to normal organ dose ratios may represent a more suitable parameter to take into consideration, providing better information than absolute tumor dose can do. These dose ratios cannot be deduced in general but need to be explored specifically for every situation. As a matter of fact, in a study comparing ^{111}In-DOTATOC versus ^{111}In-DOTATATE—as surrogates for ^{90}Y-DOTATOC and ^{177}Lu-DOTA-TATE—the two peptides appeared to be nearly equivalent for therapy when accounting for the risk/benefit balance on tumors and organs. For the patients included in the study, the mean absorbed dose to the red marrow was nearly identical, and tumor-to-kidney dose ratio slightly more advantageous for ^{90}Y-DOTATOC (91). In any case, this conclusion does not necessarily apply in general, being related instead to the type, dimension, and localization of tumors in patients. Ongoing clinical studies with ^{177}Lu-DOTATATE will hopefully provide more information, likely indicating ^{177}Lu-DOTATATE as more favorable for smaller tumors and, conversely, ^{90}Y-DOTATOC for larger tumors. New perspectives pursue the use of cocktails of [177]Lu- and ^{90}Y-radiopeptides, promising for the treatment of differently sized lesions. Preclinical animal studies showed encouraging data, and the radiobiological value of these cocktails will be hopefully addressed in patients in the very near future (92).

As a further observation comparing radionuclides, there is evidence that different physical characteristics may have greatest influence on the nephrotoxic potential and, consequently, on the risk benefit balance. Incidence of renal pathology did manifest in ^{90}Y-peptide therapy; on the contrary, despite cumulative doses up to 45 Gy, the incidence had resulted low and sporadic in Octreoscan and ^{177}Lu-TATE therapies (77,93). This can be explained by the differences in the particle range of the radionuclides and by the peptide prevalent accumulation in the radioresistant proximal tubular cells (which are able to repair and regenerate, and represent the source) compared to the more radiosensitive glomeruli (which do not regenerate, and represent the target). Especially the Auger electrons of ^{111}In-peptides, but also the short range β-particles of ^{177}Lu-peptides, selectively irradiate the tubular cells, and do not, or just partially, reach the glomeruli. The β particles of ^{90}Y-peptides may easily irradiate the cells of glomeruli increasing the potential risk of toxicity (16,64–67).

PHYSICAL AND RADIOBIOLOGICAL FACTORS RELATED TO KIDNEY DAMAGE

The experience in oncological radiotherapy provided ample evidence that the absorbed dose may be used to predict the biologic response. Unexpectedly, an overall analysis on the PRRT clinical trials demonstrated a wide inter-patient difference in the occurrence of kidney toxicity during the follow-up, This was observed in trials based on standard administered activities as well as on trials based on activities planned by individual dosimetry to define the dose to the kidney.

In most cases side effects were unforeseen or not clearly correlated with the administered activity or with the evaluated kidney dose. In other cases, such as in therapy with Octreoscan or ^{177}Lu-TATE, despite the high kidney doses comparable to those with ^{90}Y-peptide therapies, alteration of renal function parameters resulted sporadic and much lower than expected. These findings were disappointing, as, apart from the variation in the radiation sensitivity of the tissues in each individual patient, the occurrence of nephritis should mainly be determined by irradiation. At present, the radiation dose that can be safely delivered to the kidneys during PRRT remains to be established. The alarming high doses to kidneys, and, most importantly, cases of late renal failure in patients who received kidneys doses below the threshold doses for the external-beam radiotherapy (94–96), suggested to reexamine the problem. It was clear that all the factors that could affect the accuracy of dose estimates and those that could influence toxicity needed to be carefully investigated. Some new models have been designed and relevant results obtained. The following paragraphs have the intent of briefly reporting the state of the art on this topic.

External Beam Radiotherapy and PRRT: Differences Related to Renal Toxicity

According to the experience gained in external beam radiotherapy (XRT), absorbed doses to the kidneys of 23 and 28 Gy are associated to 5% ($TD_{5/5}$) and 50% ($TD_{50/5}$) of probability to cause deterministic late side effects within five years. It is also known from the XRT experience that doses > 25 Gy may lead to acute radiation nephropathy with a latent period of 6–12 months, while at lower doses chronic radiation nephropathy may occur, becoming clinically apparent one to five years after irradiation (40,90,97).

Considering internal radionuclide therapies, there is no evidence to date that these findings generally apply with the same dose values and period of manifestation. Renal toxic doses still remain undefined (98), the radiation dose delivered during radionuclide therapy differs in many respects from a dose delivered by external beam irradiation. Consequently, significant discrepancies in the radiobiological effects might be expected, especially to the kidneys, which are so intensely involved in the mechanisms of elimination during PRRT.

The major differences between XRT and PRRT can be summarized as follows: (98–101)

- The radiation dose rate in XRT is high (1–3 Gy/min) and the total prescribed dose is delivered in some tens of fruactions (typically, 2 Gy/fraction); on the contrary, radiation dose rate in PRRT is low (< 3 mGy/min) and variable, with a continuous exponential decrease related to the biological and physical decay.
- PRRT takes advantage of the radiation properties of particles having typically shorter penetration range and varying ionization density, compared to the well-defined photon or electron beams of XRT.
- Irradiation by XRT usually involves only limited regions of the body, while PRRT is characterized by WB exposures, more localized in some tissues.
- To avoid possible kidney damage, fractionation, shielding and collimation of the beam can be used in XRT, while PRRT is at present routinely performed with a coinfusion of positive charged molecules to reduce the physiological renal uptake.
- The dose distribution in external beam is "simple," the dose to the kidney being delivered fairly homogeneously throughout the parenchyma; possible non-uniformities are spatial, due to the geometry of the radiation fields, and

not to biological factors. For radionuclide therapy, dose distributions are related to temporal and spatial variability, and to the individual renal function involved in the metabolism of the specific radiopharmaceutical. Consequently, the range, the half-life, and the time-dependent biodistribution of the radionuclide result in a non-uniform distribution of both absorbed dose and dose–rate. In particular, radiocompounds for PRRT show preferential uptake in the cortex, with a consequent subregional renal dose also dependent on the type of the radionuclide.

New Models to Include Factors Influencing the Radiobiological Effect on Kidneys

Non-homogeneous Activity Distribution in the Kidneys

Until recently, the methods generally used to estimate the absorbed dose to the kidneys conventionally assumed a homogeneous activity distribution over the entire parenchyma. However, recent autoradiography studies have demonstrated that radiopeptides distribute non-uniformly in the cortex and the medulla of human kidneys, predominantly concentrating in the cortex (68). In this study, the activity in the cortex showed a stripped configuration, with a main localization in the inner cortical zone. These results eventually provided accurate measurement of the regional radioactivity, and indicated that the standard MIRD scheme may give non-adequate dose and dose rate estimates in the substructures of the kidney after PRRT.

Actually, to face the problem of kidney dishomogeneity in general nuclear medicine procedures, the MIRD Committee already developed a new multiregion model for a suborgan kidney dosimetry (102). In this model, six new age-dependent, mathematical phantoms of the kidney are used to allow suborgan dose assessment, and four uniform regions (cortex, medulla, pelvis, and papillae) as source/target are included. The S values accounting for the energy loss in the medulla from the cortex have been assembled for radionuclides of potential interest in suborgan kidney dosimetry, including ^{90}Y, ^{111}In, and ^{177}Lu. In the new model, the renal cortex dose is considered representative of the mean dose to the glomeruli and the proximal or distal collecting tubules. This model allows more patient-specific dose estimates of the kidneys by rescaling the four renal regions on the basis of the actual kidney volume and of the activity distribution assigned to the renal cortex and medulla of the kidney (15). Although the spatial resolution of PET and SPECT scanners does not allow an intracortex radiopharmaceutical distribution, it may estimate the activity proportion in the cortex and the medulla with acceptable approximation. Moreover, the detailed findings obtained by the ex vivo autoradiograms of renal tissue sections may also provide reasonable basis for kidney dose estimates.

A simple application of this model to ^{90}Y-compounds retained within the renal cortex showed that, for the adult, the absorbed dose to the cortex subregion and to the medulla is ~ 1.3 and 0.3 times that predicted by the single-region kidney model, respectively. For rapidly filtered radio-pharmaceuticals, as those for PRRT, the dose to the renal cortex and to the medullar pyramids resulted approximately 0.5 and 1.5–1.8 times that predicted by the single-region model (102). Of course, when more accurate distribution can be determined, voxel-based methods provide a more accurate estimate of dose distribution (103). The accurate pattern of the dose volume histograms offered by autoradiograms with Octreoscan could be transposed in a voxel-based model to extend to ^{177}Lu- and ^{90}Y-derivatives the dose distribution estimates in the renal areas. Results showed two fold increase in the dose estimates in $\sim 30\%$ of the cortex volume compared with the estimates produced by a single-region model (104).

Besides the new MIRD kidney model, the impact of dose nonuniformity has been examined also by means of other mathematical models (99,100,105). In particular, some precious information was obtained from a linear-quadratic (LQ) approach based on the biological effective dose (BED) concept and on a factor accounting for the effect of dose–rate and of dishomogeneity. First, a non-uniform dose distribution becomes proportionately less effective as the absorbed dose increases. That is, with less uniform absorbed dose distributions, the surviving fraction increases with the absorbed dose; therefore, a simple "dose escalation" may not lead to a significant increase in response. Moreover, the difference in survival fraction from uniform versus non-uniform dose distribution becomes more pronounced as the radiosensitivity of the cells increases. These observations are consistent with some clinical findings suggesting that the radiation dose deliverable to the kidneys is likely to be higher than the limit derived by external beam radiotherapy (76,79,93). The dishomogeneity of the radiopharmaceutical distribution in renal tissues, and the relatively lower radiosensitivity compared to tumor cells, should play favorably, giving lower kidney damage compared to the XRT uniform irradiation.

Dose and Dose-Rate: The Linear Quadratic Model from XRT to PRRT and First Applications

The dose–rate is a most important factor to be taken into consideration from the radiobiological point of view. It may differently alter the ability of tissues to recover from radiation damage, as in the case of dishomogeneity. This has been widely investigated and demonstrated in XRT.

In general, cells survival curves show an exponential trend, with a strong reduction of the surviving fraction with increasing doses. Early-responding tissues (such as most tumors) are characterized by cell-survival curves with small shoulders, and late-responding normal tissues (including kidneys, which contain slowly proliferating cells) show larger shoulders (99). Their shape is determined by the cell metabolism, the ionization density, and the dose rate. With regard to the kidney, for example, it is well known that at equal dose, fractionation of XRT lowers toxicity. The influence of the dose rate on producing different sparing or damaging effects in different tissues may even play a more important role in radionuclide therapy, where not only the dose rate is not constant, but also the dose distribution is not homogeneous (106). This generates reparable sub-lethal damage and dose–response curves sensitive to the dose rate, with lower dose rates yielding to a lower damage.

These considerations applied to PRRT suggest that, as in XRT, the fractionation of the dose allows to reduce the radiation damage in healthy tissue, with higher cumulative absorbed dose required to cause a comparable biologic effect. Therefore, the sparing effect is likely to play favorably especially to the tumor to kidney dose ratio, the kidney being a late-responding tissue (106).

Based on this background, to transpose the XRT tolerance dose for the kidneys to a corresponding limit in PRRT represented the first challenge. The idea to adapt the knowledge to radionuclide therapy has been more and more attractive. Recently, some authors examined these aspects using a mathematical formalism, quantifying the concepts of the dose–rate sparing by means of the LQ model (106,107).

The LQ model describes the biological effect in irradiated tissue by the surviving fraction (S) of cells that received a radiation dose D:

$$S = \exp(-\alpha D - \beta D^2) \quad (\text{or, equivalently} \quad -\ln SF = \alpha D + \beta D^2)$$

where the linear component αD accounts for the double-strand breaks induced by a single ionizing event, and the quadratic component βD^2 accounts for the cell kill by multiple sub-lethal events (accumulated and reparable damage).

The concept of "biological effective dose" (BED = -1/α ln S) has been introduced and defined as an extension of the absorbed dose, to mathematically interpret the changes in cell survival related to the duration and cycling of the dose delivering and to the α/β ratio. The BED represents, therefore, the dose producing the same biological effect obtained under different irradiation conditions.

For any tissue, an increased BED indicates an increased biological effect (i.e., a reduced surviving fraction).

The α/β ratio is a parameter relating the intrinsic radiosensitivity (α) and the potential sparing capacity (β) for a specified tissue or effect. In general, tissues with low α/β values (typically normal tissues, with α/β in the range of 2–5 Gy) are characterized by dose–response curves steeper and more influenced by the dose rate, as compared to tissues with high α/β (typically tumors, with $\alpha/\beta \sim 10$ Gy). In facts, larger values of β indicate an increased potential of the repairable ionizing events. Consequently, tissues with smaller α/β ratios exhibit a greater dose–rate sparing effect, which is even much more pronounced at longer half-lives, as the sub-lethal damages have more time to recover. This has interesting consequences for the kidneys in particular, whose tissue is characterized by a quite low α/β ratio—estimated to be ~ 2.4 Gy (94) (in the range of 1.5–4 Gy (100)), and a radiation response sensitive to small changes in the dose rate.

In order to apply to radionuclide therapy, some modifications have been suggested to the LQ model. In this case, an appropriate equation should account for the repair mechanism occurring when the dose is not delivered instantaneously but is protracted over a period of time (low dose-rate continuous irradiation). An additional parameter included in the LQ equation has the role to consider the effect of the repair potential and the dose rate. When a dose is delivered over a period of time and divided in multiple cycles, the biologic effective dose (BED) can be estimated by the following equation (69):

$$BED = \sum_i D_i + \beta/\alpha \cdot T_{1/2\ rep}/(T_{1/2\ ref} + T_{1/2\ eff}) \cdot \sum_i D_i^2, \text{ where}$$

D_i: dose delivered for cycle i ("committed dose per cycle");
$T_{1/2\ eff}$: effective half-life of the radiopharmaceutical; and
$T_{1/2\ rep}$: repair half-time of sub-lethal damage.

This represents a refined expression that has been suggested with the purpose of assigning a more meaningful "biological value" to absorbed doses, and, hopefully, to improve the interpretation of the radiation effects by means of increased dose–response correlation in radionuclide therapy.

Here briefly reported are the results obtained by some authors who applied the LQ model focusing on the kidney concern in PRRT.

1. Animal experiments were carried out to study the radiation effect on kidney damage and to validate the LQ model (100) (X-rays). The results remarqued the following key points: the LQ model for XRT seems to adequately describe the kidney response to fractionated irradiation for doses > 1 Gy approximately, while is not reliable for doses < 1 Gy; the α/β parameter for radiation nephropathy has been estimated to be in the range of 1.5–4 Gy, and the repair of radiation damage in kidney seems to be adequately described by a mono-exponential curve with a half-time of 1–3 hours. Kidney radiation injury shows a latent time to expression which is dose–dependent, decreasing as the dose increases.

2. The modified LQ model has been applied to clinical data of patients who underwent ^{90}Y-DOTATOC therapy (18,69,108) with the intent to identify a kidney dose limit equivalent to the TD extrapolated from the XRT experience [TD$_{50/5}$ = 23 Gy given in fractions of 1.5–2 Gy (109)]. The following assumptions were made in relation to the parameters guiding the therapy: initial dose rate of 3 mGy/min, exponentially decaying with an effective half-life of 30 hours; therapy completed in 3 cycles of at time intervals of 6–8 weeks; committed dose to the kidneys: 8–9 Gy/cycle; α/β = 2.4 Gy for renal tissues.

   According to the LQ model for low dose–rate continuous irradiation, the results indicated a shift for the 5% level of probability of nephrotoxicity from the tolerated dose value of 23 Gy in XRT to the threshold of 35 ± 7 Gy (108) for PRRT with ^{90}Y-DOTATOC. This is a significantly higher dose limit that could explain the lack of side effects in some patients. However, this threshold limit also takes into account the non-uniform dose distribution in the kidneys. Assuming the activity totally concentrated in the kidney cortex, and according to the multiregional MIRD model, a ~40% increase to the cortex dose should be considered. Although sparing effects by partial irradiation of the kidneys with PRRT are possible, it was observed that more data are needed to establish if the apparent lower renal toxicity with low dose–rate continuous irradiation represents an effective increase in the tolerance or a delay in the damage manifestation instead (108).

3. In a retrospective analysis on 18 patients who received ^{90}Y-DOTATOC therapy, the contribution of some patient-specific adjustments in the evaluation of the absorbed dose to the kidneys was investigated in view of a possible dose–effect correlation (69). For each patient, kidney dosimetry included the evaluation of: (i) the absorbed dose based on standard renal volume (15); (ii) the absorbed dose including the individual renal mass (from CT) and the activity concentration into prevalently the cortex (cortex volume: 70% of the total kidney volume) (102); and (iii) the biologic effective dose according to the LQ model previously described, accounting for dose rate and number of PRRT cycles. As for the parameters to insert in the equation, an effective half-life approximately 30 hours for ^{90}Y-DOTATOC ($T_{1/2 \, eff}$) was derived from biodistribution data (108); the half-time for sublethal damage repair and the α/β ratio were derived from the literature [$T_{1/2 \, rep} = 2.8$ hours; $\alpha/\beta = 2.6$ Gy (110)].

The interesting results of this study strongly indicated that improvements in dosimetry (including individual parameters, dose rate, and cycling of the activity administration) reflect into improved predictivity of radiation effects. Differences among estimates (i), (ii), and (iii) were significant. Accounting for the total activity administered in these patients, the kidney-absorbed doses range of (26–39) Gy, obtained with the standard kidney mass, changed to (19–40) Gy, when considering the actual kidney mass and the activity localized in the cortex. The BED range was evaluated to be (28–59) Gy (mean, 40 ± 11 Gy). Follow-up data on the renal functionality were also evaluated by means of loss of creatinine clearance per year. Interestingly, a correlation was found between BED and renal impairment, as opposed to the absorbed dose values (i) or (ii). Moreover, patient clinical data on the rapidity of renal impairment supported the hypothesis of 45 Gy as possible threshold BED value for radiation nephrotoxicity, although also other factors— such as pre-existing hypertension, diabetes, and chemotherapy—were supposed to accelerate the radiation damage.

As a further important issue, it emerged that the treatment of patients with high BED and more serious kidney side effects was completed in a low number of cycles. These findings are consistent with other preliminary results reported in the literature (58,77), similarly suggesting an improved repair possibility for kidney tissues in case of a higher number of cycles. Therefore, based on the different sensitivity of most tumor tissues (α/β: 5–25 Gy) and kidney (α/β: 1.5–4 Gy) to the dose rate and number of cycles, treatment protocols based on multiple cycles could represent a powerful strategy to lower toxicity, and, possibly, to improve the therapeutic outcome. Total administered activities could be increased accordingly. It is concluded that there is a need of clinical randomized trials to definitively compare the therapeutic efficacy of equal therapeutical activities administered in multiple cycles versus single or very few cycles.

PRACTICAL CONSIDERATIONS AND CONCLUSIONS

– Patient variability is a characteristic of radionuclide therapies, observed even in the same group of patients undergoing analogue therapeutical procedures. Dosimetric evaluations do not provide homogeneous values, and data are not all in agreement among different studies. This may be disappointing when the amount of activity to be administered in a PRRT therapy has to be established. Differences might be attributed to several influencing factors, including the different patient metabolism but also the different dosimetric methods used.

– The patient variability precludes the concept of a maximum tolerated activity to be identified by dose escalation studies and to be administered in all patients. The cumulative activity to be administered in any single patient should be evaluated after a specific dosimetric analysis.

– Dosimetry has to be performed, being it simpler or more sophisticated. Of course it is essential to be aware of the methodological limits and of the possible error sources. This opens the way to data analysis and comparison among centers and to the fulfilment of new models.

– The crude value of absorbed dose is not sufficient to predict immediate, delayed, or chronic kidney toxicity. Other important factors should be specified, including the specific tissue repair capability and radiosensibility, the dose rate, the dishomogeneous radioactivity distribution in the kidney tissue, the therapy fractionation, and the corresponding biological effectiveness.

– The clinical history of patients may have a key role in the toxicity prevention/occurrence.

Many efforts have been made to increase knowledge and improve dosimetric evaluations. Suitable perspectives should aim to the easy availability of more user-friendly and low time-consuming tools for complete treatment planning. These should include data availability, radiobiological models, softwares, fused images, and Monte Carlo codes.

REFERENCES

1. Reubi JC, Mäcke HR, Krenning EP. Candidates for peptide receptor radiotherapy today and in the future. J Nucl Med 2005; 46:67S–75S.
2. Breeman WA, de Jong M, Kwekkeboom DJ, et al. Somatostatin receptor-mediated imaging and therapy: basic science, current knowledge, limitations and future perspectives. Eur J Nucl Med 2001; 28:1421–4129.
3. de Jong M, Krenning E. New advances in peptide receptor radionuclide therapy. J Nucl Med 2002; 43:617–620.
4. de Jong M, Kwekkeboom D, Valkema R, Krenning EP. Radiolabeled peptides for tumor therapy: current status and future directions. Plenary lecture at the EANM 2002. Eur J Nucl Med Mol Imaging 2003; 30:463–469.
5. Capello A, Krenning EP, Breeman WA, Bernard BF, de Jong M. Peptide receptor radionuclide therapy in vitro using [111In-DTPA0]octreotide. J Nucl Med 2003; 44:98–104.
6. Bodei L, Kassis AI, Adelstein SJ, Mariani G. Radionuclide therapy with iodine-125 and other auger-electron-emitting radionuclides: experimental models and clinical applications. Cancer Biother Radiopharm 2003; 18:861–877.
7. Breeman WA, de Jong M, de Blois E, Bernard BF, Konijnenberg M, Krenning EP. Radiolabeling DOTA-peptides with [68]Ga. Eur J Nucl Med Mol Imaging 2005; 32:478–485.
8. Maecke HR, Hofmann M, Haberkorn U. ^{68}Ga-Labeled peptides in tumor imaging. J Nucl Med 2005; 46:172S–178S.
9. Hofmann M, Maecke H, Borner R, et al. Biokinetics and imaging with the somatostatin receptor PET radioligand ^{68}Ga-DOTATOC: preliminary data. Eur J Nucl Med 2001; 28:1751–1757.
10. Lubberink M, Tolmachev V, Widstrom C, Bruskin A, Lundqvist H, Westlin JE. 110mIn-DTPA-D-Phe1-octreotide for imaging of neuroendocrine tumors with PET. J Nucl Med 2002; 43:1391–1397.
11. Siegel JA, Thomas SR, Stubbs J, et al. Techniques for quantitative radio-pharmaceutical biodistribution data acquisition and analysis for use in human radiation dose estimates. MIRD Pamphlet No.16. J Nucl Med 1999; 40:S37–S61.
12. Foster D, Barret P. Developing and testing integrated multicompartment models to describe a single-input multiple-output study using the SAAM II software system. In: Proc. Sixth International Radiopharmaceutical. Dosimetry Symposium, Oak Ridge Institute for Science and Education, 1998.
13. Stabin MG. MIRDOSE: personal computer software for internal dose assessment in nuclear medicine. J Nucl Med 1996; 37:538–546.
14. Stabin MG, Sparks RB, Crowe E. OLINDA/EXM: the second-generation personal computer software for internal dose assessment in nuclear medicine. J Nucl Med 2005; 46:1023–1027.
15. RADAR (RAdiation Dose Assessment Resource) Stabin M, Siegel J, Lipsztein J, et al. www.doseinfo-radar.com; www.ieo.it/radar.

16. Stabin MG, Siegel JA. Physical models and dose factors for use in internal dose assessment. Health Phys 2003; 85:294–310.

17. Ljungberg M, Frey E, Sjogreen K, Liu X, Dewaraja Y, Strand SE. 3D absorbed dose calculations based on SPECT: evaluation for 111In/^{90}Y therapy using Monte Carlo simulations. Cancer Biother Radiopharm 2003; 18:99–107.

18. Pauwels S, Barone R, Walrand S, et al. Practical dosimetry of peptide receptor radionuclide therapy with ^{90}Y-labeled somatostatin analogs. J Nucl Med 2005; 46:92S–98S.

19. Valkema R, De Jong M, Bakker WH, et al. Phase I study of peptide receptor radionuclide therapy with [In-DTPA]octreotide: the Rotterdam experience. Semin Nucl Med 2002; 32:110–122.

20. Krenning EP, Bakker WH, Kooij PP, et al. Somatostatin receptor scintigraphy with indium-111-DTPA-D-Phe-1-octreotide in man: metabolism, dosimetry and comparison with iodine-123-Tyr-3-octreotide. J Nucl Med 1992; 33:652–658.

21. Stabin MG, Kooij PP, Bakker WH, et al. Radiation dosimetry for indium-111-pentetreotide. J Nucl Med 1997; 38:1919–1922.

22. de Jong M, Bakker WH, Krenning EP, et al. Yttrium-90 and indium-111 labeling, receptor binding and biodistribution of [DOTA0,D-Phe1,Tyr3]octreotide, a promising somatostatin analogue for radionuclide therapy. Eur J Nucl Med 1997; 24:368–371.

23. Otte A, Jermann E, Behe M, et al. DOTATOC—a new powerful tool for receptor-mediated radionuclide therapy. Eur J Nucl Med 1997; 24:792–795.

24. Smith-Jones PM, Bischof C, Leimer M, et al. DOTA-lanreotide: a novel somatostatin analog for tumor diagnosis and therapy. Endocrinology 1999; 140:5136–5148.

25. Virgolini I, Britton K, Buscombe J, Moncayo R, Paganelli G, Riva P. In- and Y-DOTA-lanreotide: results and implications of the MAURITIUS trial. Semin Nucl Med 2002; 32:148–155.

26. Mansi L. From the magic bullet to an effective therapy: the peptide experience. Eur J Nucl Med Eur J Nucl Med Mol Imaging 2004; 31:1393–1398.

27. Forster GJ, Engelbach MJ, Brockmann JJ, et al. Preliminary data on biodistribution and dosimetry for therapy planning of somatostatin receptor positive tumors: comparison of ^{86}Y-DOTATOC and ^{111}In-DTPA-octreotide. Eur J Nucl Med 2001; 28:17450.

28. Kwekkeboom DJ, Kooij PP, Bakker WH, Macke HR, Krenning EP. Comparison of ^{111}In-DOTA-Tyr3-octreotide and ^{111}In-DTPA-octreotide in the same patients: biodistribution, kinetics, organ and tumor uptake. J Nucl Med 1999; 40:762–767.

29. Barone R, Jamar F, Walrand S, et al. Can ^{111}In-DTPA-Octreotide (IN-OC) predict kidney and tumor exposure during treatment with ^{90}Y-SMT487 (Octreother®)? JNM 2000; 41:110P.

30. Helisch A, Förster GJ, Reber H, et al. Pre-therapeutic dosimetry and biodistribution of ^{86}Y-DOTA-Phe 1-Tyr 3-octreotide versus ^{111}In-pentetreotide in patients with advanced neuroendocrine tumors. Eur J Nucl Med Mol Imaging 2004; 31:1386–1392.

31. Virgolini I, Szilvasi I, Kurtaran A, et al. Indium-111-DOTA-lanreotide: biodistribution, safety and radiation absorbed dose in tumor patients. J Nucl Med 1998; 39:1928–1936.

32. Otte A, Herrmann R, Heppeler A, et al. Yttrium-90 DOTATOC: first clinical results. Eur J Nucl Med 1999; 26:1439–1447.
33. Cremonesi M, Ferrari M, Zoboli S, et al. Biokinetics and dosimetry in patients administered with ^{111}In-DOTA-Tyr[3]-octreotide: implications for internal radiotherapy with ^{90}Y-DOTATOC. Eur J Nucl Med 1999; 26:877–886.
34. Virgolini I, Traub T, Leimer M, et al. New radiopharmaceuticals for receptor scintigraphy and radionuclide therapy. Q J Nucl Med 2000; 44:50–58.
35. Kwekkeboom DJ, Krenning EP, de Jong M. Peptide receptor imaging and therapy. J Nucl Med 2000; 41:1704–1713.
36. Waldherr C, Pless M, Maecke HR, Haldemann A, Mueller-Brand J. The clinical value of [^{90}Y-DOTA]-D-Phe1-Tyr3-octreotide (^{90}Y-DOTATOC) in the treatment of neuroendocrine tumors: a clinical phase II study. Ann Oncol 2001; 12:941–945.
37. Forrer F, Mueller-Brand J, Maecke H. Pre-therapeutic dosimetry with radiolabeled somatostatin analogues in patients with advanced neuroendocrine tumors. Eur J Nucl Med Mol Imaging 2005; 32:511–512.
38. Reubi JC, Schar JC, Waser B, et al. Affinity profiles for human somatostatin receptor subtypes SST1-SST5 of somatostatin radiotracers selected for scintigraphic and radiotherapeutic use. Eur J Nucl Med 2000; 27:273–282.
39. de Jong M, Bakker WH, Breeman WA, et al. Pre-clinical comparison of [DTPA[0],Tyr[3]] octreotide and [DOTA[0],D-Phe1,Tyr[3]] octreotide as carriers for somatostatin receptor-targeted scintigraphy and radionuclide therapy. Int J Cancer 1998; 75:406–411.
40. Boerman OC, Oyen WJ, Corstens FH. Between the scylla and charybdis of peptide radionuclide therapy: hitting the tumor and saving the kidney. Eur J Nucl Med 2001; 28:1447–1449.
41. Waldherr C, Pless M, Maecke HR, et al. Tumor response and clinical benefit in neuroendocrine tumors after 7.4 GBq ^{90}Y-DOTATOC. J Nucl Med 2002; 43:610–616.
42. Walrand S, Jamar F, Mathieu I, et al. Quantitation in PET using isotopes emitting prompt single gammas: application to yttrium-86. Eur J Nucl Med Mol Imaging 2003; 30:354–361.
43. Buchholz HG, Herzog H, Forster GJ, et al. PET imaging with yttrium-86: comparison of phantom measurements acquired with different PET scanners before and after applying background subtraction. Eur J Nucl Med Mol Imaging 2003; 30:716–720.
44. Pentlow KS, Finn RD, Larson SM, Erdi YE, Beattie BJ, Humm JL. Quantitative imaging of yttrium-86 with PET. The occurrence and correction of anomalous apparent activity in high density regions. Clin Positron Imaging 2000; 3:85–90.
45. Rosch F, Herzog H, Stolz B, et al. Uptake kinetics of the somatostatin receptor ligand [[86]Y]DOTA-DPhe1- Tyr[3]-octreotide ([[86]Y]SMT487) using positron emission tomography in non-human primates and calculation of radiation doses of the ^{90}Y-labeled analogue. Eur J Nucl Med 1999; 26:358–366.
46. Jamar F, Barone R, Mathieu I, et al. [86]Y-DOTA0)-D-Phe1-Tyr[3]-octreotide (SMT487)—a phase 1 clinical study: pharmacokinetics, biodistribution and renal protective effect of different regimens of amino acid co-infusion. Eur J Nucl Med Mol Imaging 2003; 30:510–518.

47. Breeman WA, de Jong M, Erion JL, et al. Preclinical comparison of ^{111}In-labeled DTPA- or DOTA-bombesin analogs for receptor-targeted scintigraphy and radionuclide therapy. J Nucl Med 2002; 43:1650–1656.

48. Kwekkeboom DJ, Bakker WH, Kooij PP, et al. [177Lu-DOTAOTyr3]octreotate: comparison with [111In-DTPAo]octreotide in patients. Eur J Nucl Med 2001; 28:1319–1325.

49. Stabin MG, Brill AB. Monoclonal antibodies in the treatment of hematologic malignancies: radiation dosimetry aspects. Curr Pharm Biotechnol 2001; 2:351–356.

50. Stabin MG, Siegel JA, Sparks RB, Eckerman KF, Breitz HB. Contribution to red marrow absorbed dose from total body activity: a correction to the MIRD method. J Nucl Med 2001; 42:492–498.

51. Stabin MG, Eckerman KF, Bolch WE, Bouchet LG, Patton PW. Evolution and status of bone and marrow dose models. Cancer Biother Radiopharm 2002; 17:427–433.

52. Siegel JA, Wessels BW, Watson EE, et al. Bone marrow dosimetry and toxicity for radioimmunotherapy. Antibody Immunoconjugates and Radiopharm 1990; 3:4.

53. Siegel JA, Stabin MG, Sparks RB. Total-body and red marrow dose estimates. J Nucl Med 2003; 44:320–321 author reply 321-323.

54. Sgouros G. Dosimetry of internal emitters. J Nucl Med 2005; 46:18S–27S.

55. Sgouros G. Bone marrow dosimetry for radioimmunotherapy: theoretical considerations. J Nucl Med 1993; 34:689–694.

56. Behr TM, Behe M, Sgouros G. Correlation of red marrow radiation dosimetry with myelotoxicity: empirical factors influencing the radiation-induced myelotoxicity of radiolabeled antibodies, fragments and peptides in pre-clinical and clinical settings. Cancer Biother Radiopharm 2002; 17:445–464.

57. Forssell-Aronsson E, Fjalling M, Nilsson O, Tisell LE, Wangberg B, Ahlman H. Indium-111 activity concentration in tissue samples after intravenous injection of indium-111-DTPA-D-Phe-1-octreotide. JNM 1995; 36:7–12.

58. Barone R, De Camps J, Smith C, et al. Amino acid (AA) solutions infused for renal radioprotection: metabolic effects. Nucl Med Commun 2000; 21:563 (abstract).

59. Walrand S, Barone R, Jamar F, et al. Red marrow [90]YoctreoTher dosimetry estimated using [86]Yoctreother PET and biological correlates. Eur J Nucl Med Mol Imaging 2002; 29(S1):P434 (abstract).

60. Hindorf C, Linden O, Tennvall J, Wingardh K, Strand SE. Time dependence of the activity concentration ratio of red marrow to blood and implications for red marrow dosimetry. Cancer 2002; 94:1235–1239.

61. Stabin MG, Siegel JA, Sparks RB. Sensitivity of model-based calculations of red marrow dosimetry to changes in patient-specific parameters. Cancer Biother Radiopharm 2002; 17:535–543.

62. Shen S, Meredith RF, Duan J, et al. Improved prediction of myelotoxicity using a patient-specific imaging dose estimate for non-marrow-targeting ^{90}Y-antibody therapy. J Nucl Med 2002; 43:1245–1253.

63. Siegel JA, Yeldell D, Goldenberg DM, et al. Red marrow radiation dose adjustment using plasma FLT3-L cytokine levels: improved correlations between hematologic toxicity and bone marrow dose for radioimmunotherapy patients. J Nucl Med 2003; 44:67–76.

64. Moll S, Nickeleit V, Mueller-Brand J, Brunner FP, Maecke HR, Mihatsch MJ. A new cause of renal thrombotic microangiopathy: yttrium 90-DOTATOC internal radiotherapy. Am J Kidney Dis 2001; 37:847–851.

65. Cybulla M, Weiner SM, Otte A. End-stage renal disease after treatment with ^{90}Y-DOTATOC. Eur J Nucl Med 2001; 28:1552–1554.

66. Otte A, Cybulla M, Weiner SM. ^{90}Y-DOTATOC and nephrotoxicity. Eur J Nucl Med Mol Imaging 2002; 29:1543.

67. Schumacher T, Waldherr C, Mueller-Brand J, Maecke H. Kidney failure after treatment with ^{90}Y-DOTATOC. Eur J Nucl Med Mol Imaging 2002; 29:435.

68. de Jong M, Valkema R, Van Gameren A, et al. Inhomogeneous localization of radioactivity in the human kidney after injection of [^{111}In-DTPA]octreotide. J Nucl Med 2004; 45:1168–1171.

69. Barone R, Borson-Chazot F, Valkema R, et al. Patient-specific dosimetry in predicting renal toxicity with ^{90}Y-DOTATOC: relevance of kidney volume and dose rate in finding a dose–effect relationship. J Nucl Med 2005; 46:99S–106S.

70. Breitz H. Clinical aspects of radiation nephropathy. Cancer Biother Radiopharm 2004; 19:359–362.

71. Behr TM, Goldenberg DM, Becker W. Reducing the renal uptake of radiolabeled antibody fragments and peptides for diagnosis and therapy: present status, future prospects and limitations. Eur J Nucl Med 1998; 25:201–212.

72. Behr TM, Sharkey RM, Sgouros G, et al. Overcoming the nephotoxicity of radiometal-labeled immunoconjugates: improved cancer therapy administered to a nude mouse model in relation to the internal radiation dosimetry. Cancer 1997; 80:2591–2610.

73. Hammond PJ, Wade AF, Gwilliam ME, et al. Amino acid infusion blocks renal tubular uptake of an indium-labeled somatostatin analogue. Br J Cancer 1993; 67:1437–1439.

74. de Jong M, Rolleman EJ, Bernard BF, et al. Inhibition of renal uptake of indium-111-DTPA-octreotide in vivo. J Nucl Med 1996; 37:1388–1392.

75. Bernard BF, Krenning EP, Breeman WA, et al. D-lysine reduction of indium-111 octreotide and yttrium-90 octreotide renal uptake. J Nucl Med 1997; 38:1929–1933.

76. Cremonesi M, Bodei L, Rocca P, Stabin M, Macke HR, Paganelli G. Kidney protection during receptor-mediated radiotherapy ^{90}Y-[DOTA]^{0}-Tyr^{3}-octreotide. Cancer Biother Radiopharm 2002; 17:344.

77. Rolleman EJ, Valkema R, de Jong M, Kooij PP, Krenning EP. Safe and effective inhibition of renal uptake of radiolabeled octreotide by a combination of lysine and arginine. Eur J Nucl Med Mol Imaging 2003; 30:9–15.

78. Bodei L, Cremonesi M, Zoboli S, et al. Receptor-mediated radionuclide therapy with ^{90}Y-DOTATOC in association with amino acid infusion: a phase I study. Eur J Nucl Med Mol Imaging 2003; 30:207–216.

79. Bodei L, Cremonesi M, Grana C, et al. Receptor radionuclide therapy with ^{90}Y-[DOTA]^{0}-Tyr^{3}-octreotide (^{90}Y-DOTATOC) in neuroendocrine tumors. Eur J Nucl Med Mol Imaging 2004; 31:1038–1046.

80. de Jong M, Breeman WA, Bernard BF, et al. Tumor response after [^{90}Y-DOTA(0),Tyr^{3}]octreotide radionuclide therapy in a transplantable rat tumor model is dependent on tumor size. J Nucl Med 2001; 42:1841–1846.

81. Kwekkeboom DJ, Bakker WH, Kam BL, et al. Treatment of patients with gastro-entero-pancreatic (GEP) tumors with the novel radiolabeled somatostatin analogue [^{177}Lu-DOTA(0),Tyr3]octreotate. Eur J Nucl Med Mol Imaging 2003; 30:417–422.

82. Kwekkeboom DJ, Mueller-Brand J, Paganelli G, et al. An overview of the peptide receptor radionuclide therapy with 3 different radiolabeled somatostatin analogues. J Nucl Med 2005; 46:62S–66S.

83. Kwekkeboom DJ, Teunissen JJ, Bakker WH, et al. Radiolabeled somatostatin analog [^{177}Lu-DOTA0,Tyr^3]octreotate in patients with endocrine gastroentero-pancreatic tumors. J Clin Oncol 2005; 23:2754–2762.

84. Breeman WA, De Jong M, Visser TJ, Erion JL, Krenning EP. Optimising conditions for radiolabeling of DOTA-peptides with ^{90}Y, ^{111}In and ^{177}Lu at high specific activities. Eur J Nucl Med Mol Imaging 2003; 30:917–920.

85. Cristy M, Eckerman K. Specific Absorbed Fraction of Energy Absorbed at Various Ages from Internal Photon Sources. I. Methods, II. One-year-old, III. Five-year-old, IV. Ten-year-old, V. Fifteen-year-old male and adult female, VI. Newborn, II. Adult Male. ORNL/TM-8381, Volumes 1–7, Oak Ridge National Laboratory, Oak Ridge, TN, 1987.

86. International Commission on Radiological Protection. Limits for intakes of radionuclides by workers. ICRP Publication 30. New York: Pergamon Press, 1979.

87. Breeman WA, van der Wansem K, Bernard BF, et al. The addition of DTPA to [^{177}Lu-DOTA0,Tyr^3]octreotate prior to administration reduces rat skeleton uptake of radioactivity. Eur J Nucl Med Mol Imaging 2003; 30:312–315.

88. Bodei L, Chinol M, Cremonesi M, Paganelli G. Facts and myths about radiopeptide therapy: SCYLLA CHARYBDIS and SIBYL. Eur J Nucl Med Mol Imaging 2002; 29:1099–1100.

89. Cassady JR. Clinical radiation nephropathy. Int J Radiat Oncol Biol Phys 1995; 31:1249–1256.

90. Emami B, Lyman J, Brown A, et al. Tolerance of normal tissue to therapeutic irradiation. Int J Radiat Oncol Biol Phys 1991; 21:109–122.

91. Forrer F, Uusijärvi H, Waldherr C, et al. A comparison of ^{111}In-DOTATOC and ^{111}In-DOTATATE: biodistribution and dosimetry in the same patients with metastatic neuroendocrine tumors. Eur J Nucl Med Mol Imaging 2004; 31:1257–1262.

92. de Jong M, Breeman WA, Valkema R, Bernard BF, Krenning EP. Combination radionuclide therapy using ^{177}Lu- and ^{90}Y-labeled somatostatin analogs. J Nucl Med 2005; 46:13S–17S.

93. Valkema R, Pauwels SA, Kvols LK, et al. Long-term follow-up of renal function after peptide receptor radiation therapy with ^{90}Y-DOTA0,Tyr3-octreotide and ^{177}Lu-DOTA0, Tyr3-octreotate. J Nucl Med 2005; 46:83S–91S.

94. Breitz H, Wendt R, Stabin M, Bouchet L, Wessels B. Dosimetry of high dose skeletal targeted radiotherapy (STR) with ^{166}Ho-DOTMP. Cancer Biother Radiopharm 2003; 18:225–230.

95. Lambert B, Cybulla M, Weiner SM, et al. Renal toxicity after radionuclide therapy. Radiat Res 2004; 161:607–611.

96. Giralt S, Bensinger W, Goodman M, et al. ^{166}Ho-DOTMP plus melphalan followed by peripheral blood stem cell transplantation in patients with multiple myeloma: results of two phase 1/2 trials. Blood 2003; 102:2684–2691.

97. National Council on Radiation Protection and Measurements (NCRPM). Misadministration of Radioactive Material in Medicine — Scientific Background. Bethesda, MD: NCRPM, 1991:27.

98. McCarthy KE, Woltering EA, Anthony LB. In situ radiotherapy with ^{111}In-pentetreotide. State of the art and perspectives. Q J Nucl Med 2000; 44:88–95.

99. Kassis AI, Adelstein SJ. Radiobiologic principles in radionuclide therapy. J Nucl Med 2005; 46:4S–12S.

100. O'Donoghue J. Relevance of external beam dose–response relationships to kidney toxicity associated with radionuclide therapy. Cancer Biother Radiopharm 2004; 19:378–387.

101. Wessels B. Summary and perspectives on kidney dose–response to radionuclide therapy. Cancer Biother Radiopharm 2004; 19:388–390.

102. Bouchet LG, Bolch WE, Blanco HP, et al. MIRD Pamphlet No 19: absorbed fractions and radionuclide S values for six age-dependent multiregion models of the kidney. J Nucl Med 2003; 44:1113–1147.

103. Green A, Flynn A, Pedley RB, Dearling J, Begent R. Nonuniform absorbed dose distribution in the kidney: the influence of organ architecture. Cancer Biother Radiopharm 2004; 19:371–377.

104. Konijnenberg MW, De Jong M, Valkema R, Krenning EP. Combined functional status and dose–volume analysis for determining renal damage threshold with radionuclide therapy. Eur J Nucl Med 2004; 31:S239.

105. ICRU Report 67. Absorbed dose specification in nuclear medicine. J ICRU 2002;2.

106. Dale R. Dose-rate effects in targeted radiotherapy. Phys Med Biol 1996; 41:1184–1187.

107. Dale R. Use of the linear-quadratic radiobiological model for quantifying kidney response in targeted radiotherapy. Cancer Biother Radiopharm 2004; 19:363–370.

108. Konijnenberg MW. Is the renal dosimetry for [90Y-DOTA0,Tyr3]octreotide accurate enough to predict thresholds for individual patients? Cancer Biother Radiopharm 2003; 18:619–625.

109. Perez A, Brady LW. Principles and Practice of Radiation Oncology. Philadelphia: Lippincott-Raven Publishers, 1997.

110. Thames HD, Ang KK, Stewart FA, van der Schueren E. Does incomplete repair explain the apparent failure of the basic LQ model to predict spinal cord and kidney responses to low doses per fraction? Int J Radiat Biol 1988; 54:13–19.

FURTHER READING

1. ICRP Publication 41. Radiation Protection. Non Stochastic Effects of Ionizing Radiation. New York: Pergamon Press, 1984.

2. ICRP Publication 52. Protection of the Patient in Nuclear Medicine. New York: Pergamon Press, 1988.

3. ICRP Publication 53. Radiation Dose to Patients from Radiopharmaceuticals. Annals of ICRP. New York: Pergamon Press, 1987.

4. ICRP Publication 73. Radiological Protection and Safety in Medicine. New York: Pergamon Press, 1996.

15

Methods to Reduce Radiation Exposure to Personnel During Radiolabelling and Infusion

Mahila Ferrari

Medical Physics Department, European Institute of Oncology, Milan, Italy

INTRODUCTION

Peptide receptor-targeted radionuclide therapy (PRRT) is a promising application of radiolabeled somatostatin analogue. The most frequently used therapeutic radionuclide in PRRT is ^{90}Y, a pure, high-energy β-emitter with suitable physical characteristics for therapy [$T_{1/2} = 2.67$ days; E_{max} 2.27MeV, $E_{mean} = 939$ keV; $R_{95} = 5.95$ mm, $R_{50} = 5.3$ mm (1) in tissue].

The energy of beta-radiation can be totally absorbed in a limited volume of tissue. The exposure can be therefore limited to the tissue to be treated. This is favorable in therapeutic application, but may cause an increased risk of partial exposure of the medical staff, especially of the hands when high activities are frequently handled in syringes or vials with insufficient radiation shielding. Beta-ray doses from a thin, unshielded source may be more than 50 times larger than the gamma-ray doses from the same source (2). Often, the operators are not always completely aware of the risks they are exposed to, especially when very high activities have to be handled. Radiation protection-specific recommendations concerning ^{90}Y are limited in the literature, which is mainly focused on important guidelines and calibration procedures, and on health care of patients and relatives. In particular, data reporting the absorbed doses to the most exposed tissues of the personnel as well as the effective doses are very rare (3,4).

One of the principal difficulties of determining beta-ray doses and their significance comes from the large variations of doses over short distances. Within tissue, this arises from the strong attenuation of beta radiation. An example is the dose distribution from beta contamination on the surface of the skin. In addition, the skin (particularly of the hands) is often irradiated by small-area sources at very short distances from the surface. Such doses may therefore be extremely non-uniform just for geometrical reasons.

As for conventional nuclear medicine, also for ^{90}Y there are three main principles concerning with radiation protection, time, distance, and shielding. Radiation exposure can be managed by one or more of these:

- Reducing the time of exposure reduces the dose proportionally
- Increasing distance reduces dose due to the inverse square law
- Adding shielding reduces radiation doses.

Practical radiation protection tends to be a job of dodging the three factors to identify the most cost-effective solution. An example of reducing radiation doses by reducing the time of exposures might be improved through the operator training to minimize the time necessary to handle a source. Distance can be as simple as handling a source with forceps rather than fingers. Shielding consist of an appropriate Plexiglas shielding for the entire β-emitting solution.

During the different phases of PRRT therapy, the hospital personnel (radiochemists, physicians, nursing staff) may be exposed to intense radiation fields, and specific radiation protection procedures need to be designed and strictly observed.

Occupational radiation exposure in PRRT may occur by direct beta radiation (electron irradiation and contamination) and by Bremsstrahlung (that is the secondary photon radiation, x-ray, produced by the deceleration of beta particles as they pass through matter). The Bremsstrahlung spectrum characteristics depend on the medium the beta particles pass through.

Three principal phases in which the radiation risk can vary significantly are identified:

1. the preparation of the radiopharmaceutical (labelling procedure and splitting in syringes/vials in the radiochemistry hot laboratory)
2. administration (locoregional or systemic injections)
3. the hospitalization of the patient.

The intensity of the radiation field varies in all of these phases. The inhalation of the radiopharmaceuticals is considered to be negligible, being ^{90}Y not volatile

Routinely, at European Institute of Oncology, an activity of $\sim$26 GBq is manipulated at the same time for the treatment of eight patients receiving a systemic injection of $\sim$3.0 GBq and of two patients receiving a locoregional injection of $\sim$0.4 GBq. Therefore, considerable activities of ^{90}Y are manipulated simultaneously by the radiochemists and the operators, who become exposed to intense electron and Bremsstrahlung radiation field. In this chapter we describe the radiation protection procedures carried out during each step of PRRT. The overall risks involved and the efficacy of the adopted radiation protection procedures are reported.

SHIELDING REQUIREMENTS

The maximum range of the electron beta particles emitted by ^{90}Y in air is 9 m, in water 11.3 mm (1); the effective path length in water, which corresponds to the radius of the sphere in which 90% of emitted energy are deposited, is of 5.3 mm.

Due to the Bremsstrahlung generated by the interaction of the high energy β particles of ^{90}Y, high-atomic-number materials, such as lead and tungsten, are not appropriate. The cross section for Bremsstrahlung production increases with beta particles energy and with the atomic number, Z, of the medium. For example, Bremsstrahlung production is much more likely in lead ($Z = 82$) than in a low atomic number medium such as water, tissue, or plastic ($Z \cong 8$). In the case of ^{90}Y, the percentage of the total β-energy that is converted to Bremsstrahlung in a material with a Z of 7.9 is only 0.6%, while in lead it is approximately 6%. The lead or tungsten shields that are commonly used in nuclear medicine are not appropriate for shielding ^{90}Y.

Materials with a low atomic number, such as plastic or acrylics, are ideal shields for ^{90}Y: the total absorption of the radiation is obtained with 4.9 mm of glass or 9.2 mm of PMMA (1). The use of acrylic or composite vial shields and syringe shields reduced the radiation levels from 2.4 mGy h^{-1} GBq^{-1} to 1 μGy h^{-1} GBq^{-1} and from 11.2 mGy h^{-1} GBq^{-1} to 3 μGy h^{-1} GBq^{-1} (5), respectively.

Beddoe (6) has performed an in-depth study on dose rate to the skin for different kinds of syringes containing ^{90}Y: the results, listed in Table 1, are expressed in terms of mGy/h per unit concentration (MBq/g) of ^{90}Y radio-pharmaceutical inside the syringe. The radii (r) and wall thickness (t) considered are those of commonly supplied polypropylene syringes.

LOCAL SKIN DOSE

The appropriate measure for local skin dose in beta-radiation fields is the personal dose equivalent, Hp (0.07); that is the equivalent dose averaged over an area of

Table 1 Basal Layer (20 μm) Dose Rates in the Skin for Unshielded Polypropylene Syringe for ^{90}Y, Considering the Radius (r) and the Thickness (t) of the Syringe

Syringe (ml)	r (mm)	t (mm)	mGy/h per MBq/g
1	2.3	1.00	770
2	4.5	0.65	1350
2.5	4.45	1.40	780
5	6.42	0.79	1320

Source: From Ref. 6.

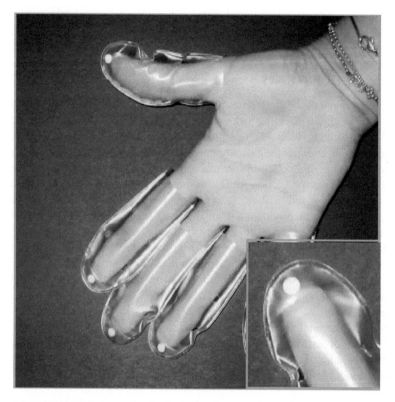

Figure 1 Fingertip monitoring: plastic thimbles containing TLD detectors (100 LiF chips) used to measure the dose to the fingertips during labelling and l.r. injection.

1 cm^2 of skin at a nominal depth of 0.07 mm and at a specified point of interest. Since irradiation of the hands can be very inhomogeneous, it is not appropriate to determine the average dose, as can be measured for instance by means of a ring containing a TLD detector, but it is indispensable to try to find and to eveluate the maximum value, usually corresponding to the fingertips. At the European Institute of Oncology, the measurement of the local skin dose during the different phases of the procedures was carried on by thermoluminescence detectors (TLD-LiF) placed in plastic thimbles (Fig. 1).

RADIOPHARMACEUTICAL PREPARATION: RADIATION PROTECTION IN THE HOT LAB

Major exposure risk occurs during the preparation of the radiopharmaceutical; the absorbed dose to radiochemist's hands, that can be very high, must be carefully monitored. It is therefore essential to optimise the shielding systems and to minimise the manipulation time. The main part of the exposure is caused by direct beta radiation from ^{90}Y.

Generally, the radiopharmaceutical preparation consists of the following steps: the verification of the provided activity of ^{90}Y with an appropriate calibrator, the labelling of the molecules with ^{90}Y, the chemical quality control of the radiopharmaceutical, and the fractionation of the product in the activities specifically prescribed for each patient.

The radiation protection principles suggest different considerations.

The labelling procedures must be performed in a dedicated hot cell for the manipulation of high energy β-emitters, whose walls must be made of materials capable of shielding both ^{90}Y β-rays and Bremsstrahlung. Typically, the observation window is made of plexiglas 10 mm thick and is further covered by 3 layers of leaded glass (equivalent to 2–3 mm of Pb), respectively to stop ^{90}Y β-rays and to minimize Bremsstrahlung. For the same reason the walls of the cell are made of a low atomic number material (PMMA) (1–2 cm thick) and covered with 2 mm of lead.

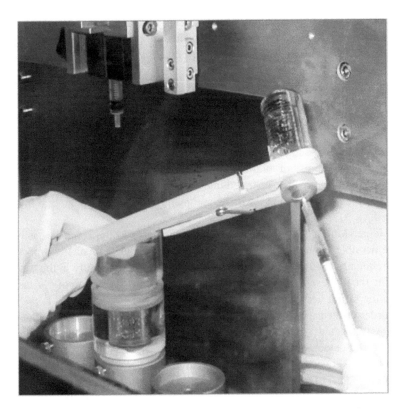

Figure 2 Labelling procedure: manipulation of the vial with the use of tongs.

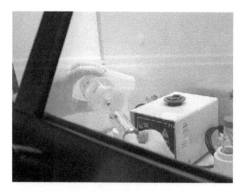

Figure 3 Labelling procedure: the vial containing ^{90}Y is shielded by a PMMA container (2 cm thick) with a hole in the lid for insertion of the needle of the syringe.

During the procedure, the radiochemist wears x-ray protection gloves made of leaded rubber (0.1 mm Pb eq.) currently used in interventional radiology to reduce the exposure to β-particles, as well as latex gloves to avoid any contamination.

Notably, tongs and adequate PMMA shields (thickness almost 1 cm) for both vials and syringes are strongly recommended during both radiolabelling and administration. In particular, long tongs (Fig. 2) have to be used to transfer the ^{90}Y vial to the dose calibrator, and then to insert it in a dedicated PMMA container (walls 2 cm thick) with a hole in the lid (Fig. 3).

For safety purposes, it's advisable that a second operator supervises the whole radiochemical procedure, in order to avoid oversights and to intervene in case of need.

Manipulation time must be minimized, and this goal can be achieved by an adequate training. The use of automatic fractionation systems is mandatory; the whole radiopharmaceutical is separated into the prescribed fractions—by weight and activity of the total solution—with an automatic system (Fig. 4), housed into the hot cell.

A Geiger-Müller survey meter should be available in the room to easily check the possible contamination of the hands of the radiochemist. It's a good habit to frequently check for possible hand contamination, especially in the case of changing the gloves, because a small drop of a concentrate solution of ^{90}Y can release to the skin a very high dose (see below).

In order to measure the absorbed dose to the fingertips, where the highest exposure is expected (Fig. 1), the radiochemist wears thin plastic thimbles containing TLD-detectors (100 LiF chips) during the whole labelling procedure.

Table 2a shows the absorbed doses to the fingertips during labelling procedures at IEO; TLDs lectures are reported according to the use/non-use of the automatic fractionation system. The measurements evidenced a wide range of doses, strongly influenced by personal skill, experience, and any slight mishap.

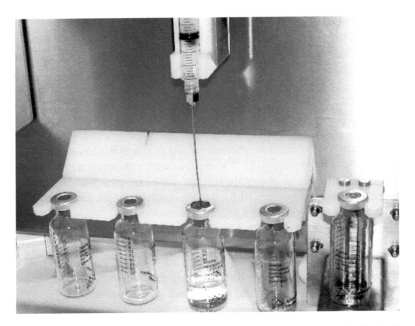

Figure 4 Labelling procedure: automatic dose fractionation system inside the hot cell. The activity of the whole volume of the solution is fractionated by weight and activity into the activities prescribed for each patient.

Therefore, the maximum values of the doses reported in Table 2a are very different from the mean values and do not represent accidents or serious problems encountered, but the occurrence of minor influencing events, and/or an incomplete respect of the radiation protection indications. In any case, the PMMA shield containing ^{90}Y- vials and syringes, the hot cell, the automatic system for fractionation, and the anti-X gloves demonstrated to be useful devices for radiation protection optimization. In particular, the dose fractionation system provided a mean 60% reduction of fingertips doses. These results pointed out that the use of standard TLD ring dosimeters does not give a correct estimation of the electron field contribution, with the consequence of a consistent underestimation

Table 2a Absorbed Dose to Fingertips (mGy) During Single Labelling Procedures

Labelling procedures	Dose (mGy)		
	Mean	Median	Max
With automatic fractionation[a]	0.6	0.4	31.2
Without automatic fractionation[a]	1.6	1.1	34.1

[a] Data normalized to the manipulation of 3.0 GBq of ^{90}Y-PRRT.

of the local absorbed dose to the parts of the hands nearer to or in contact with the sources. Therefore, we suggest the regular monitoring of the fingertip doses.

The effective dose to the radiochemist, measured with the standard film-badge, is negligible (<10 μSv/labelling), as expected.

DOSE CALIBRATOR

During the preparation of the radiopharmaceutical attention has to be paid to the dose calibrator; accurately assaying ^{90}Y requires appropriate calibration setting for ^{90}Y for each different geometry. In fact, the dose calibrator measurement of emitting radionuclides is influenced by the Bremsstrahlung produced from the interaction of the β particles with the source matrix, its container, and the calibrator chamber wall. The use of different volumes or containers may result in measurement errors. The dose calibrator must be calibrated for ^{90}Y by using the actual geometry and volume of the administered dose. Even if a particular dose calibrator does feature a setting for ^{90}Y, the dial in the manufacturer's instruction manual might not have been determined with the same geometry of the vial/syringe that will be used for patients in that facility. In any case, there are several articles that explain how to deal with this problem (7–10).

DOSE TO SKIN DUE TO CONTAMINATION

Skin dose due to contamination is very difficult to measure directly and is usually estimated. As a suggestion, we report one of the methods proposed in the literature (11). The dose is referred to the basal layer of the skin (depth 70 μm). The contribution of Bremsstrahlung to the dose rate, of the order of few percent, is generally neglected. The contamination is supposed to be uniformly and thiny spread over the skin. The equation is:

$$H_{T(skin)} = \frac{C_{skin} \cdot CF_{Beta-skin} \cdot t}{SF_{Beta}}$$

Where

$H_{T(skin)}$ = Equivalent dose to the skin (μGy)
C_{skin} = Average surface concentration of radionuclide on skin or clothing (Bq/cm^2);
$CF_{Beta-skin}$ = Conversion factor: skin beta dose rate (for ^{90}Y is equal to 2.0 (μGy/h)/(Bq/cm^2));
SF_{Beta} = Shielding factor for beta radiation due to clothing; representative values of shielding factors are approximately 3–5 for light clothing and 1000 for heavy clothing
t = Time of exposure (h).

The beta dose rate to the skin expressed in terms of average surface concentrations of a radionuclide on the skin gives more reliable estimates for this exposure pathway. However, the data in the literature vary as much as an order of magnitude.

RADIATION PROTECTION DURING THE INFUSION

The administration of the radiopharmaceutical is normally carried out in a Nuclear Medicine Department, where standard radiation protection procedures are enforced and are generally respected.

The radiopharmaceutical can be administered systemically (i.v.) or locoregionally into the brain (l.r.) by a slow infusion or a bolus injection. The radiation field outside the patient is due only to the Bremsstrahlung produced in the patient (i.v. and l.r.) and in catheters (i.v. only).

SYSTEMIC INFUSION

In the i.v. injection, slow infusion (10 to 30 minutes) is prescribed for high activities. The radiopharmaceutical is infused by means of an appropriate catheter system previously connected. The physician does not handle any "hot" tubing, connecting all the catheters when are cold and starting the infusion keeping tabs on the injection one meter from the patient.

The vial containing ^{90}Y has to be properly shielded; it has to be inserted inside the PMMA shield and further surrounded by a lead shield to reduce the Bremsstrahlung produced in glass and plexiglas PMMA (Fig. 5). Protective aprons (0.5 mm Pb equivalent) are efficient to reduce low energy components in the Bremsstrahlung spectrum (the spectrum is characterised by a maximum at ~ 80 keV and very few photons > 300 keV).

With this infusion set up, radiation dose for the personnel who administer the radiopharmaceutical or assist the patient is very low (absorbed doses: physician's hands < 0.1 mGy/patient; nurse's thorax < 5 μGy/patient).

LOCOREGIONAL INFUSION

In the l.r. administrations, the physician injects, in few seconds, small volumes of radiopharmaceutical using the shielded syringe (PMMA), wearing anti-X gloves, and handling tongs to hold the filter between syringe and injection site (Fig. 6).

The locoregional administration has been identified as one of the procedures at highest risk, so the absorbed doses to finger tips of the physician were measured by TLD-LiF dosimeters placed in plastic thimbles (Fig. 1). Table 2b reports the corresponding absorbed doses. Results show a significant 75% dose reduction when tongs and shielded syringes were used.

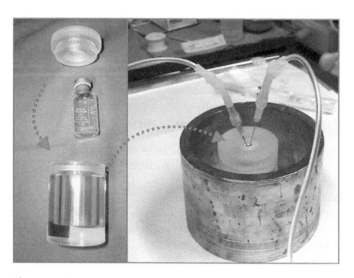

Figure 5   Systemic administration: the radiopharmaceutical is provided in a vial shielded by a PMMA sleeve (1 cm thick), further surrounded by lead (1 cm thick). A double catheter system is used, one going from the cold physiological serum to the ^{90}Y vial, and the other from the ^{90}Y vial to the patient.

The maximum values of the doses reported in Table 2b, as for the data in Table 2a, do not represent accidents or serious problems encountered, but the occurrence of minor influencing events.

PATIENT HOSPITALIZATION

After injection, patients are hospitalised in special rooms of the radio-immunotherapy ward until they reach the discharge conditions established by local radiation protection laws. Inpatient rooms did not require fixed radiation monitors or particular shielding, but the toilets were connected to a tank system for the collection and decay of contaminated excreta, containing a very large amount of radioactivity. Adult relatives, excluding pregnant women, were allowed to assist the patients.

The PRRT therapies are characterised by a very rapid elimination from the body by the urine pathway. More than 70% of injected activity is usually excreted within the first 24 hours.

The low-intensity radiation field mainly due to Bremsstrahlung emerging from the patient after the injection represents a consistent advantage from the point of view of radiation protection. This can also be inferred from the specific Bremsstrahlung constant for ^{90}Y in soft tissue ($\sim 1.4 \times 10^{-4}$ $C \cdot kg^{-1} \cdot cm^2 \cdot MBq^{-1} \cdot h^{-1}$ (12)). For this reason, restrictive radiation precautions for patient management (as in the case of ^{131}I) are not required. The only precaution required

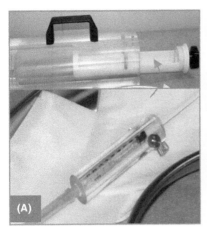
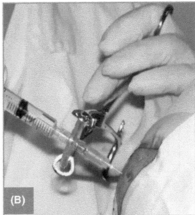

Figure 6 Locoregional administration (l.r.). (**A**) The radiopharmaceutical is provided in a PMMA shielded syringe (1 cm thick), subsequently inserted inside a PMMA case (2 cm thick) for transport. (**B**) The radiopharmaceutical is gently injected into the brain cavity through a catheter. Tongs are used to hold the filter.

is to avoid contamination from biological fluids, which can be easily done with the use of disposable coverings (e.g. latex gloves).

The air kerma rate measured around patients (Fig. 7) indicates low risk even shortly after the administration, lower than the air kerma rates related to the most common nuclear medicine examinations. The air kerma rate data can be used to estimate the effective dose to the relatives, based on the specific situation. Effective dose limits of 3 mSv (family members) and of 0.3 mSv/yr (population, as suggested by EC Radiation Protection 1997) were guaranteed as patients were hospitalized for almost six hours (l.r. PRRT) and for 48 hours (i.v. PRRT).

The prescription of almost two days of hospitalization, adopted in our center, is basically related not to real safety requirements but to the Italian regulation (13), which is very restrictive on the amount of radioactivity disposable in the environment. The recent radiation protection criteria presented in the publication ICRP 94 (14) offer detailed indications for the release of patients after

Table 2b Absorbed Dose (mGy) to Fingertips During Brain l.r. Injection

	Dose (mGy)		
Locoregional injection[a]	Mean	Median	Max
With the use of all devices	0.5	0.3	4.8
Without syringe shielding and tongs	1.9	0.9	30.7

[a] Data normalized to a single l.r. injection of 0.4 GBq of ^{90}Y-PRRT.

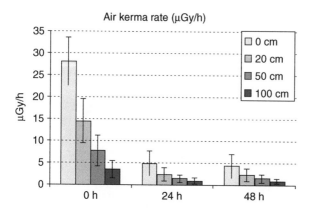

Figure 7   Air kerma rate around patients treated with systemic PRRT. The histogram shows the mean values ± 1 SD of the air kerma rate (µGy/h) at different distances from the patient and at different times from the injection. Data refer to 50 patients IV administered with 3.0 GBq for ^{90}Y-PRRT.

radionuclide therapy. This publication should represent the proper reference to establish the limits required, hopefully to be considered in a widely accepted radiation protection regulation.

CONCLUSIONS AND RECOMMENDATIONS

The manipulation of ^{90}Y may lead to high doses to the hands, particularly to the fingertips, if specific procedures and tools are not properly applied.

When all radiation protection devices are provided, the results confirm that radiolabelling, administration and hospitalization can be carried out under safe conditions, and that methods can be adopted which strongly reduce the radiation doses to the involved personnel.

Major attention has to be paid in the preparation and administration phases, due to the possible irradiation by a very intense high energy electron fluence. The use of an automatic fractionation system and of thick PMMA shields is strongly recommended, as well as the regular use of dedicated fingertip TLD dosimeters.

The data and the considerations reported may give useful information concerning the radiation protection optimization of the procedures to be adopted during different radionuclide therapies, with ^{90}Y and other beta-emitting radionuclides.

In the near future we foresee an increase in the number of therapeutical procedures with ^{90}Y-conjugates. Thus, a centralised radiopharmacy and/or a completely automatic labelling system is certainly advisable. This would allow a safe, widespread clinical use of radionuclide therapies with ^{90}Y-compounds.

REFERENCES

1. Delacroix D, Guerre JP, Leblanc P, Hickman C. Radionuclide and radiation protection data handbook 2002 (2nd edition). Radiat Prot Dosimetry 2002; 98:1–168.
2. International Commission on Radiation Units and Measurements. ICRU Report 56: Dosimetry of External Beta Rays for Radiation Protection 1997 Maryland (USA).
3. Aubert B, Guilabert N, Lamon A, Ricard M. Which protection against radiation for new protocols of internal radiotherapy by ^{90}Y. In: 6th European Alara Network workshop. Occupational Exposure Optimisation in the Medical Field and Radiopharmaceutical Industry. Proceedings, Madrid, 2002.
4. Tosi G. Report on one accident occurred in a nuclear medicine department in Italy. In: 6th European Alara Network workshop. Occupational Exposure Optimisation in the Medical Field and Radiopharmaceutical Industry. Proceedings, Madrid, 2002; 225.
5. Zimmer AM, Carey AM, Spies SM. Effectiveness of specific vial and syringe shields in reducing radiation exposure from Y-90 Zevalin. J Nucl Med 2002; 43:45.
6. Beddoe AH, Kelly MT. Absorbed dose in the skin from beta emitters in medical and laboratory containers. Br J Radiol 1994; 67:54–58.
7. Siegel JA, Zimmerman BE, Kodimer K, Dell MA, Simon MA. Accurate dose calibrator activity measurement of 90Y-ibritumomab tiuxetan. J Nucl Med 2004; 45:450–454.
8. Salako QA, DeNardo SJ. Radioassay of yttrium-90 radiation using the radionuclide dose calibrator. J Nucl Med 1997; 38:723–726.
9. Zimmerman BE, Cessna JT, Millican MA. Experimental determination of calibration settings for plastic syringes containing solutions of 90Y using commercial radionuclide calibrators. Appl Radiat Isot 2004; 60:511–517.
10. Zimmerman BE, Cessna JT. Experimental determinations of commercial dose calibrator settings for nuclides used in nuclear medicine. Appl Radiat Isot 2000; 52:615–619.
11. RADAR (Radiation Dose Assessment Resource) Stabin M, Siegel J, Lipsztein J, et al. www.doseinfo-radar.com; www.ieo.it/radar.
12. Zanzonico PB, Binkert BL, Goldsmith SJ. Bremsstrahlung radiation exposure from pure beta-ray emitters. J Nucl Med 1999; 40:1024–1028.
13. Decreto Legislativo 26 maggio 2000, n. 187. Attuazione della direttiva 97/43/EURATOM in materia di protezione sanitaria delle persone contro i pericoli delle radiazioni ionizzanti connesse ad esposizioni mediche.
14. International Commission on Radiological Protection. Release of Patients after Therapy with Unsealed Radionuclides. ICRP publication 94. New York: Pergamon Press 2005. www.elsevier.com.

16

Regulatory Requirements for Therapy Trials

Giampiero Tosi

Medical Physics Department, European Institute of Oncology, Milan, Italy

INTRODUCTION

The need of a widely accepted regulation in the field of medical and biomedical research has become more and more evident after the Second World War.

The first ethical code may be considered *The Code of Nuremberg* (1) (1946) that was written as an answer to the terrible violations of the human rights reported and discussed during the homonymous trial. This Code described the "permissible Medical Experiments" and their main ethical criteria:

1. The voluntary consent of the human subject is absolutely essential.
2. The experiment should be such as to yield fruitful results for the good of society, unprocurable by other methods or mean of study, and not random and unnecessary in nature.
3. The experiment should be so designed and based on the results of animal experimentation and a knowledge of the natural history of the disease or other problems under study that the anticipated results will justify the performance of the experiment.
4. The experiment should be conducted as to avoid all unnecessary physical and mental suffering and injury.
5. No experiment should be conducted where there is an a priori reason to believe that death or disabling injury will occur, except, perhaps, in those experiments where the experimental physicians also serve as subjects.

6. The degree of risk to be taken should never exceed that determined by the humanitarian importance of the problem to be solved by the experiment.

7. Proper preparations should be made and adequate facilities provided to protect the experimental subject against even remote possibilities of injury, disability, or death.

8. The experiment should be conducted only by scientifically qualified persons. The highest degree of skill and care should be required through all stages of the experiment of those who conduct or are engaged in the experiment.

9. During the course of the experiment the human subject should be at liberty to bring the experiment to an end if he has reached the physical or mental state where continuation of the experiment seems to him to be impossible.

10. During the course of the experiment the scientist in charge must be prepared to terminate the experiment at any stage, if he has probably cause to believe, in the exercise of the good face, superior skill, and careful judgement required to him, that a continuation of the experiment is likely to result in injury, disability, or death to the experimental subject.

The following step was represented by the *World Medical Association Declaration of Helsinki* (2): *Ethical principles for medical research involving human subjects*, adopted by the 18th WMA General Assembly, Helsinki, Finland, June 1964, and amended in the following years, until 2000, by the 29th, 35th, 41st, 48th, 52nd Assemblies by the same organization. This Declaration is structured into three parts (A. Introduction, B. Basic Principles for all Medical Research, and C. Additional Principles for Medical Research combined with medical care).

Part C lists the general principles to be respected for all medical research involving directly the treatment of patients:

Additional Principles for Medical Research Combined with Medical Care

28. The physician may combine medical research with medical care, only to the extent that the research is justified by its potential prophylactic, diagnostic, or therapeutic value. When medical research is combined with medical care, additional standards apply to protect the patients who are research subjects.

29. The benefits, risks, burdens, and effectiveness of a new method should be tested against those of the best current prophylactic, diagnostic, and therapeutics methods. This does not exclude the use of placebo or no treatment, in studies where no proven prophylactic, diagnostic, or therapeutic method exists.

30. At the conclusion of the study, every patient entered into the study should be assured of the access to the best proven prophylactic, diagnostic, and therapeutic methods identified by the study.
31. The physician should fully inform the patient which aspects of the care are related to the research. The refusal of a patient to participate in a study must never interfere with the patient-physician relationship.
32. In the treatment of a patient, where proven prophylactic, diagnostic, and therapeutic methods do not exist or have been ineffective, the physician, with informed consent of the patient, must be free to use unproven or new prophylactic, diagnostic, and therapeutic measures, if in the physician's judgement it offers hope of saving life, re-establishing health or alleviating suffering. Where possible, these measures should be made the object of research, designed to evaluate their safety and efficacy. In all cases, new information should be recorded and, where appropriate, published. The other relevant guidelines of this Declaration should be followed.

JUSTIFICATION AND OPTIMIZATION IN THE USE OF IONIZING RADIATION FOR MEDICAL PURPOSES

Both the *Code of Nuremberg* and the *Declaration of Helsinki* state the general principles of the medical research involving human beings, but do not specifically deal with the use of ionizing radiation sources.

The use of ionizing radiation, including the use of radionuclides, on human beings has been the subject of specific recommendations; the first were prepared by WHO (World Health Organization), who in 1977 published a technical report (3). The main document on this topic was issued in 1992 by ICRP (International Commission on Radiological Protection), with *ICRP Publication 62: Radiological Protection in Biomedical Research* (4). In the first four chapters of this publication, the nature, types, and magnitude of radiation risks are described, the estimates for the threshold for deterministic effects in the adult human testes, ovaries, lens, and bone marrow are given, and the methodology of risk assessment both in external and internal irradiation is treated. Thereafter, the principles of research design involving use of ionizing radiation and the factors related to project evaluation are illustrated. Moreover, three categories of risk (trivial: $\leq 10^{-6}$; minor to intermediate: 10^{-5}–10^{-4}; moderate: 10^{-3} or more), the corresponding *effective dose* range (<0.1 mSv; 1–10 mSv; >10 mSv respectively), and the level of social benefit (minor, intermediate to moderate, substantial) are defined.

Based on the general principles of radiation protection stated by ICRP, the EU promulgated on 30 June 1997 the Council Directive 97/43/Euratom on health protection of the individuals against the dangers of ionizing radiation in relation to medical exposures (5): This Directive applies to the following medical exposures:

1. the exposure of patients as part of their own medical diagnosis or treatment.
2. the exposure of individuals as part of occupational health surveillance.
3. the exposure of individuals as part of health screening programs.
4. the exposure of healthy individuals or patients voluntarily participating in medical or biomedical, diagnostic or therapeutic, or research programs.
5. the exposure of individuals as part of medico-legal procedures.

The Directive states that the basic principles to be respected are those of *justification* and of *optimization*:

1. *Justification*: medical exposures shall show a sufficient net benefit, weighing the total potential diagnostic or therapeutic benefits it produces, including the direct health benefits to an individual and the benefits to society, against the individual detriment that the exposure might cause, taking into account the efficacy, benefits, and risks of available alternative techniques having the same objective but involving no or less exposure to ionizing radiation.
2. *Optimization*: For all medical exposure of individuals for radio-therapeutic purposes, exposures of target volumes shall be individually planned, taking into account that doses to non-target volumes and tissues shall be as low as reasonably achievable and consistent with the intended radiotherapeutic purpose of the exposure.

MEDICAL TRIALS WITH THE USE OF IONIZING RADIATION

According to the Directive 97/43, "in the case of patients who voluntarily accept to undergo an experimental diagnostic or therapeutic practice and who are expected to receive a diagnostic or therapeutical benefit from this practice, the target level of doses shall be planned on an individual basis by the practitioner and/or prescriber." For these patients, moreover, another "rule" must be respected: "medical exposure for biomedical and medical research shall be examined by an *ethics committee*, set up in accordance with national procedures and/or by the competent authorities."

Patients treated with radionuclides become themselves a "radiation source," thus giving rise to a radiation field around them, whose intensity depends on the type of radionuclide, on the injected activity, and on the time elapsed after the injection, and that can be dangerous for people close to these patients. In order to guarantee an adequate level of safety for these people (relatives, caregivers and any other persons coming in contact with the treated patient), the Directive states that:

1. *dose constraints* are established for exposure of those individuals knowingly and willingly helping (other than a part of their occupation) in the support and comfort of patients undergoing medical diagnosis or treatment, where appropriate
2. in the case of patients undergoing a treatment or diagnosis with radionuclides, where appropriate the practitioner or the holder of the radiological installation provides the patient or legal guardian with *written instructions*, with a view to the restriction of doses to persons in contact with the patient, as far as reasonably achievable, and to provide information on the risks of ionizing radiation.

This last statement is an example of the application of another general principle of radiation protection, the so-called *ALARA principle*, according to which "any justified exposure must be maintained *As Low as Reasonably Achievable*," taking into account economic and social factors.

On the basis of Article 14 of the Directive "Member States shall bring into force the laws, regulations, and administrative provisions necessary to comply with this Directive before 13 May 2000. They shall forthwith inform the Commission thereof." The Directive 97/43 was applied in Italy with the Decreto Legislativo 26 maggio 2000, n. 187 "Attuazione della Direttiva 97/43 Euratom in materia di protezione sanitaria delle persone contro i pericoli delle radiazioni ionizzanti connesse ad esposizioni mediche" (6).

With regard to the therapy trials, this Italian law states that "le esposizioni di persone a scopo di ricerca scientifica clinica possono essere effettuate soltanto con il consenso scritto delle persone medesime, previa informazione sui rischi connessi con l'esposizione alle radiazioni ionizzanti" (The exposure of persons for sake of clinical scientific research can be carried out only with the written consent of the same persons, who must be informed in advance about the risks connected to the exposure to ionizing radiation). Moreover, in the Annex 1 to this law, it is established, among other things, that:

1. the *effective dose constraints* for each treatment cycle for the people assisting and comforting the treated patient are the following:
2. for adult people with an age <60 years: 3 mSv
3. for people with an age ≥ 60 years: 10 mSv
4. each cycle of treatment during a therapy trial must be carried out in a "protected department," with collection of the excreta of the patient.

According to the Directives of the European Community, a completion of the cited Decreto Legislativo 187/200 was promulgated in Italy in 2002, within the "Legge 1° marzo 2002, n. 39" (7). The article n. 39 of this law states, among other general rules concerning the exposure of persons for medical purposes, what follows:

General Principles and Consensus

Medical and biomedical research with ionizing radiation must be carried out in the respect of the general rules stated by the laws in the field of biomedical research; it must also comply with the principles of ICRP Publ. n. 62.

The exposure to ionizing radiation of volunteers participating to medical and biomedical research programs is allowed only after a freely expressed consent.

Authorization

Before starting a program of medical or biomedical research, the binding evaluation of the Committee of Ethics must be acquired. In its evaluation the Committee of Ethics shall take into account the general principles of ICRP 62 and the indications of the EC, given in the Publication Radiation Protection 99, *Guidance on medical exposures in medical and biomedical research* (8). The research plan, with enclosed the approval of the Committee of Ethics, must be notified to the ministry of Health at least thirty days before the beginning of the research.

The cited Publication 99 of the EC can be considered as the "bible" for everything that is concerned with the exposure to radiation for medical diagnosis and treatment and for medical and biomedical research with ionizing radiation. In particular, the 3rd Paragraph deeply treats the *Ethical Aspects*, and the 4th the *Risk Assessment*. From this point of view, great attention has to be given to item 42 and to the items from 48 to 53.

42. *Internal dosimetry* is necessary when using radiopharmaceuticals. For some radiopharmaceuticals there are established biokinetic models and published data enabling mean organ doses and effective doses to be derived from knowledge of the administered activity (ICRP 53 & ICRP 62). However, disturbed organ function in disease must be taken into account. For new radiopharmaceuticals, dosimetry may be based on animal experiments, but should be tested in pilot research on humans (also subject to requirements of paragraph 28) before any extensive investigation is planned. Even when using radioactive substances in tracer amounts the absorbed dose should still be assessed. Dosimetry calculation should always be performed and taken into account so that risks are known and not unduly dismissed.

RISK CATEGORIZATION (BASED ON ICRP 62)

48. To assist those planning research, and also research/ethics committees and/or competent authority, categorization of projects depending on the radiation dose to be received by each subject is useful. This is given by Table 1.

Table 1 Categories of Levels of Benefits and Corresponding Level of Risk for Healthy Adults Under 50 Years (Based on International Commission on Radiological Protection 62)

Level of social benefit	Risk level corresponding to the benefit	Risk category		Corresponding effective dose range (adults)—mSv[a]
Minor	Trivial	Category I	$\approx 10^{-6}$ or less	<0.1
Intermediate to moderate	Minor to intermediate	Category II		
		IIa	$\approx 10^{-5}$	0.1–1
		IIb	$\approx 10^{-4}$	1–10
Substantial	Moderate	Category III	$\approx 10^{-3}$ or more	$>10^{b}$

In the case of children they should be reduced by a factor of 2 or 3.
[a] To be kept below deterministic threshold except for therapeutics experiments.
[b] These figures can be increased by a factor of 5–10 for those over 50 years.

49. *Category I: Effective doses less than 0.1 mSv (adults)*: This category involves a risk (total risk from radiation exposure) for normal subjects of the order of one in a million or less. This level of risk is considered to be trivial; the level of benefit needed as the basis for approval for such investigation will be minor and would include those investigations expected "only to increase knowledge."

50. *Category IIa: Effective dose range 0.1–1 mSv (adults)*: This category involves risks of the order of one in a hundred thousand. In order to justify such risks the benefit of a research project should probably be related to "increases in knowledge leading to health benefit."

51. *Category IIb: Effective dose range 1–10 mSv (adults)*: This category involves risks to the irradiated individual of the order of one in ten thousands. The degree of benefit to society from studies in this category should be "moderate"; the benefit would be expected to be "aimed directly at the diagnosis, cure or prevention of the disease."

52. *Category III: Effective doses greater than 10 mSv (adults)*: Here the risks of the irradiated individual are estimated at greater than one in a thousand. This is a moderate risk for a single exposure but might be considered as verging on the unacceptable for continued or repeated exposure. To justify investigations in this category the benefit would have to be "substantial and usually directly related to the saving of life or the prevention or mitigation of serious disease." Doses should be kept below the threshold for deterministic effects, unless these are necessary for the therapeutic effect.

53. Table 1 applies to adults under 50 years of age. For each of the above categories the dose figures could be increased by a factor from 5 to 10

for people aged 50 years or over. In the unlikely event of approval being granted for research on children, the corresponding dose figures should probably be reduced by a factor of 2 or 3.

REFERENCES

1. The Nuremberg Code [from Trials on War Criminals before the Nuremberg Military Tribunals under Control Council Law No. 10—Nuremberg. October 1946–April 1949. Washington D.C. U.S.G.P.O., 1949–1953].
2. Declaration of Helsinki, Ethical Principles for Medical Research Involving Human Subjects, Adopted by the 18th WMA General Assembly, Helsinki, Finland, June 1964, and amended by the, 29th WMA General Assembly, Tokyo, Japan, October 1975, 35th WMA General Assembly, Venice, Italy, October 1983, 41st WMA General Assembly, Hong Kong, September 1989, 48th WMA General Assembly, Somerset West, Republic of South Africa, October 1996, and the 52nd WMA General Assembly, Edinburgh, Scotland, October 2000, available at the following address: www.wma.net.
3. World Health Organization. Use of Ionising Radiation and Radionuclides on Human Beings for Medical Research, Training, and Non-medical Purposes. Technical Report Series No. 611, WHO, Geneva (1977).
4. International Commission on Radiological Protection (ICRP). Radiological Protection in Biomedical Research. ICRP Publ. 62, Annals of ICRP, 1993, 22; 22 Pergamon Press, Oxford, 1994.
5. Council Directive 97/43 Euratom of 30 June 1997 on health protection of individuals against the dangers of ionizing radiation in relation to medical exposure, and repealing Directive 84/466/Euratom, Official Journal of the European Communities No. L 180/22 (9.7.97).
6. Decreto Legislativo 26 maggio 2000, n. 187. Attuazione della Direttiva 97/43 Euratom in materia di protezione sanitaria delle persone contro i pericoli delle radiazioni ionizzanti connesse ad esposizioni mediche. Supplemento ordinario alla Gazzetta Ufficiale della Repubblica Italiana n. 157 del 7 luglio 2000.
7. Legge 1° marzo 2002, n. 39. Disposizioni per l'adempimento di obblighi derivanti dall'appartenenza dell'Italia alle Comunità Europee. Legge Comunitaria 2001—art. 39. Supplemento ordinario alla Gazzetta Ufficiale della Repubblica Italiana n. 72 del 26 marzo 2002.
8. EC Radiation Protection 99. Guidance on medical exposures in medical and Biomedical Research.

Pretargeted Peptide Delivery with Irreversible Antibody

David A. Goodwin

Stanford University, Stanford and VA Palo Alto Health Care System, Palo Alto, California, U.S.A.

Claude F. Meares

Chemistry Department, University of California Davis, Davis, California, U.S.A.

INTRODUCTION

Radiopeptide Therapy

Studies on the biology of cell signaling have led to the discovery of a large number of extra-cellular peptide signaling molecules (1). These small molecules act on multiple targets in the human body at a distance in the circulation at very low concentrations ($<10^{-8}$ M). They are tightly bound to their receptors ($K_a \geq 10^8$), and they control and modulate the function of almost all key organs and metabolic processes (2). In many cases the regulatory peptide action is mediated through specific membrane-bound receptors, often of the G-protein coupled type, with seven trans-membrane helical domains. This cell receptor specificity gives these peptides great potential usefulness in cancer diagnosis and therapy (3). Related potential targeting molecules include interleukins (4), integrin ligands (5), and regulatory molecules like fibroblast growth factor.

One of these peptides, somatostatin, has been engineered and commercially developed as the metabolically stable tumor imaging agent ^{111}In-DTPA-octreotide (6). It has been used successfully in humans to visualize neuroendocrine tumors expressing a high number of somatostatin receptors. Because a large number of the pathological conditions clearly visualized with ^{111}In-octreotide are malignant, an urgent need has arisen for a therapeutic beta-emitting form such as octreotide labeled with the ultra-stable chelate ^{90}Y-DOTA. ^{90}Y-DOTATOC is one such agent now being developed (7). This work clearly demonstrates the potential value of other radiolabeled receptor-specific peptides in cancer imaging and therapy.

Compared to mAbs, radiolabeled peptides have several advantages. They are simple, easily synthesized, and cheap. They are rapidly excreted, giving fast blood clearance and low normal tissue background so that early imaging is possible with short $t_{1/2p}$ radionuclides (8). Their low molecular weight and rapid diffusion from the blood into the tumor give quick uptake and homogeneous distribution of radiation in the tumor. Receptor specific binding may be followed by internalization resulting in prolonged retention and increased radiation dose.

Challenges for Radiopeptide Therapy

Two problems currently prevent radiopeptides from reaching their full potential in cancer therapy: (1) Low absolute tumor concentrations, and (2) High and prolonged renal uptake. Compared to these the other disadvantages are minor.

Rapid blood disappearance of radiopeptides gives very high tumor to blood ratios but makes high concentrations in the tumor difficult to attain. Peptides are metabolized in the cortex of the kidney, with up to 10% of the injected dose sequestered for a prolonged period delivering a relatively high radiation dose (9). Administration of large amounts of D-lysine lowers renal uptake but does not completely eliminate it (10). For octreotide and other radiopeptides to be more useful for therapy it will be necessary to find a way to increase the tumor uptake and decrease normal organ concentration, especially kidneys, to avoid renal toxicity (11).

Here we describe a potential pretargeting solution to the two main problems facing radiopeptide therapy noted above. It consists of a new 3-step peptide pretargeting platform: irreversible antibodies (iAb) to capture the payload (12), peptides for targeting (13), branched poly(ethylene)glycol (bPEG) for delivery (14), and specially reactive bifunctional chelates (*L) for carrying the radioactive payload (15). The incorporation of iAbs with infinite affinity is a major advance over anti-hapten Abs and avidin/streptavidin to capture and help to bind the payload irreversibly to cancer cells (16).

EVOLUTION OF PRETARGETING SYSTEMS

Pretargeted Monoclonal Antibodies

Pretargeting was introduced in 1986 to reduce normal tissue irradiation incurred during conventional radioimmunoimmaging (17,18). The method gave a dramatic increase in the tumor/background ratio over directly labeled mAb (Fig. 1) (19).

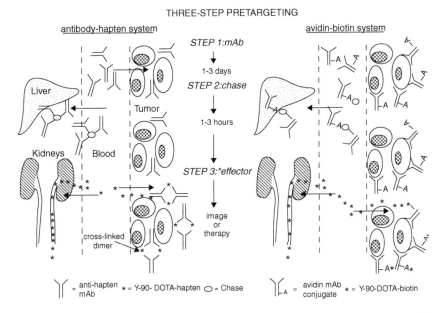

Figure 1 (*Left*): The antibody-hapten system: anti-hapten mAb, bivalent hapten. (*Right*): the avidin-biotin system: avidin-anti-tumor-mAb conjugate. The physiological compartments of importance to pretargeting are: the intravascular plasma compartment, represented by the central column with leaky capillary walls (dotted lines), the extracellular fluid as the spaces surrounding both the normal organs and tumor cells, and the intracellular compartment of the liver and kidneys.

A key kinetic feature shown in Figure 2 is the long circulation time (days) of the mAb targeting moiety giving sustained high blood concentration to drive diffusion of the targeting molecule from the blood into the target (20). This is a property shared by all agents that attain the highest target concentrations. Targeting molecules must have sufficient time in the blood to allow the slow process of diffusion to occur. This has prompted the use of various carriers and adjuvants for both small and large molecules that disappear too quickly from the blood, like stealth liposomes laced with PEG to escape the reticuloendothelial system (21), and PEGylated enzymes to reduce their immunogenicity (22). Conjugation of small chemotherapeutic drug molecules to large polymers like polylysine or polyethylene glycol is another example. In all cases the half-life in the blood is lengthened to give long-circulating derivatives (23).

Since 1986, over 235 papers have been published on pretargeting (PubMed, search term: 'pretarget*,' Feb. 22, 2006), making it one of the most intensely investigated new therapeutic antibody approaches. The hapten/ligand-antibody system (24) and the biotin-avidin system (25,26) comprise the majority of the reports published to date. Other investigators in several different mouse tumor models using a variety of pretargeting protocols have now verified the original

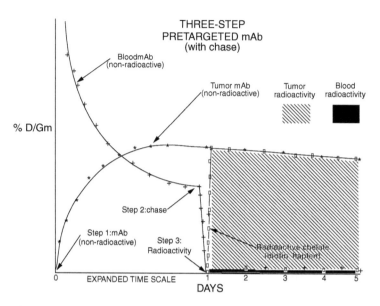

Figure 2 Diagram of the pharmacokinetics of 3-step pretargeting. At 21 hours (1 hour after chase) bivalent ^{90}Y -hapten was injected and the organs sampled at 24 hours 2, 3, 4, 5 days. Rapid uptake in tumor was seen at 3 hours and slow release of hapten from the tumor was demonstrated out to 5 days (shaded area). Note the large difference between the rates of diffusion of ^{90}Y into and out of the tumor: very rapid uptake (hours) compared to very slow loss (days) from the tumor. Blood levels were low at all times. *Source*: From Ref. 20.

reports of greatly improved therapeutic ratios (27–30). All the published methods use a long circulating conjugate to get high target uptake followed by a diffusible, rapidly excreted effector molecule, and they all give higher target to normal tissue ratios with less toxicity than conventional radioimmunotherapy.

Since cell membrane targets are present in extremely low concentrations ($\sim 10^{-9}$ M), the binding affinities for capture of effector molecules in pretargeting must be very high: Ab/hapten $K_a \sim 10^9$, Avidin/biotin $K_a \sim 10^{15}$ (31). Even with such high affinities the bound lifetime of the effector molecule is still not optimal for therapy. A solution to this problem has been provided by the creation of ligand/receptor pairs that associate irreversibly i.e., with infinite affinity (32) (see below).

Peptide Pretargeting

Radiolabeled peptides and mAbs have different advantages and weaknesses for therapy (10,33). Specifically, the long circulation time of mAbs is an advantage for producing high absolute tumor uptake. This feature of mAb targeting can be incorporated into peptide delivery by means of peptide conjugation to a suitable pretargeting carrier molecule. To use the targeting specificity of peptides, the proposed pretargeting method has multiple peptides conjugated to a long circulating bPEG molecule (34). Potentially this can produce high target concentrations comparable to mAbs.

For high target/background ratios, which is a major advantage of radiopeptides (35), a rapidly excreted radiochelate is used as the effector molecule, rather than directly labeled peptides. This method minimizes renal radiation, since radiolabeled chelates are not metabolized in the kidney. The properties of the chelates are listed in Table 1 (36).

Having several peptides per bPEG gives a multivalent targeting function with high avidity (37). Labeled peptides and pretargeted peptides are compared in Table 2.

Finally, a novel, irreversible chelate-binding antibody (iAb) is employed to capture and permanently bind the radiochelate in the tumor. The special features of this innovation are discussed briefly below.

Pretargeting depends on accessible, stable, and specific cell surface receptors for binding the pre-targeting molecule during the 24–48 hours localization phase (step 1). Some regulatory peptide receptors internalize in seconds after binding the cognate peptide (e.g., SSR and octreotide) (38,39), and if these are to be used successfully for pretargeting, ways must be found to slow or prevent this process. Conjugation of the peptides with bPEG may retard internalization, but on the other hand cross-linking on the cell surface is known to initiate or accelerate internalization in some cells. Non-internalizing cell surface markers include: CEA = carcinoembryonic antigen, TAG-72 = Tumor Associated Glycoprotein, CD20 = a B lymphocyte determinant, Fc R = Fc receptor, IL2R = interleukin 2 receptor, and the integrin ligands RGD and YIGSR. Rapidly internalizing receptors include: SSR = somatostatin receptor, VIPR = vasoactive intestinal peptide receptor, CD44R = Cell surface glyco-protein adhesion molecule, TNFR = Tumor Necrosis Factor Receptor and EGFR = Epithelial Growth Factor Receptor (40).

Table 1 Desirable Properties of Small Toxic Effector Molecules for Step 3 in Pretargeting

Chemical	Physiological
Low reactivity in plasma high in iAb	Binds irreversibly to iAb
Low molecular weight (small < 10 kDa)	Renal excretion exclusively
Hydrophilic	Solely GFR, no tubular binding
Rapidly diffusible	Extracellular distribution
Net negative charge	No protein binding in blood
High specific activity (≥ 100 Ci/mM)	No intracellular uptake
Choice of radionuclide	Non immunogenic
(bifunctional chelate)	

Table 2 Labeled Peptide Compared to Peptide-Branched Poly(Ethylene)Glycol-
Irreversible Antibodies Pretargeting

Directly labeled peptide	Pretargeted peptide
Very rapid blood disappearance ($T_{1/2}$ minutes) *High target/background ratio, high contrast imaging*	Slow blood disappearance ($T_{1/2}$ days) *High target uptake, high RAD*
Receptor specific, high affinity	Multivalent increased avidity, uptake, and retention
Low molecular weight, rapid diffusion into target	Effector molecule small, rapidly diffusing
Easy synthesis, genetically engineered, large libraries	Requires three reagents, multiple *i.v.* injections
High nontarget uptake in kidney (octreotide), lung (VIP)	Low non-target uptake, rapid renal excretion
May be physiologically toxic at *pM* concentrations	Conjugation may decrease toxicity
Low immunogenicity	Low immunogenicity
Cheap	Receptors that rapidly internalize may not work

Nevertheless, success in pretargeting a rapidly internalizing neurotensin receptor (NTR1) has been reported by de Boisferon et al. (41,42). Their in vitro cell-binding results showed a large fraction of the peptide bound to NTR1 was internalized: $>80\% \pm 4\%$. A similar fraction of the bound peptide was internalized when bivalent binding was allowed: $>90\% \pm 10\%$. In spite of these findings, dual targeting of NTR1 and CEA in human colorectal cancer xenografted nude mice, preinjected with anti-DTPA (indium) x anti-CEA BsmAb 24 hours *before* ^{111}In-labeled [Lys(DTPA)]-NT injection, had increased tumor uptake. ^{111}In-labeled [Lys(DTPA)]-NT was significantly higher ($p < 0.01$) than controls at 1, 3, and 24 hours post peptide injection (25, 27, and 48 hours post BsmAb). In addition, BsmAb pretargeting gave protracted tumor retention. The authors note the advantage of increased persistence in the tumor for radionuclide therapy. In the light of these findings, receptor internalization in vitro cannot be considered an absolute contraindication to pretargeting in vivo, especially with multivalent targeting conjugates. Pre-clinical mouse tumor studies will be necessary to assess these conjugates.

IRREVERSIBLE ANTIBODIES

Importance in Peptide Pretargeting

Antibodies developed earlier do not hold the radiometal long enough for therapeutic use. The anti-chelate antibody CHA255, initially developed for this purpose, possesses a high binding constant for (S)-benzyl-EDTA-indium and exquisite specificity for this hapten. On CHA255, the bound lifetimes of various indium chelates at 37°C were found to be in the 10–40 minutes range (43). While this is (barely) long enough to obtain good images for diagnosis, it is inconveniently short relative to other physiological time scales for the biodistribution of the chelate for therapy. The multivalent binding of antibody IgG molecules to cell surfaces can lead to bound lifetimes of several days, and modern bifunctional chelating agents hold their metals for even longer periods, so the most important challenge is to increase the antibody-chelate bound lifetime.

This requirement has led to the use of the long-lived avidin-biotin interaction, employing biotinylated metal chelates. However, avidin and strepta-vidin are both nonhuman proteins with immunogenic properties, and biotin is present in normal tissue. In contrast to avidin or streptavidin, which bind only biotin or its close analogs, antibodies can be prepared to bind specifically to one of a staggering variety of antigens. Thus, the original antibody-chelate association of CHA255 with indium chelates is an excellent basis for a new approach to extend the bound lifetime of the radiolabeled hapten by making the binding irreversible.

Using a structurally characterized antibody/ligand pair as an example, Meares et al. engineered complementary reactive groups in the antibody binding pocket and the chelate ligand so that they would be in close proximity in the antibody/ligand complex (Fig. 3).

The ligand's low reactivity prevents cross-reactions with other molecules in the medium. However, in the antibody/ligand complex the effective local concentrations of the complementary reactive groups are immense, allowing for a covalent reaction to link the two together. By eliminating the dissociation of the ligand from the antibody, the affinity becomes infinite, while the specificity is retained. This represents a major advance over both Ab/ligand and Avidin/biotin systems for capture and retention of the therapeutic effector molecules in pretargeting protocols (44).

The specially reactive irreversible ligand *L (^{111}In-AABE) had optimal biological properties for an effector molecule (Table 1). It was stable, hydrophilic, rapidly diffusible into the extracellular fluid (ECF), had high specific activity ($>$ 100 Ci/mmol), was rapidly excreted almost solely by the kidneys, had no protein binding in blood, little uptake in normal organs, and was non-immunogenic. We have previously described these properties for biotin-DOTA (45).

iAb can be used in pretargeting to replace the anti-hapten or avidin components but do not involve any foreign proteins, nor any interference or competition from binding with endogenous ligands (46). The Irreversible Antibody-bPEG-peptide platform (Fig. 4) is based on PEGylated human proteins, potentially eliminating problems with the immune system response to previous generations of drugs (47). Further, the radiolabeling linkage is much more stable than the streptavidin-biotin linkage. These add up to a substantial set of improvements which, we expect, will lead to much broader use of targeted imaging and therapy and the development of a broad range of unique and effective peptide based drugs in the future.

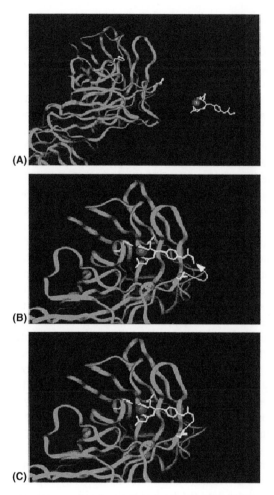

Figure 3 Requirements for an antibody with infinite affinity. (**A**) When the antibody and ligand are apart, their complementary reactive groups do not react significantly with other molecules in the blood. (**B**) When the ligand binds to the antibody, the effective concentrations of their complementary groups are sharply elevated, and a covalent link is formed. (**C**) The covalently linked antibody/ligand complex cannot dissociate. *Source*: From Ref. 32.

PEGYLATION

Branched Poly(Ethylene)Glycol

PEG conjugates are widely used in drug formulations to increase hydrophilicity, prolong circulation time (48), and decrease immunogenicity (49). It gives minimal interference with in vivo localization, enzyme function (50), or receptor binding.

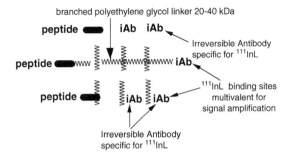

Figure 4 Branched 20–40 kD PEG-peptide platform for pretargeted therapy.

It also provides a long flexible spacer with low steric hindrance for binding reactions. The branched form of poly(ethylene)glycol (PEG) 20–40 kDa bPEG has eight equally spaced arms to provide linkers for the attachment of iAb, targeting peptides and optional synergistic functions (51). Smaller PEGs are available, but published results suggest these are not preferred for this application.

Addition of a branched 40 kDa PEG, or up to two 40 kDa branched PEG to a $F(ab')_2$, increased the serum half-life from 8.5 hours to 48 hours compared to the non-PEGylated $F(ab')_2$ (52). In reports of 271 randomly assigned patients with chronic hepatitis C and cirrhosis, once-weekly branched PEG (40 kDa) interferon alfa-2a conjugate (PEGASYS®)[a] (53) was significantly more effective than standard interferon alfa-2a administered three times weekly (54). PEG (40 kd) interferon alfa-2a was also non-toxic and non-immunogenic in 27 renal cell carcinoma patients with a similar safety profile to IFN alfa-2a (55). The proposed 3-step peptide pretargeting radionuclide therapy protocol is shown in Figure 5.

As already noted, the kidney is a major site of metabolism for peptides and uptake has correlated with the size of the peptide or polypeptide rather than its function. For example, antibody fragments, cytokines, and receptor-specific peptides are all concentrated in the kidney roughly in inverse proportion to their size (11,56). We believe the pretargeting methods using 20–40 kDa branched eight arm PEG conjugates and rapidly cleared effector molecules outlined here may reduce the renal uptake and potential toxicity seen with the use of peptides and mAb fragments in therapy. Long circulation of the iAb-bPEG-peptide conjugates may also increase the absolute amount and retention of therapeutic radionuclide in the target tumor.

CONCLUSIONS

1. The proposed method and system of 3-step iAb-bPEG-peptide pretargeting should retain the proven advantages of mAb pretargeting.

---

[a] Hoffman-La Roche, Nutley, NJ.

3-STEP PEPTIDE PRETARGETING

peptide-bPEG-iAb system

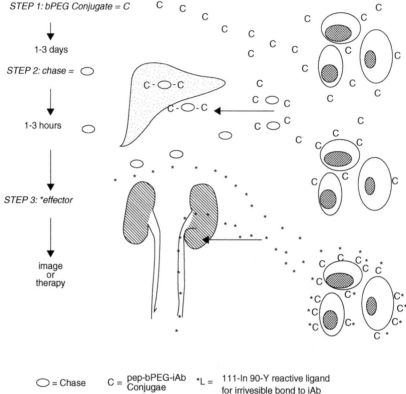

Figure 5 Proposed 3-step peptide pretargeting radionuclide therapy protocol.

The platform provides a long circulating carrier with the potential of high target concentration, rapid selective delivery of effector molecules, prolonged tumor retention, low renal uptake, and high target/background ratios

2. Synthesis of the peptide-bPEG-iAb platform uses readily obtainable, economical components and standard bioconjugate chemistry techniques

3. The bPEG carrier molecule and AABE-^{111}In have optimum pharmacokinetics for pretargeting. Non-, or slowly internalizing peptides are preferred, although preclinical mouse tumor biodistribution studies will be needed to properly assess rapidly internalizing peptides and to optimize the peptide-bPEG-iAb pretargeting parameters

4. Peptide pretargeting has great potential versatility because of the large choice of cell receptor specific peptides for targeting.

REFERENCES

1. Reubi JC. Peptide receptors as molecular targets for cancer diagnosis and therapy. Endocr Rev 2003; 24:389–427.
2. de Jong M, Krenning E. New advances in peptide receptor radionuclide therapy. J Nucl Med 2002; 43:617–620.
3. Chini B, Chinol M, Cassoni P, et al. Improved radiotracing of oxytocin receptor-expressing tumors using the new [111In]-DOTA-Lys8-deamino-vasotocin analogue. Br J Cancer 2003; 89:930–936.
4. Kobayashi H, Carrasquillo JA, Paik CH, Waldmann TA, Tagaya Y. Differences of biodistribution, pharmacokinetics, and tumor targeting between interleukins 2 and 15. Cancer Res 2000; 60:3577–3583.
5. Haubner R, Wester HJ, Burkhart F, et al. Glycosylated RGD-containing peptides: tracer for tumor targeting and angiogenesis imaging with improved biokinetics. J Nucl Med 2001; 42:326–336.
6. Kwekkeboom DJ, Krenning EP. Somatostatin receptor imaging. Semin Nucl Med 2002; 32:84–91.
7. Bodei L, Cremonesi M, Zoboli S, et al. Receptor-mediated radionuclide therapy with 90Y-DOTATOC in association with amino acid infusion: a phase I study. Eur J Nucl Med Mol Imaging 2003; 30:207–216.
8. Krenning EP, de Jong M, Kooij PP, et al. Radiolabelled somatostatin analogue(s) for peptide receptor scintigraphy and radionuclide therapy. Ann Oncol 1999; 10:S23–S29.
9. Rolleman EJ, Valkema R, de Jong M, Kooij PP, Krenning EP. Safe and effective inhibition of renal uptake of radiolabelled octreotide by a combination of lysine and arginine. Eur J Nucl Med Mol Imaging 2003; 30:9–15.
10. Bernard BF, Krenning EP, Breeman WA, et al. D-lysine reduction of indium-111 octreotide and yttrium-90 octreotide renal uptake. J Nucl Med 1997; 38:1929–1933.
11. Hammond PJ, Wade AF, Gwilliam ME, et al. Amino acid infusion blocks renal tubular uptake of an indium-labelled somatostatin analogue. Br J Cancer 1993; 67:1437–1439.
12. Meares CF, Chmura AJ, Orton MS, Corneillie TM, Whetstone PA. Molecular tools for targeted imaging and therapy of cancer. J Mol Recognit 2003; 16:255–259.
13. Kok RJ, Schraa AJ, Bos EJ, et al. Preparation and functional evaluation of RGD-modified proteins as alpha(v)beta(3) integrin directed therapeutics. Bioconjug Chem 2002; 13:128–135.
14. Goodwin DA, Song C, Meares CF. Pharmacokinetics of a Branched PEG Carrier for 3-Step Peptide Pretargeting of Tumors (Abstract), 11th International Symposium on Radiopharmacology. St. Louis, Missouri (USA): Quarterly Journal of Nuclear Medicine, 1999.
15. Chmura AJ, Schmidt BD, Corson DT, Traviglia SL, Meares CF. Electrophilic chelating agents for irreversible binding of metal chelates to engineered antibodies. J Control Release 2002; 78:249–258.
16. Goldenberg DM, Chang CH, Sharkey RM, et al. Radioimmunotherapy: is avidin-biotin pretargeting the preferred choice among pretargeting methods? Eur J Nucl Med Mol Imaging 2003; 30:777–780.
17. Goodwin DA, Mears CF, McTigue M, David GS. Monoclonal antibody hapten radiopharmaceutical delivery. Nucl Med Commun 1986; 7:569–580.

18. Goodwin DA, Meares CF, McTigue M, McCall MJ, David GS. Rapid localization of hapten in sites containing previously administered antibody for immunoscintigraphy with short half-life tracers (Abstract). J Nucl Med 1986; 27:958.

19. Goodwin DA, Meares CF, McCall MJ, McTigue M, Chaovapong W. Pre-targeted immunoscintigraphy of murine tumors with indium-111- labeled bifunctional haptens. J Nucl Med 1988; 29:226–234.

20. Goodwin DA. Pretargeting: almost the bottom line. J Nucl Med 1995; 36:876–879.

21. Janssen AP, Schiffelers RM, ten Hagen TL, et al. Peptide-targeted PEG-liposomes in anti-angiogenic therapy. Int J Pharm 2003; 254:55–58.

22. Cheng TL, Chen BM, Chan LY, Wu PY, Chern JW, Roffler SR. Poly(ethylene glycol) modification of beta-glucuronidase-antibody conjugates for solid-tumor therapy by targeted activation of glucuronide prodrugs. Cancer Immunol Immunother 1997; 44:305–315.

23. Veronese FM. Peptide and protein PEGylation: a review of problems and solutions. Biomaterials 2001; 22:405–417.

24. Janevik-Ivanovska E, Gautherot E, Hillairet de Boisferon M, et al. Bivalent hapten-bearing peptides designed for iodine-131 pretargeted radioimmunotherapy. Bioconjug Chem 1997; 8:526–533.

25. Hnatowich DJ, Fritz B, Virzi F, Mardirossian G, Rusckowski M. Improved tumor localization with (strept)avidin and labeled biotin as a substitute for antibody. Nucl Med Biol 1993; 20:189–195.

26. Hnatowich DJ, Virzi F, Rusckowski M. Investigations of avidin and biotin for imaging applications. J Nucl Med 1987; 28:1249–1302.

27. Paganelli G, Riva P, Deleide G, et al. In vivo labeling of biotinylated antibodies by radioactive avidin: a strategy to increase tumor localization. Int J Cancer 1988; 2:121–125.

28. Paganelli G, Chinol M. Radioimmunotherapy: is avidin-biotin pretargeting the preferred choice among pretargeting methods? Eur J Nucl Med Mol Imaging 2003; 30:773–776.

29. Le Doussal JM, Chetanneau A, Gruaz-Guyon A, et al. Bispecific monoclonal antibody-mediated targeting of an indium-111- labeled DTPA dimer to primary colorectal tumors: pharmacokinetics, biodistribution, scintigraphy and immune response. J Nucl Med 1993; 34:1662–1671.

30. Boerman OC, van Schaijk FG, Oyen WJ, Corstens FH. Pretargeted radio-immunotherapy of cancer: progress step by step. J Nucl Med 2003; 44:400–411.

31. Paganelli G, Pervez S, Siccardi AG, et al. Intraperitoneal radio-localization of tumors pre-targeted by biotinylated monoclonal antibodies. Int J Cancer 1990; 45:1184–1189.

32. Chmura AJ, Orton MS, Meares CF. Antibodies with infinate affinity. Proc Natl Acad Sci USA 2001; 98:8480–8484.

33. Subbiah K, Hamlin DK, Pagel JM, et al. Comparison of immunoscintigraphy, efficacy, and toxicity of conventional, and pretargeted radioimmunotherapy in CD20-expressing human lymphoma xenografts. J Nucl Med 2003; 44:437–445.

34. Veronese FM, Sacca B, Polverino de Laureto P, et al. New PEGs for peptide and protein modification, suitable for identification of the PEGylation site. Bioconjug Chem 2001; 12:62–70.

35. Pavlinkova G, Batra SK, Colcher D, Booth BJ, Baranowska-Kortylewicz J. Constructs of biotin mimetic peptide with CC49 single-chain Fv designed for tumor pretargeting. Peptides 2003; 24:353–362.

36. Moi MK, DeNardo SJ, Meares CF. Stable bifunctional chelates of metals used in radiotherapy. Cancer Res 1990; 50:789s–793s.

37. Rossi EA, Sharkey RM, McBride W, et al. Development of new multivalent-bispecific agents for pretargeting tumor localization and therapy. Clin Cancer Res 2003; 9:3886S–3896S.

38. De Jong M, Bernard BF, De Bruin E, et al. Internalization of radiolabelled [DTPA0]octreotide and [DOTA0,Tyr3]octreotide: peptides for somatostatin receptor-targeted scintigraphy and radionuclide therapy. Nucl Med Commun 1998; 19:283–288.

39. Parker SL, Kane JK, Parker MS, Berglund MM, Lundell IA, Li MD. Cloned neuropeptide Y (NPY) Y1 and pancreatic polypeptide Y4 receptors expressed in Chinese hamster ovary cells show considerable agonist- driven internalization, in contrast to the NPY Y2 receptor. Eur J Biochem 2001; 268:877–886.

40. Sundberg AL, Blomquist E, Carlsson J, Steffen AC, Gedda L. Cellular retention of radioactivity and increased radiation dose. Model experiments with EGF-dextran. Nucl Med Biol 2003; 30:303–315.

41. Hillairet De Boisferon M, Raguin O, Thiercelin C, et al. Improved tumor selectivity of radiolabeled peptides by receptor and antigen dual targeting in the neurotensin receptor model. Bioconjug Chem 2002; 13:654–662.

42. Buchegger F, Bonvin F, Kosinski M, et al. Radiolabeled neurotensin analog, 99mTc-NT-XI, evaluated in ductal pancreatic adenocarcinoma patients. J Nucl Med 2003; 44:1649–1654.

43. Meyer DL, Fineman M, Unger BW, Frincke JM. Kinetics of the dissociation of indium-(p-substituted-benzyl)ethylenediaminetetraacetic acid hapten analogues from the monoclonal anti-hapten antibody CHA255. Bioconjug Chem 1990; 1:278–284.

44. Green NM. Avidin. Adv Prot Chem 1975; 29:85–133.

45. Goodwin DA, Meares CF, Osen M. Biological properties of biotin-chelate conjugates for pretargeted diagnosis and therapy with the avidin/biotin system. J Nucl Med 1998; 39:1813–1818.

46. Rusckowski M, Fogarasi M, Fritz B, Hnatowich DJ. Effect of endogenous biotin on the applications of streptavidin and biotin in mice. Nucl Med Biol 1997; 24:263–268.

47. Goodwin DA, Meares CF. Pretargeted peptide imaging and therapy. Cancer Biother Radiopharm 1999; 14:145–152.

48. Lee LS, Conover C, Shi C, Whitlow M, Filpula D. Prolonged circulating lives of single-chain Fv proteins conjugated with polyethylene glycol: a comparison of conjugation chemistries and compounds. Bioconjug Chem 1999; 10:973–981.

49. Caliceti P, Chinol M, Roldo M, et al. Poly(ethylene glycol)-avidin bioconjugates: suitable candidates for tumor pretargeting. J Control Release 2002; 83:97–108.

50. Sawa T, Wu J, Akaike T, Maeda H. Tumor-targeting chemotherapy by a xanthine oxidase-polymer conjugate that generates oxygen-free radicals in tumor tissue. Cancer Res 2000; 60:666–671.

51. Monfardini C, Schiavon O, Caliceti P, Morpurgo M, Harris JM, Veronese FM. A branched monomethoxypoly(ethylene glycol) for protein modification. Bioconjug Chem 1995; 6:62–69.

52. Koumenis IL, Shahrokh Z, Leong S, Hsei V, Deforge L, Zapata G. Modulating pharmacokinetics of an anti-interleukin-8 F(ab')(2) by amine- specific PEGylation with preserved bioactivity. Int J Pharm 2000; 198:83–95.

53. Bailon P, Palleroni A, Schaffer CA, et al. Rational design of a potent, long-lasting form of interferon: a 40 kDa branched polyethylene glycol-conjugated interferon alpha-2a for the treatment of hepatitis C. Bioconjug Chem 2001; 12:195–202.

54. Heathcote EJ, Shiffman ML, Cooksley WG, et al. Peginterferon alfa-2a in patients with chronic hepatitis C and cirrhosis. N Engl J Med 2000; 343:1673–1680.

55. Motzer RJ, Rakhit A, Ginsberg M, et al. Phase I trial of 40-kd branched pegylated interferon alfa-2a for patients with advanced renal cell carcinoma. J Clin Oncol 2001; 19:1312–1319.

56. Lee KH, Song SH, Paik JY, et al. Specific endothelial binding and tumor uptake of radiolabeled angiostatin. Eur J Nucl Med Mol Imaging 2003; 30:1032–1037.

Targeted Chemotherapy: New Approaches to Treatment of Various Cancers Based on Cytotoxic Analogs of Luteinizing Hormone-Releasing Hormone (LH-RH), Somatostatin and Bombesin

Andrew V. Schally, Attila Nagy, and Ana Maria Comaru-Schally

Department of Medicine, Endocrine, Polypeptide, and Cancer Institute, Veterans Affairs Medical Center and Section of Experimental Medicine, Tulane University School of Medicine, New Orleans, Louisiana, U.S.A.

BACKGROUND

In the past 15 years remarkable progress has been made on the localization of tumors and their metastases expressing receptors for somatostatin using scintigraphy with radiolabeled analogs (1–4). The clinical use of analogs of somatostatin and bombesin linked to various radionuclides for cancer therapy is also rapidly advancing, as described in the preceding chapters of this book. We have used the concept of targeted therapy for the synthesis of cytotoxic analogs of hypothalamic peptides (1–4). The demonstration of specific high affinity binding sites for LH-RH, somatostatin, and bombesin in diverse surgical specimens of human cancers provided a rationale to conjugate selected cytotoxic radicals to agonists of LH-RH, antagonists of bombesin, and analogs of somatostatin (1–4). Our concept was that since cytotoxic analogs are preferentially targeted to receptors for these peptides on cancer cells, peripheral toxicity should be greatly reduced. Thus, targeted chemotherapy with cytotoxic peptide analogs should be more effective and less toxic for the treatment of various malignancies than conventional systemic chemotherapy (1–4).

Various cytotoxic drugs are being used as single agents or in combination regimens for the systemic treatment of advanced or metastatic cancers (3). The most widely used chemotherapeutic agent with the broadest spectrum of antineoplastic activity is the DNA-intercalating antibiotic, doxorubicin (DOX). This agent has been used clinically for more than three decades, demonstrating its importance in fighting cancer. However, the experience with DOX also revealed many drawbacks of systemic chemotherapy. Among them are the intrinsic or acquired resistance of cancerous cells which often require higher doses of cytotoxic drugs for effective therapy. Unfortunately, dose elevation is limited by harmful side effects, including gastrointestinal, cardiac, hepatic, renal, neurologic, and respiratory toxicities as well as the myelosuppression (3). In the case of DOX, the dose limiting toxicity is cardiomyopathy, caused by reactive oxygen species generated by the drug (5). In addition, DOX can kill all types of rapidly proliferating normal cells in the body, including cells of the bone marrow, causing severe myelotoxicity. Thousands of derivatives of DOX have been synthesized to reduce its cardiotoxicity and improve its efficacy against DOX-resistant cancers (6). These efforts led to the development of certain daunosamine-modified derivatives of DOX, which are non-cardiotoxic and non-cross-resistant with DOX. These agents include Nemorubicin, which is in phase II/III clinical trials, and an analog of DOX developed in our institute, called 2-pyrrolino-DOX (AN-201) (7). AN-201 was found to be 500–1000 times more potent than DOX in vitro, and about 100 times more active in certain experimental cancer models in vivo. However, the myelotoxicity, and a narrow therapeutic window of this agent, does not allow its use in systemic chemotherapy (1–4,8,9). Nevertheless, its extremely high efficacy as an antiproliferative agent, and its non-cross-resistance with DOX, as well as its lack of cardiotoxicity, make AN-201 an excellent candidate for targeted chemotherapy.

The fact that radionuclide analogs of somatostatin and bombesin were found to accumulate in somatostatin or bombesin receptor-positive primary and metastatic lesions in patients (10) serves as a strong rationale to use these peptide hormones as carriers for AN-201. Thus, we prepared a cytotoxic somatostatin analog, AN-238, consisting of 2-pyrrolino-DOX linked through a glutaric acid spacer to the amino terminal of a somatostatin octapeptide carrier, RC-121 (D-Phe-Cys-Tyr-D-Trp-Lys-Val-Cys-Thr-NH$_2$) (8,11). Similarly, a cytotoxic bombesin analog, AN-215, was synthesized by linking 2-pyrrolino-DOX-14-O-hemiglutarate to the amino terminal of a bombesin-like octapeptide analog, Gln-Trp-Ala-Val-Gly-His-Leu-Θ(CH$_2$-NH)-Leu-NH$_2$ (12). In addition, because the receptors for were also found on a wide variety of malignant tumors, including breast, prostate, ovarian, and endometrial cancers, we synthesized a cytotoxic LHRH analog, AN-207, by linking AN-201 to the epsilon amino group of [D-Lys^6]LHRH (9,13). DOX was likewise coupled to these peptide hormone carriers, to form cytotoxic somatostatin analog AN-162 (11), cytotoxic bombesin conjugate AN-160 (12), and cytotoxic LHRH analog AN-152 (9,13). Somatostatin analog AN-238, bombesin analog AN-215, and LHRH conjugate AN-152 have been selected for clinical development based on numerous preclinical studies performed in various laboratories world-wide and in our institute.

PRECLINICAL STUDIES WITH CYTOTOXIC SOMATOSTATIN ANALOG AN-238

More than 60% of prostate cancer specimens bind radioiodinated RC-160 with high affinity and express mRNA for somatostatin receptor subtype 5 (sst_5) (14). Metastatic lesions have been detected in patients with prostate cancer using Octreoscan scintigraphy (15). Therapy with AN-238 had a strong antitumor effect, higher than 80%, on the very aggressive androgen independent rat Dunning R-3327-AT-1 prostate cancers (16). The rats tolerated AN-238 at doses about 3 times higher than those of the non-targeted cytotoxic radical AN-201, which had no significant effect at a sub-lethal dose. AN-238 was also highly effective in inhibiting the growth of the DU-145 (17) and PC-3 (18) models of human androgen independent prostate cancers xenografted into nude mice. Orthotopically grown PC-3 tumors formed metastatic lesions in regional and distant lymph nodes of control animals, but not in mice treated with AN-238 (18).

About 70% of renal cell carcinoma (RCC) specimens express receptors for somatostatin octapeptides (10). RCC is often diagnosed at a metastatic stage and conventional chemotherapy is ineffective due to chemoresistance of this disease. A high efficacy of targeted chemotherapy in nude mice bearing SW-839 and metastatic 786-0 human RCC lines indicates that patients with metastatic lesions may benefit from therapy with AN-238 (19).

Receptors for somatostatin are also found in breast cancers, and AN-238 shows a good therapeutic efficacy in estrogen independent MDA-MB-231 and MX-1 human mammary cancers xenografted into nude mice (20). Five of ten animals bearing the DOX-resistant MX-1 cancers were cured after treatment with AN-238.

Low-grade glioblastomas (astrocytomas) express receptors for somatostatin, and treatment with AN-238 of U-87 MG and U-118 MG human glioblastomas xenografted into nude mice demonstrated a high inhibitory efficacy. AN-162, which is the DOX-containing counterpart of AN-238, had no effect on U-87 MG tumors showing the advantages of targeting AN-201 instead of DOX in certain cancers (21).

Primary small cell lung cancers (SCLC) and their metastases can be visualized by scintigraphic imaging with Octreoscan (10). In patients with non-SCLC tumors, the radioactivity accumulates in the peritumoral blood vessels after the injection of Octreoscan (10). Treatment of somatostatin receptor positive

H-69 SCLC in nude mice with AN-238 resulted in a >50% tumor growth inhibition (22). Although we detected no mRNA for $sst_{2,3,5}$ or receptors for radiolabeled RC-160 on H-157 non-SCLC cells, receptors for radiolabeled RC-160 were found on membrane preparations from tumor tissue, indicating that the somatostatin binding sites in this type of cancer may be expressed by angiogenic endothelial cells of the host (22). In H-157 xenografts in nude mice, AN-238 had a tumor inhibitory effect higher than 80%. The results of this study showed that not only epithelial cells can be targeted in tumors by cytotoxic somatostatin analog AN-238 to achieve a strong growth inhibition.

Ductal pancreatic cancers do not express mRNA for sst_2, which is the main receptor subtype mediating the cytostatic effects of somatostatin octapeptides such as octreotide, but lanreotide and vapreotide, mRNA for sst_5 and sst_3 has been found in pancreatic cancer specimens (3,4). Some ductal pancreatic cancers can be detected in patients by radiolabeled lanreotide, which may bind to sst_3 receptors. In a study with SW-1990 human pancreatic cancers that express sst_5 and sst_3, but not sst_2, we determined that AN-238 was a highly efficacious inhibitor, suggesting that this analog may be useful for the treatment of patients whose cancers can be visualized with radiolabeled lanreotide (23). AN-238 was also effective in golden hamsters bearing the PC-1.0/sst_2 ductal pancreatic cancer cell line, which was produced by a stable transfection of the sst_2 gene into the chemically induced PC-1.0 hamster pancreatic cancer cell line (24).

A loss of sst_2 was also reported in colorectal cancers, but sst_5 is present. Chemotherapy of colorectal cancers is also hampered by chemoresistance due to the expression of a mutant form of the tumor suppressor (apoptotic) protein, p-53 (25). AN-238 was highly effective in the HCT-15 and HT-29 human colon cancer models in nude mice, which express a mutant p-53, indicating that AN-238 may be useful for the treatment of patients with chemoresistant colorectal cancers (25).

Low affinity, high capacity receptors for somatostatin were also reported in gastric cancer specimens, and we demonstrated by immunohistochemistry that the AGS, Hs-746T, and NCI-N87 human gastric cancers grown in nude mice express sst_2 and sst_5 (26). The best effects were observed in the NCI-N87 model, which has the highest concentration of somatostatin receptors.

More than 60% of surgical specimens of epithelial ovarian cancers bind radiolabeled RC-160 with high affinity (27). Although receptors for LHRH are found on more than 80% of ovarian cancer specimens, some ovarian cancers, represented by the UCI-107 cell line, have no LHRH receptors, but express binding sites for somatostatin. Accordingly, AN-238 significantly inhibited the growth of subcutaneous xenografts of UCI-107 tumors (28). In contrast, cytotoxic LHRH analogs AN-152 and AN-207 had no effects on this model (4). Both cytotoxic LHRH analogs were highly effective in LHRH receptor-positive OV-1063 and ES-2 human ovarian cancers grown in nude mice, demonstrating the necessity for the presence of specific receptors on tumors (3,4).

Ongoing studies with AN-238 indicate that this analog may be useful for the treatment of a very wide variety of cancers including non-Hodgkin's lymphomas and melanomas.

PRECLINICAL STUDIES WITH CYTOTOXIC BOMBESIN ANALOG AN-215

Bombesin/GRP receptors were found on a high percentage of prostate cancer specimens, especially in early stages of the disease, and a ^{99m}Tc-labeled analog of bombesin (7–14) was shown to accumulate in prostate cancers in patients (10,29). AN-215 caused about a 70% decrease in the volume of PC-3 human androgen independent prostate cancers xenografted subcutaneously into nude mice (30).

A high concentration of bombesin receptors found on SCLC tumors in patients support the view that GRP is an autocrine growth factor in the development and progression of SCLC (2,3). Based on these findings, we tested AN-215 on H-69 human SCLC in nude mice, and found a significant inhibition of tumor growth with the targeted analog (31). Although the presence of binding sites for bombesin on H-69 cells was established with radioiodinated [Tyr^4]bombesin, mRNA for the GRP receptor subtype could not be detected. Results from other investigators indicate that receptors for substance P might provide a high affinity binding site for AN-215 on H-69 tumors (4,31). Thus, it is possible that AN-215 can bind with high affinity to receptors on tumors other than the GRP/bombesin receptor subtype. Such receptors would include the substance P receptor, which is also present on various cancers.

As about 85% of human glioblastomas express receptors for bombesin, we tested AN-215 in U-87 MG human glioblastomas in nude mice (32). AN-215 significantly inhibited the growth of U-87 MG tumors and this effect could be blocked by injection of a high concentration of the well known bombesin antagonist RC-3095 prior to administration of AN-215.

Some gastric cancers also have bombesin receptors. When we tested AN-215 in AGS, Hs-746T and NCI-N87 human gastric cancers grown in nude mice, we found that only the AGS tumors responded to therapy (26). In accord with this result, among these three cell lines only the AGS cancers had bombesin receptors.

As breast cancers can be localized in patients with a radiolabeled bombesin/GRP analog (10), we are testing AN-215 in human breast cancer cell lines xenografted into nude mice.

CLINICAL REMARKS

Biopsies of primary tumors as well as their metastases for measurement of receptors for peptide analogs will greatly facilitate the selection of patients who may benefit from the administration of peptide analogs linked to various cytotoxic radicals. Conventional chemotherapy of many cancers may have reached an upper limit for improving the survival of patients. It is expected that cytotoxic peptide analogs will cause less systemic toxicity than the current chemotherapeutic methods and consequently lead to a prolongation of survival with a good quality of life. This new targeted approach to cancer therapy should improve the current outcome of patients with various tumors considered untreatable.

CONCLUSIONS

Receptors for peptide hormones such as somatostatin, bombesin/GRP, and LHRH are suitable targets for chemotherapy based on cytotoxic conjugates of these peptides. The concentration of receptors for somatostatin and bombesin on various tumors was demonstrated to be high enough for a selective accumulation of radioactive analogs in these tumors, as compared to healthy tissues. LHRH receptors are found on tumor cells, but not in normal tissues. Based on these findings, we designed targeted cytotoxic somatostatin, bombesin and LHRH analogs AN-238, AN-215, and AN-207, respectively, all containing superactive DOX derivative AN-201. These agents showed a remarkable antitumor activity in a wide variety of experimental human cancers xenografted into nude mice. We also evaluated the benefits of therapy with AN-152, an LHRH analog containing DOX, the most widely used antineoplastic agent. Clinical phase I/IIa trials with targeted cytotoxic LHRH analog AN-152 are scheduled for the fall of 2004 in patients with ovarian and breast cancers. Clinical trials are also planned with AN-238 and AN-215 in the near future.

These advances on targeting peptides conjugated to radionuclides and on the synthesis and evaluation of targeted cytotoxic peptides have put the concept of targeted therapy on firm foundations.

REFERENCES

1. Schally AV, Nagy A. Cancer chemotherapy based on targeting of cytotoxic peptide conjugates to their receptors on tumors. Eur J Endocrinol 1999; 141:1–14.
2. Schally AV, Nagy A. New approaches to treatment of various cancers based on cytotoxic analogs of LHRH. Somatostatin and bombesin. Life Sci 2003; 72:2305–2320.
3. Schally AV, Nagy A. Chemotherapy targeted to cancers through tumoral hormone receptors. Trends Endocrinol Metab 2004; 15:300–310.
4. Nagy A, Schally AV. Targeting cytotoxic conjugates of somatostatin, luteinizing hormone-releasing hormone and bombesin to cancers expressing their receptors: A "smarter" chemotherapy. Curr Pharm Des 2005; 11:1167–1180.
5. Doroshow JH. Doxorubicin-induced cardiac toxicity. N Engl J Med 1991; 24:843–845.
6. Weiss RB. The anthracyclines: will we ever find a better doxorubicin? Semin Oncol 1992; 19:670–686.

7. Nagy A, Armatis P, Schally AV. High yield conversion of doxorubicin to 2-pyrrolinodoxorubicin, an analog 500 to 1000 times more potent: Structure-activity relationship of daunosamine-modified derivatives of doxorubicin. Proc Natl Acad Sci USA 1996; 93:2464–2469.

8. Nagy A, Schally AV. Targeted cytotoxic somatostatin analogs: a modern approach to the therapy of various cancers. Drugs Fut 2001; 26:261–270.

9. Nagy A, Schally AV. Cytotoxic analogs of luteinizing hormone-releasing hormone (LHRH); a new approach to targeted chemotherapy. Drugs Fut 2002; 27:359–370.

10. Reubi JC. Peptide receptors as molecular targets for cancer diagnosis and therapy. Endocr Rev 2003; 24:389–427.

11. Nagy A, Schally AV, Halmos G, et al. Synthesis and biological evaluation of cytotoxic analogs of somatostatin containing doxorubicin or its intensely potent derivative 2-pyrrolinodoxonubicin. Proc Natl Acad Sci USA 1998; 95:1794–1799.

12. Nagy A, Armatis P, Cai R-Z, Szepeshazi K, Halmos G, Schally AV. Design, synthesis and in vitro evaluation of cytotoxic analogs of bombesin-like peptides containing doxorubicin or its intensely potent derivative, 2-pyrrolinodoxorubicin. Proc Natl Acad Sci USA 1997; 94:652–656.

13. Nagy A, Schally AV, Armatis P, et al. Cytotoxic analogs of luteinizing hormone-releasing hormone containing doxorubicin or 2-pyrrolinodoxorubicin, a derivative 500-1000 times more potent. Proc Natl Acad Sci USA 1996; 93:7269–7273.

14. Halmos G, Schally AV, Sun B, Davis R, Bostwick DG, Plonowski A. High expression of somatostatin receptors and ribonucleic acid for its receptor subtypes in organ-confined and locally advanced human prostate cancers. J Clin Endocrinol Metab 2000; 85:2564–2571.

15. Nilsson S, Reubi JC, Kalkner KM, et al. Metastatic hormone-refractory prostatic adenocarcinoma expresses somatostatin receptors and is visualized in vivo by [^{111}In]-labeled DTPA-D-[Phe^1]-octreotide scintigraphy. Cancer Res 1995; 55:5805–5810.

16. Koppan M, Nagy A, Schally AV, Arencibia JM, Plonowski A, Halmos G. Targeted cytotoxic analogue of somatostatin AN-238 inhibits the growth of androgen-independent Dunning R-3327-AT-1 prostate cancer in rats at nontoxic doses. Cancer Res 1998; 58:4132–4137.

17. Plonowski A, Schally AV, Nagy A, Sun B, Halmos G. Effective treatment of experimental DU-145 prostate cancers with targeted cytotoxic somatostatin analog AN-238. Int J Oncology 2002; 20:397–402.

18. Plonowski A, Schally AV, Nagy A, Sun B, Szepeshazi K. Inhibition of PC-3 human androgen-independent prostate cancer and its metastases by cytotoxic somatostatin analogue AN-238. Cancer Res 1999; 59:1947–1953.

19. Plonowski A, Schally AV, Nagy A, Kiaris H, Hebert F, Halmos G. Inhibition of metastatic renal cell carcinomas expressing somatostatin receptors by a targeted cytotoxic analog of somatostatin AN-238. Cancer Res 2000; 60:2996–3001.

20. Kahan Z, Nagy A, Schally AV, et al. Inhibition of growth of MX- 1, MCF-7, MIII and MDA-MB-231 human breast cancer xenografts after administration of a targeted cytotoxic analog of somatostatin, AN-238. Int J Cancer 1999; 82:592–598.

21. Kiaris H, Schally AV, Nagy A, Sun B, Szepeshazi K, Halmos G. Regression of U-87MG human glioblastomas in nude mice after treatment with a cytotoxic somatostatin analog AN-238. Clin Cancer Res 2000; 6:709–717.

22. Kiaris H, Schally AV, Nagy A, Szepeshazi K, Hebert F, Halmos G. A targeted cytotoxic somatostatin (SST) analogue AN-238 inhibits the growth of H-69 small cell lung carcinoma (SCLC) and H-157 non-SCLC in nude mice. Eur J Cancer 2001; 37:620–628.

23. Szepeshazi K, Schally AV, Halmos G, et al. Targeting of cytotoxic somatostatin analog AN-238 to somatostatin receptor subtypes 5 and/or 3 in experimental pancreatic cancer. Clin Cancer Res 2001; 7:2854–2861.

24. Benali N, Cordelier P, Calise D, et al. Inhibition of growth and metastatic progression of pancreatic carcinoma in hamster after somatostatin receptor subtype 2 (sst2) gene expression and administration of cytotoxic somatostatin analog AN-238. Proc Natl Acad Sci USA 2000; 97:9180–9185.

25. Szepeshazi K, Schally AV, Halmos G, et al. Targeted cytotoxic somatostatin analogue AN-238 inhibits somatostatin receptor-positive experimental colon cancers independently of their p53 status. Cancer Res 2002; 62:781–788.

26. Szepeshazi K, Schally AV, Nagy A, Wagner BW, Bajo AM, Halmos G. Preclinical evaluation of therapeutic effects of targeted cytotoxic analogs of somatostatin and bombesin on human gastric carcinomas. Cancer 2003; 98:1401–1410.

27. Halmos G, Sun B, Schally AV, Hebert F, Nagy A. Human ovarian cancers express somatostatin receptors. J Clin Endocrinol Metab 2000; 85:3509–3512.

28. Plonowski A, Schally AV, Koppan M, et al. Inhibition of the UCI-107 human ovarian carcinoma cell line by a targeted cytotoxic analog of somatostatin, AN-238. Cancer 2001; 92:1168–1176.

29. Sun B, Halmos G, Schally AV, Wang X, Martinez M. The presence of receptors for bombesin/gastrin-releasing peptide and mRNA for 3 receptor subtypes in human prostate cancers. Prostate 2000; 42:295–303.

30. Plonowski A, Nagy A, Schally AV, Sun B, Groot K, Halmos G. In vivo inhibition of PC-3 human androgen-independent prostate cancer by a targeted cytotoxic bombesin analogue AN-215. Int J Cancer 2000; 88:652–657.

31. Kiaris H, Schally AV, Nagy A, Sun B, Armatis P, Szepeshazi K. Targeted Cytotoxic analog of bombesin/gastrin-releasing peptide inhibits the growth of H-69 human small-cell lung carcinoma in nude mice. Br J Cancer 1999; 81:966–971.

32. Szereday Z, Schally AV, Nagy A, et al. Effective treatment of experimental U-87MG human glioblastoma in nude mice with a targeted cytotoxic bombesin analogue, AN-215. Br J Cancer 2002; 86:1322–1327.

Index

T - #0106 - 111024 - C370 - 229/152/17 - PB - 9780367453558 - Gloss Lamination